BRET CONTRERAS & KE

STRONG CURVES

A WOMAN'S GUIDE TO BUILDING A BETTER BUTT AND BODY

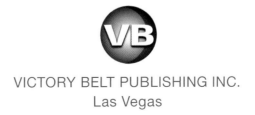

VICTORY BELT PUBLISHING INC.

Las Vegas

First Published in 2013 by Victory Belt Publishing Inc.

ISBN 13: 978-1-936608-64-5

This book is for educational purposes. The publisher and authors of this instructional book are not responsible in any manner whatsoever for any adverse effects arising directly or indirectly as a result of the information provided in this book. If not practiced safely and with caution, working out can be dangerous to you and to others. It is important to consult with a professional fitness instructor before beginning training. It is also very important to consult with a physician prior to training due to the intense and strenuous nature of the techniques in this book.

Printed in the USA
RRD 04-14

Disclaimer

Strong Curves: A woman's Guide to Building a Better Butt and Body was written with the needs of women in mind, but the *Strong Curves* workout program can also greatly benefit men. Women aren't the only ones who have weak and underactive glutes—men do as well. I've used all of the methods in this book with male clients, and whether they were retirees or professional athletes, each one saw incredible improvements in strength, physique, and mechanics.

The mainstream male workout programs do not adequately strengthen the glutes through their full range of motion. If you're a man and you purchased this book, don't pass it along to the woman in your life without giving the program a try. I believe that most men should stick to the *Strong Curves Program* as well. After all, it's very similar to the way I regularly train.

Table of content

Foreword
by Cassandra Forsythe,
PhD, RD, CSCS, FMS

Since Lou Shuler and I wrote *The New Rules of Lifting for Women* in late 2007, women have finally begun to understand and embrace the fact that lifting heavy weights does *not* make us big and bulky and will *not* turn us into men.

Instead, today's women recognize that getting under the bar, so-to-speak, and lifting, pressing, and/or pushing heavier weights than they ever thought possible actually makes their bodies look the way they really want them to look—strong, sexy, and lean. Lifting weights gives us a feeling of empowerment and strength when so many parts of our lives are still minimized or weakened. So, women are now freely stepping away from the treadmill and moving into the weight room, which was formerly a taboo place for us. (As a teenager, I remember being the only woman in the weight room; I hated cardio machines but loved the feeling that lifting weights gave me. If I ever saw another woman in there, I made her my new best friend because we were the only ones aware at that time of this great secret.)

With *Strong Curves*, Bret has moved past the need for convincing women to lift. Instead, he's put together a book that shows women *how* to lift weights in a way that makes all of their curves stand out. And trust me, there's nothing "pink" or "little" about anything in this program.

Bret is one of the most intelligent, wise, and in-tune guys I've ever met. He doesn't have to interview other people to get the answers he needs; he already knows it because he has the amazing ability to synthesize research and real-world information into something we can all use. And he does it with style. He may be a man, but he knows what women's bodies need in order to look and feel great, and it's far from guesswork. He understands the mechanics of the female body in a way that not many people will ever grasp, and he knows how to translate this information into directions and explanations that all women will understand, not just fellow science nerds.

As you will read, Bret spent years building great glutes in women, and he developed and marketed the hip-thrust and glute-bridge exercises. But then, he did something not many people could or would do: He tested it using credible scientific methods (EMG). You'd be hard-pressed to find any trainer who puts his or her money where their mouth is, but Bret did. This is why you should and will trust that Bret's methods work and that this program isn't just something he threw together to get his name on a published book.

Bret also isn't just some new kid on the block. In his 36 years on this planet, he has accomplished and learned more than most of us put together. He isn't just a workaholic; he's a "help-aholic." His experiences in the real world and in the lab have helped hundreds, if not thousands, of women to transform their glutes to perfection and the rest of their bodies into something that other women envy and work to duplicate. The good news is that with Bret's help, these inquisitive women can and do duplicate the results.

Every woman can take part in the program that Bret has outlined in *Strong Curves*, which he co-authored with the lovely, talented, and outstanding writer, Kellie Davis. He and Kellie didn't write this book only for the super strong, the ultra skinny, the childless, or unmarried. This program can easily be followed by your sister, your mother, your niece, and beyond. In fact, I'm taking on this program myself and loving every second of it. Why? Because it makes me feel strong, capable, and beautiful, and it's written in a way that's easy to comprehend, thanks to Bret's extensive research and Kellie's relatability.

For me, a nice booty has been a long-time goal. I was a gymnast in my younger years (not anything spectacular, but I gave it my best), and I always admired women who had well-muscled bodies, including a fantastic, round butt. Thankfully, I was blessed with a backside (you can look at my mom to know what I mean), but without exercise, it wasn't a backside I wanted anyone to see, especially not in a bikini. It was droopy and flabby, and it definitely produced some saddle bags in my jeans. So, I made it my goal to make my butt perky, pretty, and rock solid. Like Bret, I looked for all the ways to make my butt round and gorgeous. I squatted, I leg-pressed, I lunged, I stepped-up, I leg-curled, I dead-lifted. In fact, I trained my legs and butt more than any other body part because I wanted and needed them to improve. And they did, but they still weren't solid. It wasn't until I started glute-bridging and hip-thrusting that my glutes started to look like the ones I admired in the fitness magazines. I finally realized that I was definitely missing these movements in my former training programs.

Now, I'm training with Bret full-time (after all, he's the glute expert), and I'm so impressed with not only his methods, but also his coaching. He's an amazing coach who knows how to help a woman set goals, challenge herself, reach new heights, and, of course, build the body (and booty) of her dreams. You're going to get all of this with the *Strong Curves Program.*

You're going to feel your glutes like you've never felt them before, and you're going to love that the rest of your body will follow suit. In other words, you'll see the body transformations that you've always wanted. Why? Because you'll finally be training the areas that need the most attention but never get it. Trust me; I've been training for as long as I can recall, hitting the gym at age fifteen, and this program is the perfect complement to *The New Rules of Lifting for Women.*

As Bret and Kellie state, they wrote this book with a long-term vision in mind. This isn't meant to be a routine that you follow for only a month; it's a way of training forever. They address everything women need to know about training, eating, and living a strong, healthy life. From cellulite, to pelvic floor strength (can you say Kegels?), to pregnancy, Bret lays it on the line. Both Kellie and I have had babies, and we both know how important strength training is for pregnancy and post-partum. And you'll learn just how amazing the training is for not only your body, but also for your mind and your soul. Being strong in the gym brings strength to all areas of your life, including your job, your marriage, your role as a parent, and your friendships with others

(with a strong booty to complement it all).

You're going to learn methods in this book that few other books even try to explain. There are some very advanced glute exercises on its pages because as Bret says, "While you might not be strong enough right now to perform these movements, you will continue to gain strength if you stick to the template and push yourself [and eventually will be doing these exercises all the time, for life.]"

But the key phrase here is that you have to push yourself. You have to be willing to make grunting noises in the gym and leave sweat angels on the floor without hesitation. You can't hold back just because someone (a guy) might look at you funny for pushing more weight than he might even attempt. Some of the strongest women I know are also the most curvy, sexy, and muscular in the most lean, feminine way. That can be you, too, as long as you commit to this program fully and give it your strongest effort. You can, and you will, and you're stronger than you think you are!

So, if you want a butt that makes women and men turn their heads when you walk by, plus one that helps move your body in ways it has never moved before, you'll soon find out that *Strong Curves* is the answer you've been looking for. Take pictures, keep notes, and track your progress, because your body is going to change before your eyes, and you won't want to miss it.

In strength, and for a great booty,
Live, Love, Laugh and Lift,
Cassandra Forsythe, PhD, RD, CSCS, FMS

Cassandra Forsythe holds a PhD in Exercise Science and Nutrition and is a Registered Dietitian. She's also a Certified Strength and Conditioning Specialist (CSCS) and a Certified Sports Nutritionist (CISSN) and is certified in the Functional Movement Screen (FMS).

Two of her books for women are, *The New Rules of Lifting for Women* and *Women's Health Perfect Body Diet.* She has also been featured in major magazines such as *Oxygen, Women's Health, Men's Health,* and *Delta Sky Magazine,* and is an Advisory Board member for *Women's Health* magazine, PrecisionNutrition.com and Livestrong.com.

In Connecticut, Cassandra runs her own group fitness facility, Fitness Revolution Vernon, which has transformed the bodies of hundreds of women and men across the state through proven exercise and nutrition methods. You can find out more about Cassandra and her fitness facility at www.cassandraforsythe.com.

Preface

Genetically speaking, I was spoiled growing up. I had the skinny kid gene. I ran around in my youth from sun up to sun down, scraping my knobby knees on the pines I scaled in my Colorado backyard. I would break from a day spent running around the Rockies to feast on giant servings of fruit and cookies, and then it was back out for more exploration.

This was pretty much how I lived for the first twenty-five years of my life—carefree, bone-thin, and completely unaware of my fitness or nutritional needs. Sure, I was athletically gifted and spent most of my time moving rather than sitting. I played sports up until my freshman year of college, and started going to the gym at age fourteen. However, after I graduated with my bachelor's degree and settled into a desk job, my lifestyle started to catch up with me. I could no longer rely on genetics to help me beat out the effects of my poor diet. When I gave birth to my daughter, I lost the weight quickly—but not for the right reasons. The stress of being a new parent and starting a new career left little time for me to eat or take care of myself. I didn't spend many sessions in the gym after she was born, and I rarely ate, unintentionally starving myself thin.

When my daughter was two, I found out I was pregnant with my son. By this time, I started to pack on a little weight but was in complete denial of this whole process. I still squeezed myself into size five jeans and covered up the fat that spilled out over the top of them. A little more than three months into my pregnancy, I started showing pretty well. There was no guessing whether or not I was expecting. I steadily gained excess weight over the months and did little to control it. I ate my lunch as soon as I arrived to work and went out for another lunch in the afternoon.

Along with uncontrolled hunger and extra pounds came a bulk of pregnancy complications. I found myself in and out of the hospital more times than I care to remember, and I ended up on bed rest by month seven. I still haven't exactly figured out what bed rest entails when you have a career and a busy toddler running around the house, but it was supposed to mean I sat on my butt all day and did nothing. I tried my best but wasn't very successful with it. My body could no longer carry my pregnancy, and I gave birth to my son on Christmas Eve, four weeks before my due date.

At this time, I thought little of my lifestyle having anything to do with pregnancy complications. I blamed nature as I sat with my son in the neonatal intensive care unit. My body just wasn't designed to carry a pregnancy to term, or so I thought. Looking back now, I know in my gut that this could have all been prevented had I taken care of my body, giving it proper nutrition and exercising regularly. I brought my son home five days after he was born, and along with my new baby came an extra fifty pounds of weight.

I was overweight for the first time in my life. I had *always* been the skinny type; the kind most people wrinkle their nose at because it was hard for me to gain weight. I'm certain if my body fat had been measured at the time, I would have fallen in the obese category with a pathetic muscle-to-fat ratio.

I learned to accept the extra weight rather than do anything about it. This was mostly driven by self-consciousness and embarrassment. After I gave my body enough time to heal, I stepped into the gym on a few occasions only to leave disappointed.

I stood in the mirrors by the dumbbell rack feeling hopeless. I couldn't run due to weakened pelvic floor muscles and poor endurance, and I couldn't lift weights because I had no strength. At that time, I was completely and utterly in the worst shape of my life. I had become the very definition of "out of shape." But to me, it was the curse of being a mom. I believed what I had been told—that babies steal your beauty and ruin your body.

The Breaking Point

Over the next two years, I slowly lost the weight I gained with my pregnancy, but like my first pregnancy, it was mostly due to stress. I wasn't eating a nutritious diet, and exercise didn't extend beyond evening walks or play time with my kids. I looked great in clothes, but without them was a different story. A major turning point was when I decided to strip down to my bikini and take progress photos—or photos I thought would show progress.

I burst into tears when I uploaded the pictures onto my computer and saw my true physique for the first time rather than what I thought I looked like. I was completely disillusioned because I only focused on the scale numbers. I hadn't seen my body for what it was. The skin on my belly sagged, and my thighs were chubby and shapeless. My glutes were completely flat and non-existent other than the fat that hung from the bottom and sides of my hips.

My outlook completely changed from that moment. The fitness magazines I devoutly read every month were filled with models who were also moms. Those women proved it was possible to have children and be in great shape. So I stopped hanging my hat on excuses and signed up for classes at my gym. I devoted two nights a week to aerobic classes and one night to yoga. I went without fail to every single class. At first, I hid in the back, barely able to make it through twenty minutes of the aerobic weight-training course. I sat out during lunges because I couldn't do a stationary lunge with my own body weight. After two months, my strength increased, and I moved to the front of the room near the instructor.

Nearly four months into my new, fitter lifestyle, I stepped foot into the weight room for the first time in six years. I remember when I could finally see a little bump of biceps pop up—a total confidence booster. I made it a point to hold things close to my chest so that my arms flexed in front of others. Pathetic, I know. But I was feeling really good by that point, and I kept striving to reach new goals by learning everything I could from fitness magazines and websites.

Raising the Bar Higher

After achieving results I never thought possible, I became addicted to the gym—but in a good way. I was in better shape than I had been in before having children,
but I felt that innate competitive drive creeping back into my life. I decided I needed to take my physique to the next level, so I committed to a local figure competition. I felt utterly lost a mere three weeks into my training. I joined online forums filled with fitness-minded women—some were competitors themselves—and made great connections.

But the information still baffled me. Frustrated and confused, I hired a coach to get me on stage. By the time I hit my quarter turns in front of the judges, I weighed less than I had in high school. I felt completely drained and over-trained from the methods my coach asked me to use. The women in my circle all joked about how this feeling was normal, but deep down, I knew it wasn't healthy.

I was hooked on competing but not on my coaching. By then, I felt confident enough to get to the stage on my own, and I did so the next time around. Physically, I felt less drained and I was more intact emotionally. I only gained back two pounds, though, because I still held onto the over-training and under-eating mentality my former coach engrained in my brain.

Finding The Glute Guy

One of my most reliable sources of fitness information at the time was T-Nation, a site that regularly published Bret's work. After reading one of his articles, I scrolled down to his byline and realized that he lived in the Phoenix valley as well. I immediately contacted him with my story. He agreed to work with me to get me back on stage. He felt that while I had a great physique, I needed to take a couple of years to build muscle for the figure stage.

I was a little heartbroken, but I trusted his instincts. Within three weeks of starting his program, my physique completely changed. I was leaner, tighter, and carried more muscle than I ever thought possible. Previously, I believed my genetic limitations were set to "skinny" and I couldn't carry enough muscle to make it as an elite competitor on stage. However, his programs proved me dead wrong. I made more progress in the first six weeks of working with him than I had in the previous year on my own.

Bret put together a compilation of my progress and sent it over after four months of working with him. I was astounded by the changes; I couldn't believe I was looking at photos of my body. I went from a slender, average physique to a powerhouse stacked with muscle from head to toe. But the most rewarding part of the entire program was my strength gains. I was performing lifts at levels I thought only possible for competitive powerlifters, and I consistently beat my own personal records every month. My husband, Josh, was so impressed with my results that he also hired Bret and worked with him for nearly a year.

Bret has served as a coach, mentor, educator, and friend for the past four years, and I attribute a large part of my success to his commitment. He saw within me the ability to reach elite athletic levels, and he wanted me to learn and grow inside the fitness industry. Since training with Bret, I've stood on the stage in three figure competitions, placing overall in one and fourth in another. In the gym, I've full-squatted nearly one and a half times my own body weight, deadlifted close to two and a half times my own weight, hip thrusted more than two and a half times my body weight, and rival most men at my facility when it comes to pull-ups.

Setting the Bar Higher

The funny part about all of this is that when I started my journey five years ago, these feats never even came to mind. We all reach that breaking point when we're tired of feeling hopeless. We either succumb to that hopelessness and give up on ourselves, or we take action. I imagine right now that you are standing some-where between where I started and where I am now. If you had gone down the other path and given up hope, you wouldn't be holding this book in your hands. You want to take action and are seeking guidance toward reaching your personal health and fitness goals.

When I stepped foot in the gym in the worst shape of my life, I had one goal in mind: to look better. It was an aimless goal, and I lacked commitment. I had no clue where it would lead me, and had I not defined my goal even more, I likely would have given up on myself. But the more results I saw, the more pinpointed my goals became.

I want you to go into this program with the same intentions. Start with a general goal, but as you progress, make it more concrete. Make it your own. We all want to get in shape, lose weight, gain confidence, grow stronger, and look good in a bikini. But those goals aren't very personal. Make this program personal. Get selfish with your goals, and do whatever it takes to achieve them. Most importantly, never look back once your momentum picks up and you're headed down that road toward a better you.

The other day, I was helping a friend with a project that forced me to pull out my before and after pictures. I found a photo taken on the day I brought home my son from the hospital. I hardly recognized myself, not just physically, but mentally as well. I couldn't imagine ever getting to that place to begin with, and I never want to go back there. It had nothing to do with my physique

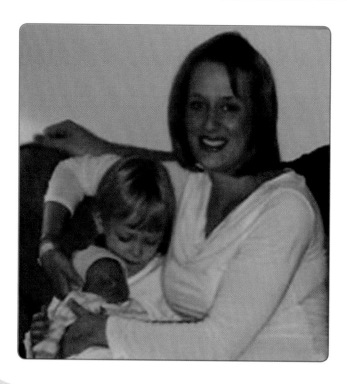

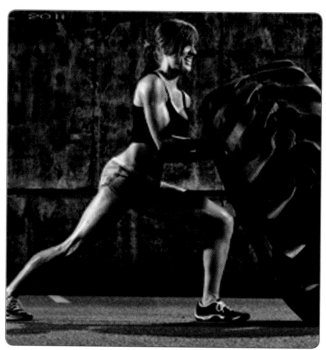

but with my confidence and emotions.

Building *Strong Curves* isn't just about creating physical changes, but emotional ones as well. Once you start achieving strength gains, shedding pounds of fat, and building the curves you have always dreamed of having, your outlook on life will completely change. As these changes take place and your confidence soars, check back with your goals and keep striving toward greater ones. You will find a great deal of improvement in all areas of your life when you take care of your body.

It has been a great honor and privilege to work with Bret on this project. He has been a tremendous asset to my life over the past four years. I feel a deep attachment to this book and the *Strong Curves* movement because I wholeheartedly believe in this program. I have never met a person with more passion and commitment to his work than Bret. That passion shines in every chapter, as they are each catered toward improving your physique, lifestyle, and self-confidence. *Strong Curves* is the culmination of Bret's research, field-testing, and practices implemented over the past fifteen years.

I can tell you first-hand that this program works and the results are nothing short of incredible. I will admit this program is tough. When I tested the Twelve-Week Gluteal Goddess Program for Advanced Lifters, I emailed Bret the first week in and asked if he was trying to kill me. He advised me not to push myself so hard. So if I can give you a slice of wisdom, it's this; don't overdo it. The program on its own is tough enough. If you try to go all-out every session, you will be cursing Bret in your sleep. Take every part of each phase in strides, and train at your current level of conditioning.

If it's too tough, cater the workout to fit your fitness level. Scale back on the amount of repetitions per set or the intensity of your repetitions. If you aren't able to perform a certain exercise, the Exercise Index offers a variety of supplemental exercises to help you reach your goals.

Bret and I put hundreds of hours of sweat into this book because we want you to commit to the program. No stone was left unturned, making it possible for you to achieve your desired results no matter where you stand today. If you feel like giving up, keep my story in the back of your mind (and carry my before and after photos with you for a little motivation). I want you to succeed for selfish reasons. I want you to know what it's like to be a confident, sexy woman. It's the most incredible feeling in the world when you can walk up to the power rack in the gym and pull more weight than the guy standing next to you. You can be that woman, and *Strong Curves* will teach you how.

Chapter 1:

Introduction

If proverbial sayings were coined in the fitness world, "Abs are made in the kitchen" would likely be the most repeated phrase. The right nutrition will deliver a far more visible six-pack than performing endless sets of core exercises. Getting rid of belly fat reveals the muscle beneath, plain and simple.

While this is certainly true for the abs, it isn't the same for the glutes. If you've ever dieted down to reveal great abs, you probably noticed at the same time that your butt flattened out. Dieting with minimal or no training doesn't do the same justice for your booty. Abs are made in the kitchen, but *glutes are made in the gym*.

Louie Simmons is a coach known for his ability to get powerlifters incredibly strong. Charles Glass home grows some of the biggest bodybuilders to ever step on stage. Celebrity trainers like Joe Dowell get the stars just right for the big screen. And coaches like Mike Boyle have mastered the art of building powerful athletes while keeping them injury-free.

I adopted the art of glute-building and have created the best program for sculpting a shapely backside while developing strong, powerful muscles. Since I've been at this so long, I can simply glance at a routine and determine whether or not it will deliver good gluteal results. Is this a program that calls for a couple sets of bodyweight lunges? Nope.

Anytime you begin an exercise program, you will see initial results, but if you give it a few weeks, the results will taper off, leaving you with lackluster results.

When a new client comes to me, I can determine in a single repetition whether or not she is properly using her glutes during the exercise. For example, squats and back extensions can be amazing glute exercises, but not the way you might be doing them. It isn't just about doing the best glute exercises and going through the motions; it's about getting incredibly strong at the best glute exercises while using perfect form and activating the glutes sufficiently.

I visit a lot of gyms around the world when I travel and can say that when many women train, they leave much room on the table for increased gluteal strength and shape. I wish I could travel to every commercial gym and show women how to properly train using the best booty-building exercises and the right programs. I would show them how to hit the glutes with the right frequency, use great technical form, and activate the glutes through a full range of motion.

Since I can't be everywhere all at once, *Strong Curves* brings my expertise and coaching right to your living room or gym. You picked up this book because you want to see changes in your physique. You want to grow stronger, more powerful, and build shapelier curves. Think of this book as one-on-one coaching from me. I put every bit of knowledge I've accumulated over the past fifteen years into these chapters so that you can walk into the gym or use your equipment at home with confidence.

My Big Break

It all started on September 16, 2009 with an article I published on the men's fitness site, T-Nation, titled *Dispelling the Glute Myth*. From that moment, I transformed from a local Arizona personal trainer into an online fitness personality. I was no longer the strength and conditioning coach secretly obsessed with the glute muscles. My obsession became public. There was no turning back because I was officially dubbed "The Glute Guy." In fact, in recent years, I'm often approached by strangers who say, "Hey, you're The Glute Guy!"

I'm okay with that, as there are far worse names. I'm just glad I didn't develop an obsession for ankle flexibility. Imagine hearing, "Hey, you're the Ankle Dorsiflexion Dude." It just doesn't have the same ring to it.

The status of "The Glute Guy" brings with it some incredible opportunities that I wouldn't have found otherwise. In the past four years, I've had the honor of speaking at some of the most highly influential strength and conditioning and sports conferences around the globe. My byline has appeared on articles for the same magazines I read so much as a teen that I wore out the pages (no, not *those* magazines, ladies), including *Muscle Mag*, *Men's Fitness*, and *Men's Health*. I've also had the honor of being an expert in the Glute Edition of *Oxygen Magazine* and have regular features on sites like T-Nation and StrengthCoach.com.

But the most rewarding part of my entire career in the strength industry has been the incredible transformation I've helped my female clients achieve. I love working with women, and it isn't just because I'm a man. If you polled fitness professionals, I think most would agree that training women is highly rewarding because they usually do exactly what you ask them to do to achieve their results. That is the very reason I wrote this book with you in mind. I knew from the moment I sat down to perfect the *Strong Curves Program* that you would do everything I ask of you in this book to achieve the body you've always wanted. Then, when all is said and done, you would email me with huge thanks. Okay, you don't have to do that, but I would seriously love to hear from you and learn about your results.

So, how did I go from the teenage kid who plastered my walls with the pages of bodybuilding magazines to the guy who molds, strengthens, and builds the best butts around the world? This story actually begins way back in 1992 with my own booty, or lack thereof. My quest to teach women how to build a perfect pair of glutes started when I realized that I didn't have any glutes to call my own.

The Candid Birth of the Glute Guy

I learned about the importance of the glute muscles first-hand back in high school. My junior year, I decided to join the football team after much coaxing from my friends who laced up their shoulder pads back when we were freshman. I was astounded by their strength in the weight room. My teammates, who had been training for a few years, could squat and power clean with such intensity, but I shied away from those big lifts. I was untrained when it came to weights and didn't have the same great mentorships that they did with the coaches.

I stuck with lifts I knew I could perform easily like the leg press, pushups, and biceps curls.

I started seeing improvements in my physique from my routine and felt pretty confident with my new hot body (it's okay to snicker at my expense), until that fateful day I walked behind my buddy, Cameron. At that moment, I happened to be escorting my crush to Physics class with my arms fully flexed while holding her books. Suddenly, she leaned into me. I thought I would finally get the chance to ask her out, but my world crashed down around me in the next four seconds. Mind you, it was high school and I was overly sensitive, so this next part may seem trivial. But stick with me. As she leaned closer, she whispered, "Cameron's butt looks so good in those jeans."

"His butt? Oh, love of my life that I thought I knew everything about?" I had no idea at the time that girls were even into the glutes. I guess I hadn't grown with the times. In elementary school, it was all about who told the funniest jokes, and in middle school, the guy who looked like a 90210 character got the most girls. So I didn't put an ounce of thought into my backside until that very moment in time. And it wasn't that Cameron had a good pair of jeans on that day or that he just had a nicer butt than me. It was that I had no butt at all. None, nada, zilch, zip. My case of gluteal development was so bad that my sister's boyfriend commented one afternoon on the golf course regarding my rather bleak situation. As I stepped up to the putting green, he blurted out, "Bret, your back goes right into your legs. You have no butt at all."

Not only did the girls in high school know that guys should have nice butts, but the guys were now telling me the same thing. Somehow I had become the poster boy for the *buttless* pandemic that swept the male population. With my ego still minutely intact, I began my quest to build the best butt possible. I realized I wasn't genetically gifted with the posterior of an NFL wide receiver, but I did not want this to be my fate.

I started reading every publication on the glutes I could get my hands on. I spent hours in the bookstores reading how the bodybuilders trained their lower bodies and how powerlifters built their posterior chains. In 1995, my cousin and training partner bought me *The Complete Guide to Butt and Legs* as a Christmas present and a way of thanking me for turning him into "Brian the Beast" over the past year of training. In his words, he'd never met someone *so obsessed* with glute training.

At age eighteen, I began squatting, but not like the squats you will see in this book. No, they were the amateurish micro-squats you see inexperienced lifters do. I loaded the bar up with two hundred seventy-five pounds of raw iron and eked down about five inches before I pushed back up. After a few bouts of this pathetic attempt to build glutes, a solid lifter in the gym approached me and told me to squat deep like a real man. I racked the weight and turned to stand up to this "puny jerk," only to see a mythical beast—if memory serves me correctly, he was in fact a centaur—making eye contact with his own reflection. I bowed my head in respect, understanding it was something I had yet to earn in the gym. I had to scale back and learn the discipline of squatting before I could lift at an elite level. I brought down my weight to about half of what I was using and squatted like a man.

I felt a good pain in my lower body the next day, so I stuck with this approach. My glutes grew slightly, but I was no Cameron from the varsity football squad. Eventually, I added in deadlifts and then lunges. The more proficient I got at lifting and the stronger I became, the better my glutes looked. Despite the intense amount of work I was putting into training, however, I never felt like my glutes were the limiting factor during a set. Other muscles burned out before my glutes, and they never felt completely taxed.

Prioritizing Exercise

By age twenty-two, I had graduated from college and prepared for my high school math teaching career. Despite the career path I chose, exercise was always a top priority with me. During this time, I also certified with ACE to be a personal trainer. I worked out with all of my friends and family at local gyms, teaching them the methods I was using for strength training.

I began printing out articles and studies on glute training on my home computer. I still need to pay back the IOUs for all the printer ink I used. My bedroom shelves soon had little room for anything but strength training material, namely focusing on gluteal development. I began collecting fitness equipment over time with any money I saved on my teacher's salary (which is nothing to boast about). Over the years, I purchased what amounted to a complete gym, which made my transition from teaching to full-time trainer much easier.

When I was twenty-eight, I left teaching for good to open Lifts, a gym I ran in Scottsdale, Arizona. This is where the bulk of my glute experimentation and testing happened.

Enter the Hip Thrust

I remember the evening I thought of the hip thrust like it was yesterday. It was October 13, 2006, and I was home watching Ken Shamrock get destroyed by Tito Ortiz in a UFC fight. I waited for Shamrock to buck Ortiz off, but he made no attempt to bridge his hips or get out from under Ortiz in any fashion.

At this time, I was already a certified strength and conditioning specialist from the National Strength & Conditioning Association, and this incident got my mind going. Why didn't these fighters do exercises to help them build explosive power? It seemed the only practical way to get out from under what is known as a full mount in the mixed martial arts arena. The wheels in my head spun rapidly, and I headed to my garage to work on some new ideas.

After that night, I started experimenting with my clients in the gym. I began with bodyweight hip thrusts, and then single-leg hip thrusts. This all eventually led to the weighted hip thrusts and bridges that you'll find in the *Strong Curves* workouts. My clients would show up to sessions asking to do these exercises, claiming that they never felt their glutes work as hard during a session than they did with the bridging exercises I introduced.

The results were positive all around. Women who had never trained before were building the strongest glutes

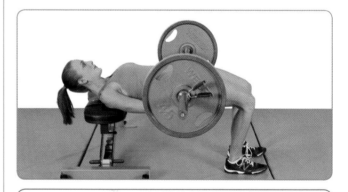

Client success story

I trained Rachel, age twenty-four, for several years before I figured out how to load up glute bridge patterns. I prescribed heavy squats, deadlifts, and lunges each week. She reached a point where she could deep squat 135 x 20 reps, deadlift 155 x 20 reps, and lunge with the thirty-pound dumbbells for forty steps. Her legs were phenomenal, but her glutes were always a bit lacking. Once I thought up the hip thrust exercise and had her start performing it, her glute size and shape took off. In just a month, her glutes looked better than ever. Clearly, the hip thrust required her to activate her glutes much more than the other exercises.

I had ever seen. Girls who previously relied solely on squats and lunges found glute bridges and hip thrusts to bring them to the next level. Of course, there is always the genetic aspect of glutes. Some women responded rapidly, seeing results right away, while others took longer. But they all walked away with a strong and perky set of glutes.

All of my friends and family were on board with my glute obsession after they saw the results of my clients at *Lifts*. I created a family of gluteal connoisseurs, and they couldn't go to the grocery store without noting the lack of rears on most people. You will probably never find another family like us who can hang out at the airport while waiting for a flight and happily analyze butt shapes and sizes together.

Finding the Proof

I had clients come in all day advertising new and improved glutes, but I wanted to learn more about why my training methods worked. Toward the end of my lease at the gym, I transitioned from trainer to writer and started investigating research for my eBook. I leased an electromyography (EMG) machine that measured the electrical activity of muscles and began working late into the night at my gym. Since my entire glute quest began with my own weak glutes, I was the perfect guinea pig for my experiments. With all the doors locked and blinds drawn, I dropped my shorts to hook up electrodes to my glutes, quadriceps, hamstrings, and adductors.

I was the mad scientist of self-gluteal studies, hiding away until 1:00 a.m. most nights trying to discover the most effective means for building glute strength and size. Most guys my age spent their free time watching baseball, playing video games, chasing girls, or hanging out with friends. But I chose to hike up my underwear and test the glute activation of various exercises at all hours of the night. I even made an appointment with a local anatomy professor so that I could spend some time examining the gluteal anatomy of a cadaver. To each his own, right?

Well, to your advantage these experiments paid off, leading to the publication of my eBook, *Advanced Techniques in Glutei Maximi Strengthening*. I received high praise from strength coaches and fitness professionals all over the world, and my methods proved well in other areas, including coaching for sprinters, patients of physical therapists, and sports athletes. Soon magazines both online and print were contacting me to pen articles on the glutes for their upcoming issues. Though I enjoy researching all aspects of strength training and biomechanics, the glutes seem to be what I do best.

My friends and colleagues thought I would finally be content with my achievements, but I decided to sell all of my worldly possessions and move halfway across the world to study at the prestigious sport science institution in New Zealand, AUT University. At AUT, I've been lucky to receive expertise and training from top researchers, scientists, and coaches who have helped me further improve upon my knowledge of the human body—especially the glutes.

The *Strong Curves* Method

Strong Curves is the apex of my research over the past fifteen years. My program designs have evolved markedly during this time, and over the past five years in particular I've blended creative art with cutting-edge science to create what I feel is the most effective female training system on the market.

Many women go into strength training with the same fears: growing big, bulky muscles that lack femininity. This program proves that the stronger you are, the curvier and more feminine your physique will become.

My clients have shown time and again that this program works. While in Auckland, New Zealand in preparation for my PhD, I trained women on the other side of the world using my methods. Each one has seen the most incredible, life-altering results. One client went on to win her fitness competition after not placing in any past shows. Another completely transformed her physique with astonishing results and recently won her very first competition. Her new confidence has improved all aspects of her life.

Now that I'm back in Phoenix, guess what I'm up to? Training figure and bikini competitors. We've developed our own language. Training your glutes is referred to as "gluting." We work our butts "on" rather than work our butts "off," and each girl consistently reaches new levels of gluteal strength and development.

Strong Curves is so effective because it doesn't take a linear approach to training. There is no single method that works best for everyone. What works for you may not work for the next woman. So in my approach, I use what is known as the "shotgun method," covering every single aspect possible to provide you with the most rewarding results.

You may respond well to high reps and moderate

load, or you may respond better to low reps and heavy load. You may do well with one method this month and another next month. A certain exercise might bring you incredible results one year, while the next year you find that focusing on a different exercise helps you reach your goal. But if you are covering all of your bases month in and month out, you will respond well to the entire program. That is what I have learned after years of experimenting.

Not only will this program teach you to fire your glutes during bridging exercises, but also during all exercises in the program. It may feel tough and awkward at first, but after a couple of months, you'll take every opportunity to squeeze your glutes throughout the day.

Though the aesthetic reward of the *Strong Curves Program* is in and of itself worthwhile, the incredible power you attain when you build strong glutes is like nothing you feel with any other muscle group. Your glutes are the center of your body. They are involved in nearly all movement patterns. I found this out for myself once I started building stronger glutes. Things in life are just easier when you have your glutes to power you through activities. You will find running is easier on your knees, your back feels less strained after a long workday, furniture is easier to move, and your kids are easier to keep up with. Your glutes are designed to be the strongest muscle in your body. Imagine how much power they will bring once you build up their strength.

These full body workouts are designed to build the most powerful muscles and leanest physique in the least amount of time. You will hit your glutes multiple times during each session to guarantee the best results. You will train under heavier load with low reps and lighter load with high reps. This program will activate your glutes to their utmost potential, it will stretch them under heavy load, and it will work them through full ranges of motion in a variety of directions and angles. It is a well-rounded program designed with every female body in mind.

How to Approach *Strong Curves*

This book is packed with information regarding strength training for women. Each section can be read on its own but was written to build your knowledge about the program. You can skip right to the workouts, but I encourage you to read the manual in its entirety from start to finish. The more knowledge you have about strength training, the more powerful you will become.

The goal of this book is to provide you with the most comprehensive look at female training so that you feel confident in your quest to build the strongest curves possible. This book offers all the right tools to help you develop a solid foundation for strength training and design your own programs for life. I want you to succeed not only with the twelve-week programs offered in these pages, but also with your commitment to training from this day forward.

The initial chapters invite you to explore why you should train differently than men. You don't necessarily need to do different exercises, but your physique is entirely unique from theirs, and you can't expect to cater to your goals if you train like your male counterparts. You will also learn about two crucial muscle groups that will improve your quality of life, how and why muscles grow, and the importance of movement quality.

Strong Curves offers a simple nutrition guide influenced by the work of nutrition expert, Alan Aragon, that is practical no matter what your goals are with this program. It was designed to complement the workouts in this book and help you achieve your goals even faster.

You will also find four twelve-week programs along with dozens of supplemental exercises in the Exercise Index. I provide more than two hundred exercises complete with detailed photos to show how the exercises should be performed.

Throughout the book, Kellie gives great advice and tips on how to accomplish your goals while using the *Strong Curves Program.* As a woman who has gone through many struggles that you may face, her insight is invaluable for your journey.

My advice before beginning your quest for *Strong Curves* is to take everything in small strides. Have that end goal in mind, but set smaller goals along the way. I often find that if you are constantly striving for that big, lofty goal, you lose sight of why you began your journey in the first place. You will achieve the results you want no matter where you stand today. Just be relentless in your pursuits, and never give up on yourself.

Kellie and I look forward to hearing about your journey. I encourage you to write us during and after this program to share your experiences with us by email.

Chapter 2:
Female Anatomy

The other day in the gym, I watched a woman working out with her husband. He took her through a series of six chest exercises, and they proceeded up the stairs to walk on the treadmill for thirty minutes. It takes every bit of restraint to not open my big mouth when I see situations like this, but the sad reality is that these workouts are all too common for women who go to the gym regularly with a male workout partner.

I shouldn't even reduce it to that. I see this all the time with women, even if they are training alone. They schedule their workout week like a typical bodybuilder, devoting an entire session to a single body part—hitting the glutes only once a week without implementing the best exercises. If I ask you to sit back and rationalize why a woman would want to spend an entire hour training her chest, you probably couldn't give me a single reason.

Sure, you want a strong chest, but do you want to add inches to your pectoral muscles? I don't think that is really a goal, so why train this way? You need to make your workouts as efficient and productive as possible, and "chest day" is not the best route to go. Neither is an arm day, a leg day (usually lacking glute-specific exercises), a shoulder day … well, you get my point. But so many women jump on board with these workout standards and fail to reach their goals. Body part splits work well for those who are near or at maximal growth and need to bring up lagging parts—like high caliber bodybuilders. These types of workouts also focus largely on the upper body, quads, and hamstrings, leaving little room for glute work. With *Strong Curves*, every training day is a glute-specialization day, since this is the most difficult and most important area for a woman to develop.

Another route I often see women traveling is the path of excessive aerobic exercise. This comes in all forms, not limited to long bouts on the treadmill. If you enter the gym with plans to hit the weights and emerge two hours and twenty-seven exercises later, you are guilty of excessive cardio. Just because you train with weights, it doesn't automatically mean you are strength training. You can train hard or long, but not both. Your training program design must be smart in order for it to be effective. Training at high volume for long periods of time actually works against your goals. The same goes for long sessions of cardio exercise. If you truly enjoy running several miles a week or any other form of distance aerobic exercise, then you must work to preserve muscle and stave off catabolism or the breaking down of muscle for energy.

This happens with strategically planned strength sessions and caloric intake. The harder you train, the more you need to eat to preserve muscle. Most women who enjoy long sessions of cardio because they feel it's the only way to burn fat and get in shape also under-nourish their bodies. The very idea that you must starve yourself to get the body you want is wrong on so many levels. There is a huge difference between caloric deficit for weight loss and starvation. But too often, the line that divides these methods is blurry, and women cross over into starvation without ever knowing it. You will learn more about that in Chapter Five.

Apples to Oranges

If you compare the physical structure of a man with a woman, you can tell why both sexes should not share the same training program. This isn't to say that women should train with different exercises or with less intensity or that they should lift less weight relative to their body structure and size. All of those factors remain constant when putting together training programs for either a man or a woman. Due to differences in anthropometry and goals, a woman's program design will differ from a man's simply because her body shape is different. In addition, her image of an ideal body differs from that of a man. For this reason, optimal training for a woman will require a considerably different program design—from the way a routine is split up, to the exercise selection and exercise order, to the frequency, volume, intensity, and density.

Men and women respond to resistance training much in the same manner. However, men and women show significant measurable differences with regard to muscle mass, strength, and hormone levels. The strength differences are largely attributable to body size and composition. Compared to women, men are larger, they carry more muscle mass, and they're leaner.

The sex hormone testosterone drives the difference in size and body composition, but sex hormone-related strength differences are mostly found in the upper body—meaning women tend to possess lower body strength levels similar to men relative to their body weight, but men have greater upper body strength relative to their body weight compared to women. However, when comparing strength per pound of fat-free mass (mostly muscles and bones), strength differences aren't so apparent. Furthermore, when assessing muscle architecture, sex becomes unimportant, and women possess the same force production capabilities as men.

On a side note, I've found that women can become as strong or even stronger than men pound-for-pound during hip thrust exercises. Currently, there are several women performing hip thrusts with two-and-a-half times their body weight! This is insane, and I don't know of any men who can do this at the moment. Clearly, with regard to glutes women do not lag behind men, provided they train properly.

Typically, men are overconfident about strength training, and they often load up too much weight on various exercises, which causes them to use poor form. Conversely, many women lack confidence in the gym and are self-conscious about their strength levels and form even if they're advanced. My colleagues in the industry often joke that men should reduce the weight they use on various exercises by ten percent, but women should increase the weight they use on various exercises by ten percent.

Shannon was 125 pounds and fairly new to my style of strength training. At first she was keeping up with her training partners, but after a few months I noticed she was getting incredibly strong—much stronger than the other women she trained with. I modified her program by just having her perform one hard set of certain exercises. Within five months of training with me twice per week, she started reaching strength levels that I could not believe, hip thrusting three-hundred eighty-five pounds for two reps, performing one-hundred pound back extensions for ten reps, deadlifting a two-hundred-three pound kettlebell for fifteen reps, and even hanging with me in a high-rep hip thrust competition. As a bikini competitor, it was nice to see her on stage as an incredibly lean athlete, but with nice round glutes.

What Women Want

Unlike Mel Gibson, I don't possess the ability to hear what women are thinking. (That was an obscure movie reference.) But if I did possess this ability, I doubt I would walk around the gym hearing women say to themselves, "If I could just get my arms to grow to the size of my neck" or "How can I add inches to my chest muscles?"

It just isn't realistic to think that if you train using the same program as your male counterpart that you will achieve the results that you want. It's like planting an orange seed and expecting an apple tree to grow. If you aren't training your glutes regularly using the right exercises, your glutes won't grow—plain and simple. If you train five days a week with body part splits, devoting a workout to your chest, shoulders, legs, back, and arms, you aren't hitting the right muscles frequently enough to see the results you want.

One huge advantage that you have over men is your recovery time. Whether this has to do with lower levels of strength and/or muscle mass or simply an inherent expedited recovery system, you fatigue less and recover faster than men do. This works to your advantage in that you can train the same muscles frequently throughout your week. That is why I designed the *Strong Curves Program* to hit every muscle group multiple times per week. Your lower body, namely your glutes, will get the most attention. With this program, if you train three to four days per week, your glutes will get the attention they deserve and reward you by growing stronger, rounder, perkier, and shapelier.

After I wrote the *Strong Curves Program* for this book, Kellie decided to test the Gluteal Goddess Program for Advanced Lifters. She sent me her results at the end of each phase with some useful feedback to help me perfect the program even more before I put it in your hands. Our communication was largely through email, but I had the chance to meet with her face-to-face when she had just begun the second phase of the program. I hadn't seen her in five months and couldn't believe how much her body had changed. I don't think she's ever looked better, and I was very impressed with her results after only five weeks in the program. Her upper body was incredibly lean and slender, yet still carried noticeable muscle. Her legs and glutes were in the best shape I'd ever seen them, and she told me she wasn't even dieting. Of course, this was around the holidays, so I wouldn't expect her to diet then. And it wasn't just me who noticed; everyone who saw her commented on how lean and shapely she looked.

The actual program she used was our beta test, so the one in this book is slightly different. However, the template is exactly the same, so she followed the methods you will learn in these pages. I think her results are a great measure to show that no matter the level or stage of your physique, this program will work. Kellie is an elite lifter in many respects, making progress harder to come by. But the progress she achieved in a short time even blew me away. She was the first seasoned test subject to use this program. I also tested this program on clients in New Zealand who achieved amazing results, and I'm currently using the system with my clients in Phoenix. Their results are absolutely phenomenal.

Strong Curves implements the most effective training methods specific to your desires with a nutrition plan that amps up your fat-burning potential to give you the best strategy for building the body you desire.

Chapter 3:

The Important Muscles No One Talks About

Strong Curves offers plenty of opportunities to work all the skeletal muscles in your body, but I want to devote an entire chapter to two key muscle groups because they play an integral role in your success. The first is the glutes (that came out of left field, huh?). But the second muscle is rarely talked about with women when it comes to strength training: the pelvic floor, which we will get to later on in the chapter.

Muscles Deserving of Your Attention

Brazilian models are known for their perky posteriors, which are often thought to be purely a genetic gift. But it isn't solely about genetics. The secret to their perfect pair of cheeks is simply their glute workouts. You see, it's all about the booty in Brazil. It isn't uncommon for these women to devote thirty to sixty minutes of time each workout session to building their glutes and nothing else. No upper body workouts, no abdominal training—just glutes.

I think they have it right. In my experience, most women should just work their butts in order to achieve the body they desire. A life-long booty-specialization program, if you will.

Leandro Carvahlo popularized the Brazilian Butt-Lift Workout several years back, and his signature moves were thought to be the ultimate path to sculpting the behind of his super model clients. But it isn't just his signature moves. It's the frequency and volume of the glute workouts that make the largest difference, and that's what is lacking in the majority of workout programs designed for women. If you've ever seen Carvahlo's videos, you will notice the exercises are purely bodyweight. This is all good and well, but some critical elements that are lacking in the Brazilian Butt-Lift Workout are load (intensity) and strength (progressive overload), not to mention focusing on the best glute activation exercises (exercise selection).

Strength creates curves, and you can only get so far in terms of strength when using only bodyweight loads. For example, a bodyweight glute bridge will activate the glutes at between twenty percent to thirty percent of their maximal ability. Many of my advanced female clients perform barbell glute bridges with over two hundred twenty-five pounds (some of them use over three hundred fifteen pounds), which activates the glutes to one-hundred percent of their maximal ability. For this reason, loaded exercises give you an advantage over bodyweight exercises, and this added tension on the muscles is what builds the sexy shape in the glutes. It is imperative that you continue to ask your glutes to do more over time, as this is the stimulus that drives adaptation.

Strong Curves addresses all the necessary elements in your workout. You hit the glutes multiple times per week with varying volume and load to build the strongest, curviest butt possible. Glute exercises effectively raise the metabolism, causing your entire body to lean out, and they do a great job of working the upper body and core muscles during the process. For example, squats and deadlifts will activate a ton of upper body and core muscle. If you choose to do so, you can also work on upper body and core strength, as well as your quads, hamstrings, and calves. Over the next twelve weeks, you will not only develop greater strength and musculature, but you will also flaunt an amazing pair of glutes as an added bonus. Okay, that might be your overall goal. Either way, it's a winning combination.

The Pelvic Floor

Your pelvic floor is a subject usually discussed with your physician—and likely when you are already having issues related to pelvic floor weakness. This is a very real topic that should be discussed more in the fitness arena, though. The reason why it isn't talked about more often is that we currently don't know that much about pelvic floor dysfunction. I've consulted the literature and had discussions with some of the top physical therapists in the world on the topic of pelvic floor dysfunction, and there really isn't much to go by. I expect this to change in the next decade, but until more is known, I'll offer you the best advice possible based on present findings.

Pregnancy, childbirth, and age all affect the strength of your pelvic floor. The *Strong Curves Program* promotes strengthening of all skeletal muscles, including the pelvic floor. Later in this chapter, I will discuss the importance of adding a few supplemental exercises to help build and maintain strength in this muscle region.

The Glutes in Their Natural Habitat

Now, onto the glutes! I promise not to get too carried away in this section, but it's important for you to understand gluteal physiology and why these strange and stubborn muscles just won't grow unless you encourage them. You will also learn why these muscles are an integral part of your overall strength and physical health.

As you learned in my introduction, I have become quite the expert at sculpting behinds. Although it may seem trivial, I must tell you that this is not an easy task. Even if you couldn't care less about the perkiness of your posterior (which I doubt is the case), your glutes are still an important factor in training no matter your purpose.

Let's take the aesthetic aspect of the glutes out of the equation altogether and focus solely on improving performance and function. If a sprinter comes to me because she wants to shed seconds off her time, I work on her glutes. If a baseball pitcher asks me to help improve his performance, I get his glutes stronger. For clients with back pain, I strengthen the glutes. For clients with poor posture, valgus collapse, anterior pelvic tilt, or any other physical impediment, I get those glutes stronger.

The glutes play an integral role in your overall functioning and wellness, but the single nagging issue that prevents you from running like a well-oiled machine is that your glutes shut down. That's right. The glutes actually stop working properly due to inactivity. World renowned physical therapist Vladimir Janda noticed this decades ago. Some muscles are quite prone to inhibition, with the glutes probably being the worst of the bunch. So, all of this sitting at a desk all day, watching television, and driving from place to place causes your glutes to retire early.

A toddler offers a good example of amazing glute activation. Yes, toddlers have chubby little bottoms, but they have really great glute muscles as well. If you ever get a chance to hang out with a toddler for a day, just sit back and watch the adorable little guy or girl move. Pay attention to how he picks things up. This toddler will likely have better squat form than ninety-nine percent of the people in your gym. Watch the kid bend, move, and manipulate around objects. This bouncing ball of energy is constantly going and taking full advantage of those glute muscles.

Our glute muscles would stay this strong throughout our lives if we continued to behave like toddlers. Well, not the tantrums and the putting small objects in our mouths, but the activity of kids is what keeps their glutes strong. Unfortunately, the older we get, the less active we become. With video games, computers, and television popping up in bedrooms all over the world, inactivity creeps up on us at younger and younger ages. The more sedentary we become, the less we use our glutes. Unlike other muscles, your glutes will be pretty lazy if you allow them to be. Rather than sticking up for themselves and saying, "Hey! We need activity, too," they go into early retirement. They just close up shop and stop working.

This causes other muscles to take over and bear the brunt of the work. Considering that your glute muscles were designed by nature to be the strongest muscles in your body, this overcompensation puts a lot of wear and tear on muscles that are not meant to handle this workload.

When the glutes shut down, you recruit other muscles to do big jobs that they are not meant to do. Your low back picks up most of the slack, as do your hamstrings, quads, and other surrounding muscles. Over time, this causes injuries. Most low back injuries are preventable, but only if strong glutes are part of the picture.

Even the slightest lower body injury will cause your glutes to shut down. This is thought to be due to our

> Donna always felt hip thrusts in her quadriceps rather than her glutes. She's a very strong squatter and is quad-dominant by nature. Whether she's doing bodyweight hip thrusts or one-hundred eighty-five pound hip thrusts, she feels them solely in her quads. I decided to give her feet-elevated glute bridges while placing her heels on the top of the bench. This took her quads completely out of the lift, placing the burden solely on the hamstrings and glutes. Though it's an easier exercise than the barbell hip thrust, for the first time Donna was able to feel a bridging movement in her glutes. In fact, she'd never felt a glute exercise burn her booty so deeply in her entire life. She squats two-hundred pounds and deadlifts two-hundred thirty-five pounds, but we stick to two sets of thirty feet-elevated glute bridges with only body weight. This does the trick and even helps her feel her glutes activating better during other lower body movements. Her glutes firmed up significantly after performing this movement for only two weeks.

prehistoric survival instincts. Since your glutes are the largest, most powerful muscle in your body and since your brain wants to protect and preserve the nagging part, shutting down the glutes is a wise strategy because it inhibits powerful locomotion, which would be counterproductive to rehabilitation. If something goes haywire or injury occurs, your body instinctively turns them off to protect the injured region. Even the smallest injury like a stubbed toe will trigger your brain to turn off your glutes, and the same has been shown for ankle, knee, hip, and low back injuries. To allow these injuries to heal, it's wise for your body to shut down the glutes so that you can't move as quickly or explosively.

While the stubbed toe and other injuries will eventually heal and return to normal, your glute activation doesn't always follow suit. Unless you are actively recruiting the glute muscles to perform tasks, they have no reason to turn back on. Think about a lion, known as the king of the African plains. These beasts are powerful, fierce hunters, but if you watch nature movies, they pretty much lie around all day and do nothing until it's time to hunt. That's because instinct tells them to preserve energy for those big tasks. If you equate your glutes to the lions (or lionesses) of the human body, you can see how they work by nature. They will lie around all day long until you recruit them for big tasks. But, unlike lions, they don't need to conserve energy to survive (at least not in this day and age when food isn't scarce). In fact, the more you activate and recruit your glutes, the stronger and more powerful they become.

Talk About Lazy

The gluteus maximus is a walking paradox. Contrary to popular opinion, it is made up of a higher proportion of slow-twitch muscle fibers that fire more slowly so that they fatigue less quickly, but the muscle behaves like it has fast-twitch muscle fibers that generate short bursts of strength for explosive movements. This means that the gluteus maximus is a stubborn muscle that would rather stay dormant and let other muscles take on the big tasks.

Daily activities such as walking, using the stairs, performing chores, and job duties can keep your other muscles functioning sufficiently, but your glutes need direct, heavy, or explosive hip movement to fire correctly. For example, someone performing a bodyweight squatting movement might activate sixty percent of maximum quadriceps contraction but only ten percent of maximum glute contraction. You can see why normal daily life keeps the quads active and strong while letting the glutes go dormant at the same time. I can bet a good majority of desk workers do not get sufficient muscle activation in their hips on a daily basis. Sitting for many hours each day can potentially damage the glute muscles by several different mechanisms. The first is the shortening of your hip flexors. When this occurs, you lose mobility, feel stiff, and pain may increase in areas like your low back, knees, and, of course, hips.

Once your hip flexors tighten up, your glutes decide it's time to hit the road, and they start to shut down. This happens because the tightening (caused by adaptive shortening) of your hip flexors doesn't allow for full hip extension at the range where your glutes work their best. Additionally, the shortened hip flexors inhibit glute firing in a complex process known as reciprocal inhibition. Basically your glutes say, "Okay, hip flexors, if you want to be short with me, I'll give you the silent treatment." Daily sitting compresses the gluteus maximus, impairing blood flow and nutrition, and interfering with neuromuscular power. Finally, as I mentioned earlier in the chapter, prior injuries and pain inhibit the glutes and prevent strong contractions.

Noted previously, several muscles can make up for weak glutes, including hamstrings, adductors, quadriceps, and erector spinae. Imagine running a moving company where your biggest, strongest worker decides he's going take it easy and let everyone else do the work for him. Your other workers would wear down much faster and begin to suffer aches, pains, and injuries. They probably wouldn't get enough work done during the day either. This is exactly what happens to your surrounding muscle and tissue when you have weak glutes.

Combine hours of sitting with a lack of daily activation, and you're missing all of the ingredients for a nice butt. This is more like a recipe for a very depressed backside that doesn't activate well and has a hard time going through its natural range of motion due to hip immobility. A very sad sight indeed. Many practitioners have coined the term "gluteal amnesia" to describe the dormant glutes that so many office workers and pretty much everyone without a physical job succumb to as they get older. Poor glutes are a virtual pandemic in our society, but *Strong Curves* is going to make sure you don't succumb to that fate.

What's the Big Deal About Glutes Anyway?

The gluteal muscle group is made up of the gluteus maximus, gluteus medius, and gluteus minimus. Physiologically, the gluteus maximus is the strongest muscle in the human body. By location alone, you can see that the gluteal muscle group is connected to your upper body, core, and lower body extremities through the pelvis, sacrum, coccyx, and femur, not to mention the tibia through the iliotibial band and the latissimus dorsi through the thoracolumbar connective tissue. The glutes are a critical component of all movement involving running, jumping, throwing, swinging, striking, maneuvering, and twisting. You never see an NFL receiver without a strong pair of glutes because they are such an integral part of his performance.

Your glutes have several large jobs that are all related to your ability to move correctly, including:

- Moving the thigh rearward, known as hip extension
- Extending the trunk, also known as hip extension
- Moving the thigh laterally, known as hip abduction
- Rotating the trunk or leg, known as hip external rotation
- Rotating the pelvis rearward, known as posterior pelvic tilt
- Stabilizing the hips isometrically in all four actions mentioned above
- Absorbing the impact (eccentrically) of hip flexion, adduction, internal rotation, and anterior pelvic tilt.
- Preventing valgus collapse (knees caving inward)
- Preventing excessive spinal motion (flexion and hyperextension)
- Preventing slouching posture and lower-cross syndrome
- Reducing incidents of hamstring and groin strains, sacroiliac joint pain that causes low back pain, iliotibial band syndrome and patellofemoral (knee) pain, anterior femoral glide syndrome that causes pain in the front of the hips, piriformis syndrome that sometimes leads to sciatica, and sports hernias.
- Reducing injury potential in all areas of the body due to its vast linkage to the body's various kinetic chains

Your glutes are also responsible for many aspects of sports performance. If you think back to high school and college, the fastest runners probably had nice glutes. The strongest servers in tennis, the highest jumpers in basketball, the most powerful weight lifters, the hardest kickers in soccer, and the best wrestlers likely carried similar attributes.

Mary initially experienced pain in her low back during hip thrusts, so I had her engage in posterior pelvic tilt when performing them. Being a personal trainer herself, she was in good shape, so I started her hip thrust at one-hundred five pounds. After two weeks, she progressed to one-hundred fifty-five pounds and put two solid inches on her glutes without gaining any extra weight. Her booty was already fantastic, but the hip thrusts took her glutes to a brand new level in a very short period of time. Her training group could not believe how quickly she progressed and even jokingly accused her of getting implants.

Gluteal Muscles

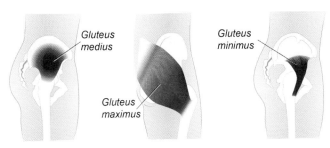

Gluteus medius

Gluteus minimus

Gluteus maximus

The Good, The Bad, and The Ugly Booty

Butts come in all shapes and sizes. Often, what differentiates a good booty from a bad one is glute strength. It's important to understand one thing before you begin your booty-sculpting mission with *Strong Curves:* You can't change your genetics. This doesn't mean that if you have a flat bottom, it will always be flat. But you can't expect to change a barstool seat cushion to a beanbag chair by adding more cotton.

Okay, that was a bad analogy. You will improve the strength, shape, and tone of your glutes no matter where you begin when you work through the *Strong Curves Program.* Still, you can only go as far as your genetics will take you. I've trained a client who went from having a weak, flat, sagging butt (her words, not mine) to having powerful, shapely glutes that others envied. But she still couldn't keep up with the Kardashians. It just wasn't in her stars, yet she loved her new shape so much so that she didn't care.

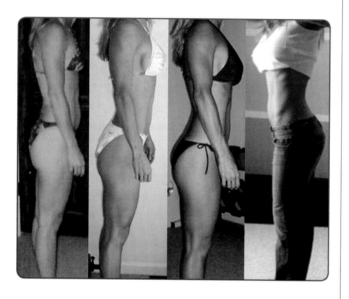

I've had other clients who went from zero to superhero glutes in a matter of weeks. It all depends on what you are genetically capable of accomplishing. Other factors—the relative percentage of Type I and Type II muscles fibers, age, natural hormone levels, somatotype (body type and build), and stubborn body parts—are also beyond your control.

Keep that in mind, but know full well that you will achieve tremendous results if you stick with the program and follow my template to the letter. Veer from the program, make your own rules, change things around, or give up, and you will be back to square *uno.*

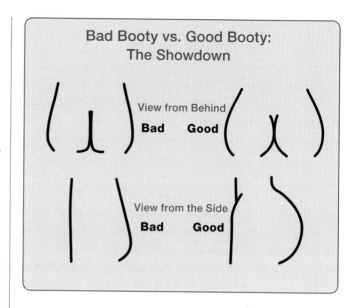

Bad Booty vs. Good Booty: The Showdown

View from Behind
Bad **Good**

View from the Side
Bad **Good**

Though my drawing is rudimentary, it clearly demonstrates the difference between a strong set of glutes and a weak set. The bad booty on the left lacks depth, fullness, and has what are known as glute folds, where the actual buttocks show excessive folds at the separation point from the hamstring. The booty on the right is perky, round, and shapely. If you were a master sculptor, you would know that you need to add matter in certain areas and take away matter in other areas in order to create the needed changes to go from gluteus patheticus to gluteus magnificus. The next logical question is, "How do I go from looking like the picture on the left to looking like the picture on the right?"

What determines a good booty over a bad booty is the amount of muscle you carry back there. Many women feel that losing weight is the answer, but when they get down to the weight they desire, their butts don't get any better. In fact, sometimes they get worse. Remember, glutes are made in the gym. You have to build that muscle and hit it from all angles to curve out your backside.

We discussed how to get from bad to good and even from good to superhero, but what about the ugly? It isn't that your bottom is physically ugly. It's that your glutes have shut down for so long that you now suffer from poor movement quality. I address the importance of movement quality in Chapter Six, so don't skip it. This chapter is directly speaking to you.

So, the ugly is when you actually suffer injury or physical symptoms from glute inactivity. I work on a regular basis with clients who suffer from poor movement patterns due to weak glutes. It's far more common than you would like to think, and fitness professionals are used to it. The only way you will overcome these issues is if you address them head on.

As I mentioned before, it's important to be honest with yourself about your abilities. If an exercise is too difficult, there is no shame in regressing the movement to a level that is more comfortable. If you find an exercise is far too difficult in the workout, refer to the Exercise Index for an exercise that is more suitable. They are categorized by exercise type and arranged in a progressively more challenging manner, so you can easily find a replacement.

This doesn't mean that the initial exercise just goes off the radar, though. Keep it as a future goal. *Strong Curves* was designed for progressive overload, so I'll bet you will progress to that level far faster than you imagine. This means that week-to-week, you will make great improvements with your workouts. Don't give up on yourself, and keep striving toward those goals.

So, rather than pushing through exercises that are too difficult, you must be able to evaluate your own movement quality and regress your workout until you are moving properly again. Weak glutes can cause your knees to cave in during a squat (valgus collapse), your posture to erode, or your low back to ache when you go about daily activities.

Don't worry; every bad or ugly booty is fixable. By the end of this program, you will have glutes that pack power and, as an added bonus, fill out your jeans just right. Your back pain may go away, your poor movement patterns may disappear, and you will be well on your way to a healthier, happier life all thanks to glute activation, strength, and good form!

Get Those Glutes Firing on All Cylinders

One of the most important factors in this program is consistent glute activation. You should activate your glutes during the entire duration of your workout, including all lower and most upper body movements. It will not happen instantly, but after two months on this program, you will really feel your glutes working with every exercise.

On days off, take ten minutes to work on glute activation. Perform different at-home glute exercises that are

Lisa was a twenty-five-year-old, athletic-looking girl who started training with me at my former gym, *Lifts*. She felt her glutes had not changed shape over a twelve-month period despite performing heavy strength training, high rep strength training, explosive strength training, and all of the best glute exercises known to mankind. Lisa lost body fat and gained muscle elsewhere, but she was always a bit frustrated with her lack of glute development. When we compared her initial training pictures with her pictures after one year of training, it was evident that her backside had indeed improved markedly. I tried to convince her that she had already made great strides, but she wanted the perfect butt.

In contrast, Alicia was a nineteen-year-old, thin girl who came to *Lifts* at around the same time as Lisa. She trained with her mother, and her butt went from "not a whole lot" to "a whole lot" in a very short period of time. Trust me when I tell you that it looked unbelievable. One day, her mother asked, "Can you believe how amazing Alicia's butt looks?" Now, if your mother notices your booty, you know you've made great improvements. I asked one of the trainers at my gym to pick up Alicia's training journal so that we could see exactly how long she'd been training with us and how many sessions she'd performed. At that time, she'd only performed six workouts in a two-week period.

Alicia's booty literally transformed with only six hours of training spanning over a fourteen-day period. To this day, I have never witnessed such rapid results and find this to be the most impressive case of genetic response.

These two scenarios illustrate just how important genetics can be with regard to glute adaptations. These two girls received the same training stimulus but showcased quite different results. These cases prove, however, that anyone and everyone can and will see results. Lisa no longer trains with me, but she went on to become a figure competitor with a great pair of glutes. She has continued to train hard using the best methods, and the effort has paid off.

On the other hand, I've run into Alicia a few times over the past couple of years, and she stopped training. Needless to say, she lost most of her behind's c-shape, even though she possesses the perfect genetics to maintain it.

offered in this book. It will make a huge difference, and you will soon feel your glutes working when you walk, when you run, and even when you stand in place. The biggest problem with glute development is that people are not activating their glutes sufficiently. The gluteus maximus is a strange muscle. It's always trying to find a reason to shut down.

Quite often, people are performing great glute exercises but aren't activating them properly throughout the movements. For example, you can squat and lunge while using mostly quad and spinal erectors, and you can deadlift and bridge by using mostly spinal erectors and hamstrings. When you learn to activate your glutes properly and master the feel of strong glute contractions, you'll begin to heavily incorporate your glutes into all of your lower body movement patterns, including squats, deadlifts, good mornings, lunges, hip thrusts, back extensions, and even planks.

You may have seen my YouTube videos of strong ladies and athletes moving heavy weight on their glute exercises. They didn't start out that way. Most of my clients started out with bodyweight squats and bridges. I worked hard to get them to sit back, keep their knees tracking over their toes, utilize proper lumbopelvic mechanics, push through the feet properly, and symmetrically activate the glutes. Once all of these happen I add load. After about six weeks of constant feedback and reminding, my clients almost always boast how well their glutes work during their sessions and how confident they are because they have already reached strength levels they previously thought were unattainable.

In studying muscle activation/EMG (electromyography), I learned a few things. First, clients commented on how they felt their glutes working more with certain tweaks. This proved true in all cases. In other words, EMG activity confirmed that they activated their glutes more when doing a movement a certain way. For example, some flared their feet outward during a bridge, and this led to much greater levels of glute activation. This testing also helped me figure out why most of my advanced clients gravitated toward rounding their upper backs when performing back extensions, which was accompanied by posterior pelvic tilting and led to greater levels of glute activation.

Second, shorter individuals who were the best squatters tended to activate more quad and less glute than their taller counterparts during squatting and lunging motions. In fact, my best squatter of all time only activates about fifteen percent of her average glute MVC (maximum voluntary contraction)!

When I teach seminars for coaches, I always run them through a glute activation test consisting of supine, prone, quadruped, and side lying movements off the floor. About a third of them give up because of severe hamstring cramps, which proves my theory that most people do not know how to activate their glutes properly—coaches included. If you have weak glute muscles, other muscles are quick to jump in and take over responsibility. Hamstrings, spinal erectors, and other surrounding muscles often bear the brunt of the work that is required by the glutes. This keeps your glutes consistently underworked, underdeveloped, and underutilized.

So, before you begin the *Strong Curves Program*, you must first learn to activate your glutes from various positions. I've had clients who can fire their glutes like crazy from one position, but not in another. Even Kellie, my Mona Lisa, struggled to activate her glutes whenever her legs were straight as in the case of planks, push-ups, and back extensions, despite the fact that her glutes fired incredibly hard during bent leg movements such as squats and bridges. It takes a good amount of work and patience to correctly fire your glutes from all positions, but these exercises will get you started.

Don't be too hard on yourself if you find you can't perform these testing exercises correctly. Most people can't at first, but you will master them over time and create that strong, enviable booty you want.

Kellie's Notes on Muscle Size vs. Muscular Strength—My Davis Versus Goliath Story

I'm not intimidating by any means. Sure, I look athletic, but most people expect me to walk into the gym and head to yoga class. The other day, I was training with the Strong Curves Program and working on my barbell glute bridges. There just happened to be a band of male pro bodybuilders across the room doing a lot more talking than working. I guess my bridges caught their attention because one of them, a top ten Mr. Olympia contender who was only a few weeks out from a show, came over and asked if he could try the exercise. I warned him that it wasn't as easy as it looked, and it took a long time to work up to the weight I was using, which was a meager three hundred fifty-five pounds. Surely, my tiny one hundred twenty-eight-pound frame was no match for this beast with forearms larger than my legs.

He inched under the bar, barely able to get it over his massive quads, and lay their trapped. Sweat poured down his forehead, and grunts bellowed out from his throat, while the bar didn't move a single centimeter. He couldn't lift it off the floor with his hips because his glutes weren't strong enough. He spent more time in the gym each week than I probably spent all month, but all that training didn't translate to hip strength. In fact, many bodybuilders train their glutes inadequately, and it shows on stage.

For a good twenty minutes after his humiliating defeat, he came up with several "tricks" that he was sure I had used to move the weight. But, rest assured, no trickery was involved. It's just good work ethic, the right programming, and learning to activate the glutes properly so they grow in strength and size. Sadly for him, my glutes are just stronger than his in that range of motion.

Testing Exercises

Get down on the floor, and perform each of these movements for about sixty seconds each. If it's a single-leg movement, perform about thirty seconds on each side.

Side lying hip abduction—From a side-lying position with the body in a straight line, use the upper glutes to raise the leg. Avoid leaning backward during the movement. You should palpate the upper glutes to feel them contracting properly during the movement.

Side lying clam—From a side-lying position, flex the hips about 45 degrees, and keep the heels in contact with one another. The gluteus maximus should contract to externally rotate and lift the leg (like opening a clamshell). You shouldn't twist the spine or sway, and you should feel your glutes contracting sufficiently.

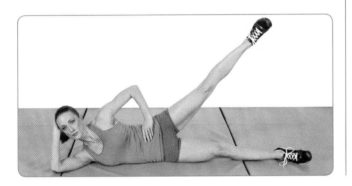

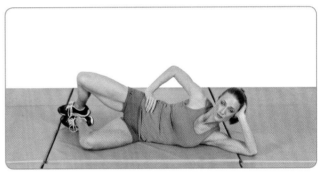

Double-leg glute bridge—From a supine position with bent legs, push through the heels, and raise the hips into the air. You should reach full hip extension and should be able to palpate the glutes, erectors, and hamstrings and find that the glutes are doing most of the work, not the erectors and hamstrings. The lumbar spine shouldn't overarch (hyperextend), the pelvis shouldn't rotate forward (anterior tilt), and the movement should occur in the hips.

Quadruped bent leg hip extension—From a quadruped (all fours) position, raise one bent leg upward. The movement should occur mostly at the hips and not much at the spine and pelvis. The glutes should produce the movement, not the low back and hamstrings.

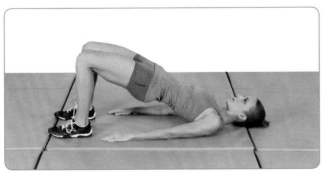

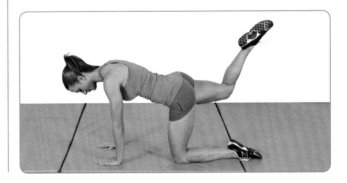

Bird dog—From a quadruped position, lift the left arm up, and kick the right leg up at the same time. Then, repeat with the right arm and left leg. Though you'll be lifting opposing limbs, you shouldn't shift or rotate in the core, and your spine should remain relatively neutral.

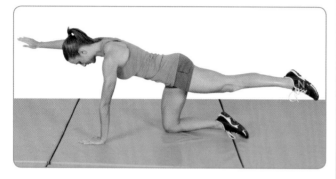

Single-leg glute bridge—From a supine position, center one bent leg, and raise the hips into the air. The non-working leg hovers in the air and can remain straight (in line with the body) or flexed with a bent knee. You shouldn't hyperextend the low back or anteriorly tilt the pelvis, and your core shouldn't shift or rotate. The glute max should contract very hard to raise your body into the air, and you should not feel any pain in the low back or sacral region.

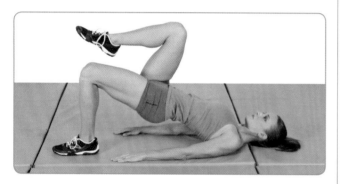

How did that feel? If your cheeks are on fire right now, that's a good thing. If your glutes cramped up, and you doubled over in pain, that's great! It means your glutes know how to work properly during movement, and you are well on your way to a perfectly strong and perky booty.

If, on the other hand, your hamstrings or lower back are tight, you need to practice these exercises on a daily basis until you feel your glutes working. Think of the posterior chain as a river of electrical current flowing from the brain and branching off into three waterfalls—the erectors, the glutes, and the hamstrings. Many individuals shuttle too much electrical current to the erectors and hamstrings and not enough to the glutes. After being on the *Strong Curves Program* for a period of time, you'll entice the brain to direct more juice to the glutes and less to the hamstrings and erec-

tors. Essentially, you'll rewire your motor patterns.

If you feel pain during any of these movements, it's a bad sign. For example, people with weak glutes sometimes feel pain in their low backs when performing the single-leg glute bridge test. Never perform any exercise that causes immediate pain. If it hurts, don't do it! You can always find movements to perform that won't cause pain. Once you get stronger, you'll be able to progress to more challenging movements, but you need to strengthen the glutes so that they keep the sacrum tight and the spine and pelvis in check in order to prevent painful patterns.

These exercises are always a good starting point if you are a beginner and lacking in the glute department. Spend ten minutes once or twice each day with these glute activation exercises, and you will be a glute master in no time.

> **Kellie's Quick Tip:** *I try to fit in various glute-activation exercises throughout my day. When I cook, I do side leg raises or kickbacks. In the morning, I perform single-leg hip thrusts on my bed. I also keep my glutes tight during all exercises, including all upper push and pull movements. After doing this for a few days, you will feel a noticeable firmness in your glutes all the time.*

Time to Get Personal

I don't know if it's the subject matter or location of the subject matter, but you rarely hear fitness professionals discussing pelvic floor strength. I will be the first to admit that though I have trained hundreds of women over the past fifteen years, not a single client has ever asked me about pelvic floor muscles.

I figure it's because I'm a guy, but many of my female colleagues report to me the same thing. I always make it a discussion point with my clients as a part of the learning process when we go over core stability. Usually, the discussion never goes beyond this, but I want to expand upon the topic with you because this might just answer some of those hard to discuss questions.

When discussing core muscles, the groups most often include larger muscles such as the rectus abdominis, internal and external obliques, and erector spinae, as well as smaller muscles such as the transverse abdominis, multifidus, diaphragm, and pelvic floor muscles. The core musculature forms a corset around your low back and hips, with your pelvic floor muscles slung like a hammock from your coccyx to your pubis.

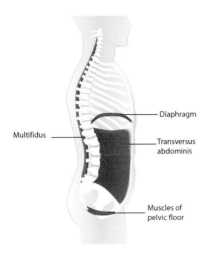

The pelvic floor (pubococcygeal or PC) muscles consist of a deep and superficial muscle layer responsible for holding all of the pelvic organs in place so that they are healthy and well-functioning. Weakened pelvic muscles can cause a number of issues, including urinary and stool incontinence, poor muscle action during labor and delivery, decreased sexual pleasure, decreased vaginal lubrication during menopause, and a prolapsed uterus.

An estimated two hundred million women worldwide suffer from urinary incontinence due to weakened pelvic muscles. As many as one-third of new mothers experience stress incontinence—the involuntary loss of urine due to physical activity like coughing, jumping, sneezing, and exercising. Women who have given birth or are going through menopause also report sexual difficulties or lack of lubrication due to weak pelvic floor muscles, resulting in painful intercourse and the inability to experience orgasm.

These are hard issues to discuss with a healthcare or fitness professional, so many women suffer from the symptoms for years without relief. The optimal solution entails a comprehensive approach. Healthcare and fitness professionals generally agree that exercising the pelvic floor muscles is an excellent way to prevent and treat these problems. Though pelvic floor exercises may not provide a complete solution to all ailments, they are often a step in the right direction. Strong pelvic floor muscles have been shown to improve these symptoms for nearly eighty-six percent of women who try them.

That said, since poor relationships between pelvic floor muscle length and tension are often created by tight and weak surrounding musculature attached to the pelvis, which is commonly accompanied by trigger points (hyperirritable spots in the muscle often referred to as "knots"), along with faulty breathing patterns, multiple components must be addressed for optimal results.

Flexibility Work

Sometimes, the pelvic floor can become too rigid due to tight musculature surrounding the pelvis, such as tight adductors, hip flexors, and abdominals. Regular stretching and strengthening of these muscles (through full ranges of motion) can benefit you by lengthening the muscles and removing the stimulus responsible for the pelvic floor rigidity.

Conversely, some therapists believe that pelvic floor laxity can be caused by weak glutes that are responsible for pulling rearward on the sacrum, keeping the "hammock" tight. By strengthening the gluteals, the "hammock" is pulled tight and no slack exists, allowing the pelvic floor muscles to function at their proper length. This theory is yet to be proven, but rest assured that the *Strong Curves Program* works to improve this issue to the fullest extent.

Trigger Point Therapy

Kegel exercises will help if the issue is laxity in the pelvic floor muscles, but in many women, the pelvic floor muscles are chronically short and experience frequent spasms. For this reason, Kegels could aggravate rather than solve the pelvic floor issues. Many women have "trigger points" in their pelvic floor muscles, and some therapists have found it beneficial to have them perform "self-myofascial release" or SMR, which is a type of massage that can be done on one's self. You may find trigger points in the inner thighs, the lower abdominals, the upper gluteals, or even the pelvic floor muscles themselves. It's possible to perform SMR for the pelvic floor muscles by placing a tennis ball on the ground and appropriately positioning your body over the tennis ball so that the ball is located right under the perineum, in between the anus and vagina.

If you're experiencing pelvic floor-related issues, I recommend that you hold this position for five minutes daily in order to cause the pelvic floor muscles to relax. This can be painful and uncomfortable at first, but you will eventually tolerate it well.

Diaphragmatic Breathing

Breathing dysfunction also often accompanies pelvic floor dysfunction. Remember that the diaphragm and the pelvic floor muscles form the top and bottom of the core stability "cylinder," and both sides need to function properly for optimal biomechanics. You need to make sure you're breathing with your diaphragm to allow your core to function properly. Here's how to focus on your breathing patterns:

1. Sit or lie comfortably wearing loose garments.

2. Put one hand on your chest and one hand on your stomach.

3. Slowly inhale through your nose for a total of four seconds.

4. As you inhale, push your belly out, and feel your stomach expand with your hand. Your belly should rise first for two seconds, followed by your chest for two seconds.

5. Exhale through pursed lips in reverse order—chest first and belly second, making sure to spend more time on exhalation than inhalation.

By learning to breathe properly and relaxing the pelvic floor muscles through trigger point therapy, the pelvic floor will be more apt to "learn." After breathing drills and trigger point therapy, you can then perform Kegels in order to "re-educate" the pelvic floor muscles how to function properly.

Pelvic Floor Exercises

Pelvic floor exercises, along with your *Strong Curves* strength training routine, will improve blood circulation and strengthen muscles to increase pelvic floor muscle function and support pelvic organs. Below are just a few ways pelvic floor muscle strengthening can improve your quality of life:

- Exercise helps to strengthen muscle around the rectal opening and urethra to prevent involuntary loss of waste.

- Pelvic floor exercises help a mother during pregnancy, delivery, and post-partum recovery from either a vaginal or cesarean childbirth.

- An increased blood flow due to exercise causes extra lubrication, which prevents discomfort during sexual intercourse.

- A firm pelvic floor allows tightening of the vaginal walls during contraction, increasing pleasure during intercourse due to the vast number of nerve endings in this area.

- Exercise helps reduce the risk of prolapsed organs such as a prolapsed uterus.

Performing pelvic floor exercises every day is only half the battle. Experts find that even when women attempt to add them to their daily regimen, they often don't understand how to activate the PC muscles properly. Physical therapists at incontinence centers are trained professionals who handle pelvic floor weakness on a daily basis. They use biofeedback monitors that help women understand how to exercise the pelvic floor muscles properly and assess them for weakness.

You don't need to go to an incontinence clinic to get your pelvic floor muscles working, but you do need to understand exactly what's working when you do this type of exercise. Studies show that an alarming number of women don't even know how to voluntarily activate their pelvic floor muscles. Many will mistakenly activate their glutes or other muscles. Among the women who do know how to voluntarily activate their pelvic floor muscles, many do so in a faulty manner by pushing out on the muscles. Proper contraction of these muscles involves a "pulling in" action, which is why it's very important to practice proper muscle contraction so that it becomes automatic.

> **Kellie's Quick Tip:** *PC muscle exercises are easy to get excited about and just as easy to forget. Most women find that they remember to do them the first few days but completely stop after about a week. Don't let that happen. Set an alarm to go off three times a day to help you stay on track with your exercises. Just like the gym, the more regularly you practice, the better you will feel.*

Though strength training—especially the *Strong Curves Program*—is one of the best methods to improve all-over strength, your PC muscles will only improve so much through full body exercise. In fact, the core stabilization requirements of many of the exercises included in *Strong Curves* will train the diaphragm, pelvic floor, transverse abdominis, and multifidis to work together like a cylinder to produce intra-abdominal pressure (IAP). IAP is created when taking in and holding a deep breath while lifting weights. A strong core region creates a natural protective "belt" during this action to protect the spine. But just like your glutes, your PC muscles might need exercises that specifically require activation—and this doesn't just go for women. Men can use exercise to strengthen their PC muscles as well. In fact, this is a very important practice for men who have undergone prostate operations.

For those suffering from pelvic floor-related dysfunction, I recommend getting in three daily sessions of ten quality PC muscle contractions each day. This will take very little time and can be done while you go about your daily activities. You might need a little more focus during your first initial sessions, but after a while you'll be able to perform them with ease.

Here are a few tips to make sure you activate your PC muscles correctly during your Kegel exercises so that you can make the most of this practice:

- Find a mental image to focus on. A college professor described them to me as trying not to pass gas or pee your pants. So, imagine meeting the President. You wouldn't want to pass gas or pee your pants in front of the President, would you? If this doesn't work, try drawing your tailbone toward your pubic bone, or imagine recoiling the pelvic floor from your underwear. It sounds strange, but you need to imagine yourself doing something that allows your mind to focus on the exercises.

- Most women find it easiest to perform Kegel exercises while lying on their backs with their feet on the floor (like the set up for a glute bridge). However, you can do them seated or standing as well.

- When you perform Kegels, the exercises should not be visible to anyone else. Your glutes and abdominal muscles should not move. You want to completely isolate your PC muscles.

- Try not to hold your breath while doing these. You may find this impossible at first because you're concentrating too hard to think about it, but after a few sessions, return your breathing patterns to normal.

- Completely relax between each contraction. You may want to take a ten-second break before starting your next one.

- Remember that quality counts over quantity. You want a few good contractions each session over ten mediocre ones. The stronger your PC muscles get, the better your contractions will be. Stick with it, and know that just like deadlifts, squats, and bridges, they will get easier.

Chapter 4:

Building Booty-ful Muscle

One of the most common reasons people give up on training and nutrition programs is expectation. They go in with a certain result in mind and want to achieve that result in a given time period—likely as promised by the program designer. After weeks of working their way toward their goal, they realize they aren't achieving the results they were striving toward. It's far easier to forget the whole idea rather than tinker with their programs until they find what works best for them.

So, it's important to note that while you will follow the same *Strong Curves Program* as other women— maybe even women you know—you won't get the exact same results as anyone else. If you do everything I say, you will achieve success with this program, but researchers haven't devised any protocols to assess what works best for each individual. Just like your hair color, eye color, height, and skin tone are unique to you, so is your response to stimuli in an exercise program.

To be successful with any workout or nutrition program, you must learn to assess your own needs and be in tune with your body. I know this is far easier said than done. That's why it's important to also keep an open mind and realize, just like those late night infomercials warn, that "results may vary." This doesn't mean you won't torch any fat or build any muscle. That's far from the truth. I can promise that by the time you complete the first twelve weeks of any *Strong Curves Program*, you will be leaner, stronger, and more confident. But never forget that many factors—genetics, age, lifestyle, body structure, metabolism, initial conditioning, and overall health, to name a few—come into play.

When I assess a new client, I come up with the best program to fit her needs and goals on that given day. Over time, her needs may change. She may respond well to certain programming one month, but plateau with it the next. Then again, she may respond so well to the program that I leave it as is.

Since I'm not there training you, I will rely on you to notice these changes within your own program. Always keep in mind that your body has the ability to adapt rapidly to new stimuli, so experiment with your workouts to achieve the best results.

Shotgun Approach vs. Rifle Approach

In everyday life, we find it better to take the rifle approach than the shotgun approach. With the rifle approach, you focus on a single activity until completed before moving on to the next task. If you choose the shotgun approach, you tend to jump around too often, leaving projects unfinished.

However, in the past decade of research and fieldwork I've grown fond of the shotgun as my weapon of choice when designing training programs. I'm a precise marksman, so even though I choose a program that spans across a wide area, I do so with the same goals in mind—to get you leaner and stronger. If, like many programs, you take the rifle approach to exercise, you focus on one goal at a time, building up each goal in a pyramid fashion. A newcomer to exercise might start with stability and endurance in the initial phase, then move on to several different phases of strength, finally ending up in a power phase months down the line.

The problem I have with this approach is that your body is usually ready to take on those big stressors (like lifts that use force and explosion) pretty early on in the game. But with the rifle approach, you don't get to that phase for a long time. What if I told you, "We are going to play it safe, so you won't see hip thrusts in your program until week twenty-four of *Strong Curves*?" You wouldn't have much confidence in my ability to coach you, and you would probably see only incremental changes in your progress each month. That's not what you want, and that isn't what I want for you from this program.

The shotgun approach to training allows you to address every need at once, leaving out the guesswork. For example, what's the best exercise for a particular muscle, and what's the best rep range for muscle growth? This hasn't been determined by researchers yet, so we must rely on anecdotal information by the many lifters out there. If you ask a variety of lifters, you'll get a variety of answers.

In addition to adding in different exercises, rep ranges, and intensities, I also find that frequent workouts introduce you to a good amount of variety. You will get proficient at many different techniques and learn what's optimal for your body—keeping in mind that it will change from time to time.

The template that I use for *Strong Curves* addresses all of these needs, allowing you to progress in stability, muscle endurance, strength, and power all at once. This will get you stronger, leaner, and shapelier in less time.

Muscle Growth (aka Hypertrophy)

Now, for the "sciency" part of the book. When I designed *Strong Curves*, I kept in mind the immense amount of knowledge given to me by my friend, Brad Schoenfeld, known in many circles as the hypertrophy specialist. I can't imagine another individual who knows and understands more about muscle growth than Brad. But don't worry; I'll try to keep it brief and somewhat simple.

Your muscle generally grows through three main types of stimuli. Though there are many redundant mechanisms and physiological pathways to muscle growth (also called hypertrophy), they generally fall within these three categories:

1. Muscle damage
2. Metabolic stress
3. Mechanical tension

Muscle Damage

Strength training is damaging to muscle tissue, and the level of damage created is worse when a muscle is lengthened (eccentrically) extensively, such as during the lowering portion of an exercise that really stretches the muscle. And the entire muscle cell experiences damage. Parts located on the cell's outer structure, the contractile elements that create muscle contractions, and parts located inside the muscle cell all receive microscopic tears in addition to the supportive connective tissue surrounding the cell.

When the cell's membranes are torn, calcium tends to leak out, and the cell's natural equilibrium is disrupted. This causes the body to respond in the same way as it would during an infection. It releases neutrophils, which work their way to the damaged tissue. More chemicals are released to attract macrophages and lymphocytes, which help remove cellular debris and maintain the cell's structure. Various cytokines and growth factors are produced that activate myoblasts and satellite cells (cells that normally lay dormant outside the cell but will lend their nuclei to the muscles when called upon). This allows the muscle cells to create more material and grow larger.

While it's true that damage can trigger hypertrophy, it doesn't mean that we should actively try to cause as much damage as possible during a workout. You want to stimulate, not annihilate. Most lifters enjoy feeling a little bit of soreness in the muscles on the days following a workout, but it isn't ideal to be extremely sore because it interferes with setting personal records and getting stronger.

The *Strong Curves Program* includes the best exercises and methods for inducing muscle damage. You will focus on full range movements that actively stretch the muscles. Exercises that require a maximal stretch for the glutes under heavy load—such as lunges, Bulgarian split squats, and full squats—are excellent movements for muscle damage. But as I previously mentioned, you don't want to get carried away. If it's hard to get out of a chair the day after a workout or you feel like you got kicked by a mule, you're training too hard. Moderate soreness is fine as long as you're getting stronger and beating your prior records. Just know that you won't set any records if you're so sore that you hobble around. My advanced female clients' workouts are sometimes volume-dense and involve heavy weight, which is very physically taxing. But I build them up gradually over time so as to not induce excess soreness.

Strong Curves offers plenty of variety to keep your body guessing. A phenomenon known as the "repeated bout effect" protects muscles from continuous damage from repeated stimuli. This means that you might get very sore the first time you perform a certain exercise, but the following session and especially the one after that are unlikely to produce as much soreness since your body prepares itself for repeated occurrences. By switching things up and rotating exercises over time, you can continue to experience ideal levels of muscle damage without compromising strength since you'll always stick to the same great movement patterns such as squat, lunge, hip hinge, and bridging motions. Finally, *Strong Curves* includes plenty of single-leg movements that anecdotally lead to more glute soreness, which (theoretically) is a good indicator of muscle damage.

Metabolic Stress

During strength training, the muscle cell also undergoes a considerable change in metabolic environment. In fact, some researchers believe that the metabolite accumulation induced by metabolic stress is more important for hypertrophy than high force (tension) development, though Brad and I believe that mechanical tension is still most important. The importance of metabolic stress does help explain why bodybuilders experience greater gains in musculature compared to powerlifters, despite the fact that powerlifters regularly experience greater absolute tension in their muscles.

Higher rep training with lower rest periods leads to greater metabolic stress due to many factors. First, it relies primarily upon anaerobic glycolysis for energy production, which creates a buildup of metabolites including lactate, hydrogen ion, inorganic phosphate, and creatine. Second, the increased time under tension leads to increased ischemia, hormonal milieu, and cell swelling. But let me try to explain this in laymen's terms.

What all of this means is that by focusing on metabolic stress in your workouts, your sets will occlude the muscles and deprive them of oxygen (hypoxia), which leads to hypertrophy through several mechanisms, including increased satellite cell activity (which, as I mentioned earlier, are muscle stem cells that sit outside the cell and donate their nuclei to the muscle cells when called upon). It also elevates anabolic hormone levels that theoretically lead to greater hypertrophy, especially in the muscles being worked. Finally, it pumps up the muscles. This increases muscularity by several mechanisms including an expansion of the muscles due to a perceived threat to the structural integrity of the cells' ultrastructures.

The *Strong Curves Program* includes the best possible methods to induce maximal metabolic stress. First, we include exercises that pump up the muscles and induce serious burn. When you learn to hip thrust properly and perform back extensions the way we recommend, you'll be blown away by the deep burn and pump in your glutes. Second, we utilize medium and high reps from time to time, and we perform multiple glute exercises from various angles and directions, both of which increase time under tension, leading to metabolic stress.

Furthermore, we execute special techniques to increase the set's intensiveness; the rest-pause method extends the set, allowing for the execution of more repetitions, and the constant tension method induces maximal cell swelling (giving you that full muscle feeling) and ischemia (restricted blood flow and oxygen).

Finally, we organized the program so that the anabolic hormone response could be maximized, allowing molecules such as testosterone, growth hormone, and IGF-1 (which actually turns into MGF in the muscles and is an extremely hypertrophic agent) to accumulate and exert an effect that will improve body composition. This is why we move at a moderate pace, take sets close to failure, train with sufficient intensity, and get you in and out of the gym in an hour or less.

Mechanical Tension

I left mechanical tension for last because I feel it's the most important aspect of muscle growth. Mechanical tension is created when a muscle either contracts or is stretched. Combine these two elements (contractions and stretch) through full range eccentric and concentric actions, and you'll see even greater results. Mechanical tension leads to increased hypertrophy through many different mechanisms, including increased growth factor and cytokine release, satellite cell activation, and activation of the incredibly important mTOR pathway (the head honcho pathway to hypertrophy).

When it comes to hypertrophy, the greater muscle tension the better. Increased tension requires increased neural drive, and this neural drive activates several pathways to hypertrophy and influences gene expression as well. High-tension, low rep training fails to deliver superior results compared to moderate-tension, moderate rep training popularized by bodybuilders. For this reason, time under tension seems to be more important.

There is a relationship between EMG and muscle activation, muscle force, mechanical tension, and hypertrophy. The greater these measures, the greater the hypertrophy. *Strong Curves* is sure to include the exercises that place the greatest amount of tension on the muscles and lead to the highest levels of activation. In fact, we employ partial range of motion exercises from time to time so that greater loads can be used to (theoretically) place greater tension on the muscles. Research shows that the gluteus maximus has a better leverage for creating torque (or turning force) at the hips and also receives greater neural drive at end-range hip extension compared to flexed-range hip extension. In other words, your glutes fire harder when squeezed (think bridges and hip thrusts) rather than when stretched (think good mornings and squats). For this reason, exercises such as barbell glute bridges are great glute-builders because you are in a stable position, you have a short range of motion focusing on end-range hip extension to activate the greatest amount of fibers, and the barbell load is centered directly over the hips to require your glutes to do most of the work.

The program in this book incorporates exercises that have long resistance moment arms (long levers), such as reverse hypers and back extensions, which increase muscle force requirements. Finally, we teach techniques that combine multiple roles of the gluteus maximus such as proper full squats (which combine hip extension with hip external rotation) and American deadlifts (which combine hip extension with posterior pelvic tilting). These techniques lead to greater muscle activation and broader tension across the vast array of gluteal fibers.

Consensus on Muscle Hypertrophy

Clearly, maximal hypertrophy is reached through a proper and well-designed combination of the three primary mechanisms of muscle growth. This is why we utilize the shotgun approach and leave no stone unturned. Your glutes deserve the best program imaginable, and I won't let your glutes down.

One huge mistake I see is the tendency to go too heavy to the point where form breaks down. This does not increase muscle activity; it creates energy leaks and places more stress on the joints rather than the muscles.

I see this all the time in the gym and just shake my head. If tension and activation increase muscle size and strength, why would you skip that part? I don't get it, but I hope you do and avoid going for those heavy lifts prior to learning proper form and muscle activation, especially with the glutes. The *Strong Curves Program* starts you at the right level to learn proper movement patterns. These should be mastered before you even think about heavy lifts.

As your strength increases, you should maintain excellent form when you add weight to your movements. If your form begins to break down at any time, decrease the weight until it is darn near perfect and you feel your muscles actively working the way they are supposed to. This is what helps you get stronger, and increased strength is the most vital component for shaping the muscle.

> If you need help with your form, I have a YouTube channel that hosts several descriptive videos to guide you. You can find it by searching for BretContreras1 in the YouTube search engine.

Don't believe me? We all know at least one person who has avidly visited the gym year in and year out. When you first met or saw this person, you envied her physique. But over time, your opinion became, "Eh, she looks all right." That's because she looks the same now as she did three years ago. She has been lifting the same weights and performing the same exercises every single week. But the more proficient you get at training, the less appealing her workouts become. That's because you have found the real secret to great results: Building strength over time through increased intensity and program variation.

Continually working out with the same weights might help you become leaner, but it won't increase muscle size or shape. This fictitious person from the gym might have a small, flat bum and thin, flabby arms. Muscle fills you out and gives you those nice curves you have always wanted. Her program will never achieve those results. Worrying about rep ranges is good, but I want you to be more concerned about increasing your strength, adding weight to your lifts, and setting new personal records.

This might not seem like a big deal now, but the first time you master an incredible feat like walking weighted lunges, squatting with heavy weight for reps, or deadlifting a barbell with a load equal to your body weight for ten reps, you will feel exhilarated.

In order to apply tension correctly you must first learn how to activate the muscles. Current researchers use electromyography (EMG) to estimate muscle force. While it is not exact—especially during dynamic movements as opposed to isometric movements or when muscles fatigue—it's the most practical method available for estimating how hard a muscle works during a given exercise. The EMG experiments I performed late into the night a few years back show that different exercises uniquely work different regions of the glutes.

Some exercises work the entire glutes evenly, some hit the lower glutes a bit better than they hit the upper glutes, and some target the upper glutes.

Researchers and practitioners don't know the exact formula for optimal hypertrophy, and the best methods for muscle growth vary extensively depending on the situation and the individual. That is what I kept in mind when creating *Strong Curves* so that it covers all possible bases. I wanted to address all components of muscle hypertrophy so that this program is centered on the most tension-creating, glute-activating exercises possible. You will use strategies to increase metabolic stress, such as higher rep ranges, high-density training, rest pause methods, and constant tension methods. You will perform exercises that induce muscular damage due to heavy stretch loading such as reverse lunges, and you will hit the glutes with integrated multi-joint movements in addition to targeted single joint movements. Your glutes will work from multiple angles and directions of resistance to stress different ranges of motion; with all types of rep ranges to vary the intertwining roles of tension, stress, and damage, while using many types of resistance to provide novel stimuli and prevent adaptation. To put it simply: Your glutes will have no choice but to grow stronger and more muscular.

Below is a chart that shows the average and maximum activation received on several popular hip-strengthening exercises:

Gluteus Maximus Average Electromyography Chart

Exercise	Upper glute max	Mid glute max	Lower glute max
Bodyweight Glute Bridge	29.1	13.1	17.3
Bodyweight Single-leg Glute Bridge	53.9	24.8	45.2
Bodyweight Side Lying Abduction	54.9	7.2	5.4
Bodyweight Side Lying Clam	70.6	8.2	6.7
Bodyweight Full Squat	27.8	7.0	30.5
Bodyweight Reverse Lunge	36.4	9.5	43.3
Bodyweight Bulgarian Split Squat	32.3	14.7	56.7
Bodyweight Single-leg Box Squat	54.4	17.7	37.2
Bodyweight High Step Up	72.0	15.4	37.0
Bodyweight Back Extension	34.0	12.1	29.6
Bodyweight Reverse Hyper	66.9	27.2	51.7
Bodyweight 45-Degree Hyper	43.9	13.9	31.7
Bodyweight Hip Thrust	39.6	17.9	47.5
Bodyweight Single-leg Hip Thrust	66.9	27.5	60.8
Barbell Full Squat	59.0	25.4	71.1
Barbell Deadlift	81.5	37.0	85.6
Barbell Hip Thrust	134.0	62.6	72.9
Seated Band Hip Abduction	93.9	24.5	24.2
Cable Hip Rotation	83.9	55.7	51.7

The Big Bulk Scare

I know what you're thinking. All of this talk about muscle-building and strength-gaining usually has women running back to the aerobics class because they don't want to get big and bulky. If you train naturally without any anabolic or hormonal concoctions to make your muscles grow, you need not fear growing muscles like Arnold Schwarzenegger.

Physiologically, you have a much harder time building muscles like a man because you have lower levels of testosterone. Though you do carry a small amount of testosterone, and strength training promotes anabolism, you are in the clear when it comes to growing muscles so large you need to cut the sleeves off your shirts.

Body recomposing expert Alan Aragon has devised a model for the rate of muscle growth. He compiled data after monitoring clients for considerable time to come to this conclusion. His model shows that for women, the average rate of muscle gain per pound per year diminishes over time, becoming hardest to gain muscle after four years of proper training. Note that this is with proper training. Someone can improperly train for four years and never gain a pound of muscle.

Going by his model, in the first year of proper strength training and nutrition, a woman may gain ten to twelve pounds of lean muscle mass. By year two, she may gain five to six pounds of lean muscle mass. In year three, she will only gain two to three pounds of lean muscle mass. The numbers in year four are less than one, so not even worth calculating. At most, over the course of four years, you may gain twenty-one to twenty-two pounds of lean muscle mass. This is your optimum potential, of course, as factors like age, lifestyle, nutrition, and genetics may limit that potential. Again, this comes only with proper training and the right cocktail of personal factors. Some individuals can train for years with no progress because their programs are not designed properly or they don't exercise correctly.

Now, if you're gasping in despair at the thought of gaining twelve pounds in a year, you haven't considered what you will be taking off. Muscle allows your body to become more metabolically efficient, so the more you have, the more fat you burn, and training for continuous strength gains ensures that the metabolism is kicked into high gear.

You may gain ten pounds of muscle in a year, but considering that you burn fat at twice the rate you put on muscle, you can lose twenty pounds or more of fat in that same time. The harder and smarter you work, the more fat you burn. The better you eat, the more fat you burn—all while building nice rounded muscle to give your body shape. The bottom line is that you won't grow excessively large glutes. Here is a typical conversation that I have with women regarding this topic:

Bret: "You're afraid that you'll wake up tomorrow and have huge glutes, right? Well strength training doesn't work that way. If it did, I would be out of a job. It takes time to develop a nice muscle, especially the glutes. But let's pretend that you're right. Let's say you'd end up with huge glutes if I were to train you the way I want to train you for two months. Wouldn't there be a point in between, say four weeks from now, where your glutes looked absolutely perfect?"

Client: "Yes, that sounds about right."

Bret: "Then I'll make a deal with you. As soon as we reach the point where you think your butt looks perfect, we'll quit trying to gain strength and just maintain a general level of fitness. Deal?"

Client: "Deal!"

Guess what? She never reaches that level. Sure, butts get rounder and perkier, but once the compliments start rolling in, it further motivates women to try even harder in hopes of seeing greater gains. All I have to do is get a client through the initial fears of excess development, and they're on board. I have never had a client say to me, "Bret, my butt looks perfect. I don't want it to get any rounder or shapelier. Let's stop trying to get stronger at hip thrusts."

Client success story: Kim, a fifty-four-year-old mother of two, came to me with the fear of her butt growing larger. She refused to do any heavy glute exercises. It took a lot of convincing to help her understand the difference between muscle mass and fat mass in the butt region.

She thought growing her glutes meant they would get even wider. On the contrary, as she started training they grew rounder, perkier, and shapelier. But she didn't admit this right away. For weeks, she stopped short on her exercise sets. I'd force her to work harder and perform more reps. The battle of wits ensued with me telling her my program was working and her telling me it wasn't.

I knew better. One day, without any coercion on my part, she set an enormous personal record (PR) on hip thrusts. I decided to call her out, saying, "What's going on, Kim? For weeks, you've been berating me for pushing you to set records, and now you're Roger Federer, setting records like crazy. You're getting compliments, aren't you?" Laughter filled the room, and her face turned candy apple red. Apparently, she had earned the nickname "Buns of Steel" at work.

Once those compliments start rolling in, I know that I never have to convince a client to push herself toward greater levels of strength.

So in theory, butts could indeed grow too large. Occasionally, there are women who do seem to pack on some serious muscle mass back there. But I have trained many women over the years, and I have personally never trained a woman who grows glutes too large (though I've trained some of the best booties around). This is quite apparent when a client leans out. I've never gotten a female client down to low body fat levels and heard her complain that she has too much glute muscle.

On the contrary, most want even more shape back there, even though we're doing everything in our power to build and maintain the glutes. So, put your mind to rest. I have seen huge success by getting every female client of mine much stronger at hip thrusts. The stronger the booty, the better the booty.

Moving in Different Directions

The majority of exercise programs designed by trainers or in popular fitness books have you moving in the same basic directions. If a program focuses on squats, lunges, bench presses, lat pulldowns, and crunches, you are only moving up, down, forward, and backward. That might seem fine, but what about moving side to side or rotational movements?

These directions are called "force vectors," and it's best to target multiple vectors during your program. By doing so, you train your body through all the intended functions and activate your muscles in multiple ways, as they were designed to do.

The gluteus maximus was designed to extend the hips, posteriorly tilt the pelvis, abduct the hips, and externally rotate the hips. To train the glutes through its multiple functions, you need to include exercises in your program that move the torso, hips, and pelvis forward and backward; exercises that move the thigh inward and outward (from side to side), and exercises that twist the hips laterally and medially. In other words, you want to perform exercises that have you moving your hips up and down (squats and deadlifts), forward and backward (hip thrusts and back extensions), and side to side (side lying abductions and band standing abductions), in addition to exercises that have you rotating the hips back and forth (cable hip rotations) and tilting the pelvis forward and back (RKC planks and American hip thrusts).

Just doing squats and lunges won't get you there. The *Strong Curves Program* has you performing all of these force vectors every week. That way, you train your

body in all of the major planes to strengthen the glutes from all directions in all ranges and prevent potential injuries that could arise from a lack of glute strength and conditioning.

Movement Quality Over Quantity

Poor movement quality is a pandemic in our society. Just hang out in a shopping center one day and watch the people around you. Take note of how people walk, get up and down from a seated position, and their posture from a seated or standing position. People are hunched over, wobbly, and stiff. This is all due to jobs that require long hours of sitting and a sedentary lifestyle.

Most movement issues relate to three factors: mobility, stability, and motor control. You can have a great handle on one factor but still have issues with the other two factors. Renowned physical therapist Gray Cook has discussed this at length for years. For instance, a person may possess sufficient hamstring flexibility to deadlift properly, but once weight is added, their form falls apart. In this instance, the individual doesn't have a mobility problem; she has a stability or motor control problem. Issues with any one of these three factors can be corrected, and corrective exercises in the form of foam rolling, stretching, mobility drills, and activation drills should be a regular part of your workout program until your form is ideal and you no longer need them.

Many of the correctives are simply conducted during the warm-up as a way to get more bang for your buck. Body temperature needs to be elevated prior to heavy lifting (hence the primary purpose of a warm-up), but why achieve this tissue temperature increase through riding a stationary bicycle or walking on the treadmill? These activities don't move your joints through a full range of motion and don't get the juices flowing optimally. Tissues can be warmed and the nervous system can be primed while you perform exercises that will help correct dysfunction, activate dormant muscles, and assist with good posture, while taking your joints through a full range. This is the strategy behind our dynamic warm-up, which I've developed over time with the help of popular strength coaches such as Mike Boyle and Mark Verstegen.

Mobility

People typically lose mobility in the same regions of the body—the hips, ankles, and thoracic spine (upper back). Your hips require movement in several directions, including external and internal rotation, flexion, extension, abduction, and adduction. Sitting all day causes hip flexors to shorten because you have limited range of motion all day. When you lose hip mobility, you are unable to perform big exercises properly.

Poor ankle mobility, especially ankle dorsiflexion (the upward movement of your foot toward your shin), causes issues with regard to squatting and lunging. If your ankles can't move beyond a certain degree, you can't squat to a full range of motion, and your back ends up overcompensating for lack of ankle mobility. In other words, you end up in a rounded-back and excessively bent-over position.

Though it seems like an innocuous issue, poor ankle dorsiflexion can cause issues in your feet, knees, hips, low back, and eventually your shoulders. The most common cause of this flexibility deficiency is your Gastroc/ Soleus complex—the calf muscles. If you have tight calf muscles, it will decrease your ankle mobility. Luckily, however, this is easily fixable. Tight joint capsules, scar tissue, and previous injuries can also restrict motion.

When squatting and lifting heavy things, you need to keep your chest up. If you cannot do this, you may have poor thoracic spine mobility, which is also often the result of sitting at a desk all day. Low back and neck pain, rotator cuff flair-ups, and the inability to twist or rotate painlessly also relate directly to thoracic spine mobility—or lack thereof. This lack of mobility is responsible for the perpetual shoulder slump we see in many people, too. Did that make you sit-up a little taller just now?

The ability to extend, rotate, and laterally flex the upper back is something you must work hard not to lose as you age. Many people overcompensate with their lumbar spine (low back) when lifting, bending, and twisting, which causes low back pain and injury. If you don't move with your hips and thoracic spine, your low back will suffer.

Stability

The core region of your body is made up of your lumbar spine (lower back), pelvis, and hips and is called the lumbopelvic hip complex (LPHC). It greatly influences upper and lower extremities, and many bones, muscles, and joints can be involved in the dysfunction of the LPHC. If something is dysfunctional in your upper or lower extremities, it may affect your LPHC function and vice versa.

Take poor ankle dorsiflexion, for example. If you are unable to bend your ankles during a deep squat, the only way you'll get low is by rounding your low back, and you'll probably rise up onto your toes and shift your weight forward, too. This ends up putting considerable stress on your lumbar spine.

If you don't have adequate hip flexion in a deadlift, you'll also have to round over at your spine in order to pick up the bar. This isn't a safe practice, especially as you get stronger. My electromyography (EMG) experiments have shown that when you lean forward too much in a squat or round too much in a deadlift, your gluteus maximus does not fire to its full extent. Poor form inhibits the glutes.

Poor form isn't always due to lack of mobility, though. You may be capable of going to full range of motion, but your body prevents you from doing so because you lack stability, not flexibility. Your body is very clever and will work against you to prevent injury. Strength always complements flexibility in exercise. Yogis may appear to be just flexible people, but they possess surprising stability that allows them to perform the movements properly.

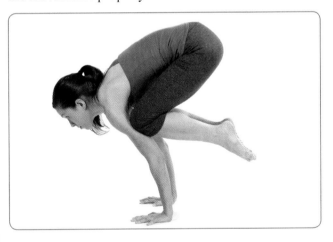

Squatting to full range isn't easy. If you watch bodybuilders in the gym, you'll notice that many of them load a considerable amount of weight onto the bar and squeak down with their squats to just above parallel at best. After years of doing this, many of them couldn't squat through a full range of motion if they wanted to. In fact, a good percentage of the population in your gym likely has the same issue. Probably not from years of bodybuilding, but from other lifestyle factors like sitting in an office chair all day.

Pulling a deadlift from the ground requires a great amount of core stability and hamstring flexibility. Most back injuries in the weight room stem from deadlift accidents. If you have poor core stability, you tend to round your back to compensate for the lack of strength, putting your low back at great risk.

The lumbar spine, pelvis, and hips need a good amount of rotary stability during single-leg exercises as well. When I add single-leg exercises to a client's program for the first time, they often fall all over the place. Don't worry; I did too, the first time I tried many of these exercises. They are challenging for even the most elite lifters until they build stability. But if you do them right, you'll quickly build up proper stability, and your knee will track properly over your mid-toes during single-leg movements, which is what prevents knee pain.

Motor Control

Motor control is when your brain puts everything together and uses stability and mobility harmoniously. Often, poor motor control stems from the inability to perform an exercise correctly due to simple lack of knowledge.

The back extension is a prime example. Perhaps because the exercise is misnamed, people often over-recruit the low back or erector spinae during this exercise. Once the trainee learns that the correct movement involves more recruitment of the glute muscles and the motion is supposed to hinge around their hip joints (and not their spine), their motor control improves. However, if they have weak glutes, they may tend to continually overcompensate with their erector spinae until their glutes strengthen.

Another issue with this exercise may be poor hamstring flexibility. As the trainee continues to gain mobility and strengthen the glutes, the exercise becomes much more effective.

Many trainers and coaches believe that poor form is always due to lack of strength or flexibility in a particular muscle, but often the solution simply involves groov-

ing proper patterning over and over until it becomes automatic. It has been suggested that thousands of repetitions are required to engrain a motor engram, which is a memorized motor pattern. In this way, "practice" doesn't make perfect—*perfect* practice makes perfect.

It's easier to learn the right way to perform a movement right off the bat than it is to correct a faulty movement pattern. So, take the time getting your form looking good from the get-go because it will be very difficult to correct it down the road.

Mobility and flexibility, stability and strength, and motor control are interrelated and work together to form sound fundamental movement patterns. New clients are typically deficient in all three areas and quickly gain proficiency in their form by simultaneous improvements in all three categories. Their core muscles get stronger, which informs the brain that it's okay to move through deeper ranges of motion. This is because the pelvis will remain stable as a result of increased core stability. Then the hip extensor muscles are strengthened in a stretched position, which increases mobility, and movements eventually feel coordinated and natural. This, in turn, allows for further increases in strength and flexibility.

Addressing the Issues

In the Warm-Up Section of *Strong Curves* (Chapter 11), you will find a good selection of drills, including self-myofascial release, static stretching, mobility drills, and activation drills. I encourage you to use these warm-ups with each of your workouts. Though strength training will greatly improve your stability, mobility, and motor control, these warm-up techniques will improve tissue quality and prime your body for training. Even if you currently have good functional movement patterns, you don't want to lose them. Spending several minutes each session activating certain muscles and controlling your joints through a full range of motion is well worth the effort because it will prevent your body from shutting down and losing functional ability as you age.

Chapter 5:

Nourishing Those
Strong Curves

I'm always amazed at how complex eating has become in our society and how little we understand food. While there is plenty we don't know because researchers haven't explored it yet, you should have a basic understanding of what is good and bad with regard to the food on your plate.

Cooking and eating used to just make sense. Our grandparents and great-grandparents ate foods because they were grown from the earth and because the foods gave them energy for the day. They didn't care about the biochemical makeup of food items. Do you think your great-grandma knew which food had the most antioxidants or whether a carbohydrate digested quickly or slowly? She just cooked what was fresh and available during a given season.

As food sciences advance, we learn why certain foods are good for us and what benefits certain nutrients can provide. But the food industry also learns how to manipulate food to make it appear healthy while making it cheaper and less perishable. As a result, we end up thinking food with little nutrition is good for us. A cereal can now be completely stripped of all nutrients and pumped full of synthetic replicas of the same ones that were stripped out. We now have a fortified product sold as a health food item, but in reality, it offers few health benefits, if any.

The food market is flooded with these items. You can purchase junk foods labeled "organic," "all natural," and "whole food." When these labels are placed on packaged, processed foods, they completely devalue the real foods that are actually nutritious. No wonder we are all so confused. A bag of potato chips should not carry the same healthy label as an apple picked fresh from an orchard, but it does.

Before you begin the *Strong Curves* nutrition plan, you must first get a few misconceptions out of your head. Fat is not bad for you. Carbohydrates are not bad for you. Neither is making us fat. The excessive consumption of calories is what has an adverse effect on your health. Just like there is no formula for a perfect workout that fits everyone, there is also no perfect diet.

Guidelines can be set to get you headed in the right direction. That is what I intend to do in this chapter, but know that your own adjustments can make your nutrition work even better. One thing is for certain, whether you thrive on high carb/low fat, high fat/low carb, or moderate carb/moderate fat, you still need to fill your diet with a nutritious variety of foods.

You must also forget about starving yourself skinny. You need to eat the right amount of calories from the right foods every day to achieve the body you want, and that body is one with full, rounded, and athletic muscles. It isn't one with soft, barely-there muscles and a fat layer resting upon bone. That's what starvation will get you.

Why You Need To Eat

Your goals determine how many calories you need to consume each day. If weight loss is your goal, then you need to create a caloric deficit—eat fewer calories. If you are trying to gain weight or add muscle, then you need a caloric surplus—eat more calories. If you just want to maintain your same body weight while improving your body composition, then you need caloric maintenance. Whether eating for maintenance, weight loss, or muscle gain, you will constantly strive to improve your body composition.

For simplicity's sake, body composition can be broken down into two categories: fat mass and fat-free mass. Fat mass is the sum of your total body fat, and fat-free mass is everything else, which includes muscle, bone, organs, blood, other tissues, and water.

Typically, your goal with body composition change is to not lose fat-free mass, but rather to slowly decrease your fat mass over time. It is much easier to lower your body fat percentage by losing fat mass than it is by adding muscle. Not only does fat loss have a greater effect on your body fat percentage, but it is also far easier to lose fat than build muscle. It can take you up to five times longer to add five pounds of muscle than to burn five pounds of fat. This is important to note because when you reach your ideal weight, you will shed fat quickly and put on muscle at a much slower rate.

So, once you reach your ideal weight, it's time to pack on more muscle in all the right places while still shedding any fat you may carry. That's when things get tricky. This process takes time, so be patient. When Kellie first came to me as a client, she was at her ideal weight. We worked on building quality lean mass while shedding fat over the course of several months.

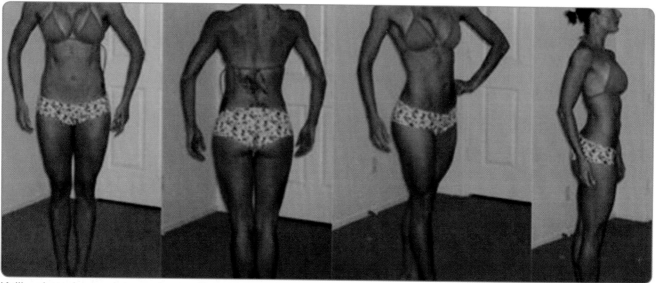

Kellie when she came to me for our first session

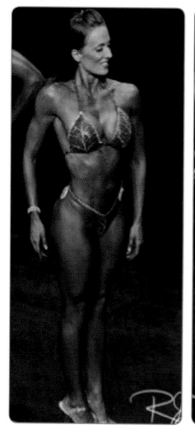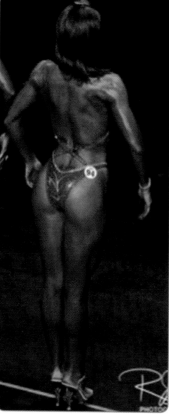

The results were incredible, and within eighteen months, she packed on close to eight pounds of lean muscle while maintaining the same weight. This means she also lost eight pounds of fat mass. Notice that at first, before she came to me, she achieved really great results through weight loss alone. Once she started training with me, she spent a considerable amount of time molding her physique while staying the same weight. She will continue to do this for years to come and is constantly striving to improve her strength, muscle maturity, and muscle quality.

Kellie eighteen months after our first session

Chapter 5: NOURISHING THOSE *STRONG CURVES*

Plenty of Food Choices

Your diet can be broken down into three primary groups of macronutrients (proteins, carbohydrates, and fats), plus vitamins, minerals, and other nutrients that are delivered in small quantities. With the macronutrients, each one is surrounded by its own controversies, but for the sake of this book, all are important for their own reasons.

I'm not going to get into the debate of whether you should eat high, moderate, low, or no carbs, fats, or proteins. Just like exercise, nutrition has many schools of thought. What I do want to provide you with is a guide that will help you determine the right daily food intake to help you reach your physique and strength goals. Whether you tinker with the amount of each macronutrient you eat each day or not, that is totally up to you. These are general guidelines and ideas to get you headed in the right direction. Before we get into how much you should eat each day to reach your goals, I want to provide a brief description of each macronutrient and an overview of what they do for your body.

Protein

Protein exists in all of the living cells in your body. These proteins are constantly broken down and re-placed. Some are nonessential, meaning that your body produces them on its own. Others are essential and come directly from dietary sources.

Protein can be found in both plant and animal sources. Animal sources are considered complete proteins because they provide all of the essential amino acids needed to carry out normal daily function. Plant sources are incomplete because they are low in one or more of the essential amino acids. Vegetarians need to eat far more plant-based protein and a far wider variety of foods to meet their nutritional needs.

Protein is found in red meat, pork, poultry, fish, game meat, eggs, nuts, tofu, legumes, dairy products, and plants (in small amounts). Many adults do not get enough protein to meet their daily dietary needs. This is largely because we consume far too many processed, packaged foods. Eating a diet rich in whole foods helps ensure you will get a quality amount of proteins because most sources of whole natural foods have essential and nonessential amino acids. Go back through that list I just gave you of foods with protein and you will see what I mean.

When deciding on sources of protein, four main factors come into play: digestibility, quality, amino acid profile, and presence (or lack) of other nutrients. Digestibility simply means how well the protein is digested and absorbed into the bloodstream. The more digestible it is, the easier your body can use the nutrients. Quality is the measurement of how well the protein is used in your body. Along with digestibility, the amino acid profile plays a key role in the quality of your source of protein.

Amino acids are the building blocks of protein. There are eighteen to twenty-two amino acids, and each is found in different proportions within your food sources. The amino acid profile can influence how your body uses the protein. In addition to amino acids, your protein sources may offer other nutrients. The presence or absence of these nutrients also plays a relevant role in your diet. For instance, grass fed beef and fatty fish are rich in omega-3 fatty acids, while other sources may lack this fatty acid.

Your best bet for protein is to vary the type and amount you eat from each resource. Eating chicken breasts and egg whites three hundred sixty-five days a year will not only bore your palate, but may also deprive you of important nutrients. The greater variety you add to your diet, the more likely you will get the right nutrients in the right amounts.

Dietary Fats

Just like protein and carbohydrates, not all dietary fats are created equal. The primary types of dietary fats are triglycerides (TGs) and cholesterol. Now, don't get these confused with blood TGs and cholesterol. These are two distinctly different things. Other dietary fats exist in small amounts, but these two make up the primary fats in your diet, so we will focus on them.

The dietary fat confusion stemmed from the whole mix-up between the fats in your blood and the fats in your food. This happened around the late 1970s and early 1980s when butter was removed from the table and egg yolks tossed in the trash. On the contrary, your body actually makes its own cholesterol in the liver—probably far more than many people eat in a given day—and your body tends to adapt how much cholesterol it makes depending on your diet.

Dietary triglycerides have a far greater effect on your blood cholesterol levels than dietary cholesterol. More importantly, the type of dietary triglycerides you eat makes all the difference. TGs consist of three fatty acid chains bound to a glycerol molecule backbone. Chain length, degree of saturation, and chemical structure distinguish one fat from the next. When most people talk about dietary fat, they're really talking about types of dietary TGs without even knowing it.

TGs are subdivided into four main categories:

- Trans fat
- Saturated fat
- Monounsaturated fat
- Polyunsaturated fat

Trans fats received a lot of bad press over the past several years, and they deserve it for the most part. Trans fats are primarily vegetable oils or man-made fats added to processed foods to given them longer shelf life. Though some trans fats exist in nature in small amounts, the real concern are the ones that come from factories. Try to avoid processed foods with known added trans fats.

Saturated fats are another story. For quite a while, these TGs have been to blame for our ever-climbing non-communicable disease rate, but counter-arguments have surfaced over recent years citing that saturated fats have no health risks. The truth likely lies somewhere in the middle of these two extremes. Saturated fats can pose some health risks, but it's probably more about the type and amount of saturated fats consumed, along with the amount of daily carbohydrate and caloric intake, the level of physical activity, and good old genetics that make up the brunt of these issues.

Saturated fats (found primarily in animal fat, but also coconut oil and palm kernel oil) can be divided into subcategories, each one behaving differently in the body. Some behave negatively, and others not so bad. For the most part, an individual who is lean, eats plenty of whole foods, and gets daily rigorous exercise really sees no danger in increasing saturated fat intake. For those who are overweight, inactive, stressed out, and/ or eating a poor diet, saturated fats might behave differently inside of the body. Context plays a huge role here, so I can't say whether these fats are good, bad, or neutral. It all depends.

Monounsaturated fats are pretty neutral. One of the best sources is extra virgin olive oil, which is always good to add to your diet when you want to consume more dietary fat. If you don't like how olive oil tastes, high oleic safflower oil is a great alternative.

Polyunsaturated fats are often known as omega-3 and omega-6 fatty acids. Alpha-linolenic acid (ALA) is omega-3 (w-3), while linoleic acid (LA) is omega-6 (w-6). If you get plenty of these two fatty acids, you could live forever without touching another type of dietary TG, assuming your body is proficient at converting ALA to EPA (eicosapentaenoic acid) and EPA to DHA (docosahexaenoic acid). Sure, some saturated fat is valuable because it's used to manufacture cholesterol, forming the backbone of important anabolic hormones like testosterone, but saturated fat isn't essential.

Many incredible things happen within your body due to the metabolism of ALA and LA. I will spare you the details because they're pretty complex. One important thing to note is that the modern diet tends to have ratios leaning toward w-6 over w-3. With regard to the metabolic effects of these two fatty acids, too little w-3 combined with too much w-6 can become problematic.

As a society, we eat a far greater amount of w-6 than w-3, which can lead to health problems that are still being studied by researchers. In order to ensure you get a sufficient amount of omega-3 fatty acid in your diet, I recommend taking at least 500mg of EPA/DHA per day. If you consume a good amount of fatty fish and free-range meat each day, your diet likely is sufficient enough in these nutrients. If not, 500mg equates to two fish oil capsules a day. Not such a bad trade-off for improved dietary balances.

Carbohydrates

Carbohydrates refer to a general class of compounds that contain carbon, hydrogen, and oxygen. This group includes monosaccharides (simple sugars), oligosaccharides (chains of 2-10 molecules), and polysaccharides (long chains of molecules like fiber).

The carb debate has ensued for decades, and dietary recommendations are all over the place. Just like the other macronutrients, I am not here to take sides, but simply inform. Your dietary needs are based on many factors with regard to carbs, but one thing holds true: You have absolutely no physiological need for dietary carbohydrates.

As for essential nutrients like essential amino acids, the question is whether they can be made in the body or whether they are needed for survival. Even though your brain and other organs thrive on glucose and the tissue in your body needs glucose in small amounts, your body is able to make as much as it needs in order to carry out these functions. Surprisingly, glucose can be made from lactate and pyruvate (during glucose metabolism), glycerol (during fat metabolism), and amino acids (during protein metabolism). In other words, if you don't consume carbohydrates, your body will create glucose on its own by converting it from fats and/or proteins.

Whether the amino acids used to create glucose come from proteins in your diet or muscle tissue depends upon whether you are eating or suffering total starvation. So long as your protein intake is high, you don't have to worry about sacrificing muscle.

There is no practical amount of carbs you need each day because it's determined by your own needs, how active you are, whether or not you function well with or without them, and a host of other factors. I know plenty of people who thrive on low to no carb diets. Conversely, I know plenty of people who can't seem to function without carbohydrates.

The *Strong Curves* nutritional recommendations are a middle ground in terms of carbohydrate intake. Start with the plan provided, and adjust accordingly. A good way to determine if you need adjustments is your energy while on this diet. If you eat a meal with carbohydrates and immediately start yawning, you may do better on a higher fat, lower carb diet. On the other hand, if you eat on the lower end of the carbohydrate spectrum and feel fatigued all day, you may choose to increase your carb intake while lowering your fat intake.

Just like the workout programs, I can't be there as your personal coach, so I need you to be the best advo-cate for your needs. Play with your diet until you find the sweet spot to help you reach your goal, but be careful how much monkeying around you do with those calories. Give yourself a good four weeks to adjust initially.

Women tend to need more time to determine whether or not a diet is working because their hormones fluctuate so much throughout the month. If, after four weeks, you aren't seeing any changes, make slight adjustments with your carbs and fat intake. Your protein should be pretty set from the beginning, and make sure you have sufficient energy to set personal records in the gym. If not, you won't build *Strong Curves*.

Setting Your Macronutrients

Now that you have a good understanding of why each type of macronutrient is important in your diet, it's time to figure out what you will eat on a daily basis. Most diets narrow food choices to so few that people grow bored within weeks. Sometimes after a few days, the dog dish starts to look appealing. Diets like these allow foods to control your life. The less options you have, the more you think about food. If you've ever held a conversation with a bodybuilding or figure competitor days before they step on stage, they are likely obsessing about food and hunger. Stick around long enough, and you'll get a list of what they want to eat the moment they step off stage. And most of them eat the entire list.

This is a slippery slope, and I don't ever want you to slide down it. Food deprivation turns into food obsession, and I want you to have a healthy relationship with food. Food is fuel for life, and eating is such an enjoyable pastime. It's one of the only times during your day when you get to sit back, relax, and take care of yourself. So, use this time wisely, and make the most of it.

More importantly, drastic dietary and exercise protocols used by many bodybuilding, figure, and bikini competitors do more harm than good over the long haul. I can't tell you how many figure and bikini girls I've trained who have permanently harmed their bodies and are left with sluggish metabolisms, thyroid dysfunction, and other issues. It doesn't have to be that way.

Your food choices can be divided up into the three macronutrient groups. You will decide how many grams of each macronutrient you need to eat based on the number of calories you need per day to reach your goal.

Protein

Chicken breast, ground chicken, dark chicken meat, canned chicken, fresh tuna, canned tuna, ground turkey, turkey breast, dark turkey meat, lean beef, steak, goat meat, lamb, white fish, salmon, canned salmon, pork, ham, wild boar, venison, bison, eggs, whey protein, hemp protein, tofu, ostrich, and more

Fat

Olive oil, butter, canola oil, nut oils, avocado, raw nuts, nut butters, coconut oil, cheese, whole milk, cream, seeds, Greek yogurt, kefir, skyr, cottage cheese

* Note that yogurt, cottage cheese, and milk can also be protein sources

Carbohydrate

Berries, apples, apricots, peaches, melons, cherries, bananas, pears, grapes, mangoes, pineapple, figs, other fruits, dried fruits, carrots, yams, winter squash, brown rice, white rice, whole grains, potatoes, oats, pumpkin

This list is just to get you started. Note that fibrous and non-starchy vegetables are an important part of your daily diet, but do not fit into any of the three groups. I would like for you to consume two to three cups of these vegetables per day. Just be careful of the "vegetables are freebies" notion because that can steer you in the wrong direction. There's no such thing as a negative-calorie food. You shouldn't fear consuming ample amounts, but if you begin consuming plates of veggies and start overeating, you will need to scale back. Also note that when cooking vegetables or eating salads, you are adding fat calories to your meals when you use oils and dressings. Be very conscious of this because I've had clients stop progressing simply because they were using too much oil in their meals.

Fibrous Vegetables

All leafy greens (lettuces, spinach, kale, arugula, dandelion greens, bok choy, collards, mustard greens, etc.)	All sprouts (alfalfa, Brussels sprouts, bean sprouts, etc.)
	Broccoli
	Cucumber
	Garlic
	All onions
All peppers	Green beans
Artichokes	Tomatoes
Asparagus	Zucchini squash
	Carrots

Can you ever eat foods that aren't good for you? Sure, it's okay from time to time as long as you work out the calories and account for the carbohydrates and fats. Just remember to consume these sparingly, perhaps two to three times per week in small amounts. Once you start eating whole foods nearly all of the time, you may lose your taste for treats. So, if you don't get the urge to splurge, you don't need to use the wild card calories.

> **Kellie's Quick Tips:** *Eat a variety of fruits and vegetables in an array of colors each day. Fuel up on plenty of eggs, fresh meats, and ample healthy fats. Food is your best friend for achieving body recomposition. Don't deprive yourself of valuable nutrients.*
>
> *Depriving yourself of all of the foods you love can send you straight to the ice cream freezer. You want to work treats into your diet, but do so with caution. Junk food tastes yummy, but it's also calorically dense. A single donut can have up to five hundred calories per serving. A plate of fresh veggies, a side of yams, and a serving of chicken equals about the same. Think about what happens in your belly when you eat each of these.*
>
> *The donut fills a tiny space, probably about one-fourth of the room in your stomach. On the other hand, the plate of delicious whole foods fills you to the brim and satisfies your appetite. This isn't intended to completely steer you away from those rewarding goodies, but keep this advice in perspective with regard to those enticing treats. Reward yourself, realizing that it's a treat, not a meal. If you intend on eating that piece of cake at the end of your meal, don't pile as many carbs and fats onto your plate for the main course. Making these small compromises in your diet will keep you on track and may prevent overindulgences.*

How Many Calories Will You Need?

While some women have a good awareness and do not need a formula for caloric intake, you may prefer to have a set system to assist you with your goals. If you absolutely dread counting calories, measuring food, and tracking what you eat, feel free to skip over this section. But if you can't seem to control your eating habits, keep reading for some good tips.

Remember that your body is unique and may require adjustments to this formula, but it's a good place to start. An excellent method for determining caloric intake is the Harris Benedict Equation. This equation estimates your total daily caloric expenditure, which is your resting metabolic rate (RMR, also known as basal metabolic rate or BMR). This is the number of calories required each day for your basic bodily functions like tissue repair, circulation, brain activities, digestion, etc. It then adds this to the number of calories you burn during exercise and activity.

$$\boxed{\text{RMR calories}} + \boxed{\text{exercise calories}} = \boxed{\text{total calories needed per day}}$$

Step 1: Calculate RMR (resting metabolic rate) calories

This formula is specific for women:

$$\boxed{655} + \boxed{\begin{array}{c}\text{weight in}\\ \text{kilograms x}\\ 9.6\end{array}} + \boxed{\begin{array}{c}\text{height in}\\ \text{centimeters}\\ \text{x 1.8}\end{array}} - \boxed{\text{age x 4.7}}$$

To convert pounds to kilograms, divide your weight in pounds by 2.2. To convert your height in inches to centimeters, multiply by 2.5. If you are 130 pounds in weight and 5 feet 6 inches tall at age 35, this will be your RMR:

Weight: 59.1 kilograms x 9.6 = 567.27
Height: 165 centimeters x 1.8 = 297
Age: 35 years x 4.7 = 164.5
RMR = (655 + 567.27 + 297)—164.5 = 1,355 calories

As a former math teacher, these equations come easily to me, but this online calculator can do the math for you: www.bmi-calculator.net/bmr-calculator.

Cheating on the Math. If you don't like using complex formulas to figure out your calories, here is a cheat sheet. To maintain your current weight, multiply your weight by fourteen. This is based on the idea that you burn fourteen calories per pound of body weight each day with an hour of activity. If you want to lose weight, multiply your current body weight by eleven or twelve so that you burn more energy than you consume.

Step 2: Calculating Calories to Support Daily Activity at Current Weight

Unless you're a test subject for sleep clinic studies, you likely don't lie around all day without moving. So, the next step is to figure out just how much you move and how many calories you need to support that movement. This is usually when things get a little tense because no one likes to admit how sedentary they truly are. A good portion of my daily work involves reading and writing, so I spend a large amount of my working hours in a chair pounding away at a keyboard. This isn't ideal, but most of us work desk jobs these days and spend much of our time in our seats.

Adding the *Strong Curves* training program to your weekly regimen will help make up for those hours you spend sitting in a chair, so the more days per week you use the program, the better off you will be. The Harris Benedict Equation calculates the number of calories you need per day by the amount of activity you perform.

To determine your total daily caloric need, multiply your RMR by the activity level factor as follows:

- Sedentary (little to no exercise, not a choice with *Strong Curves*): RMR x 1.2

- Light activity (light exercise/sports 1-3 days/week): RMR x 1.375

- Moderate activity (moderate exercise/sports 3-5 days/week): RMR x 1.55

- High Activity (hard exercise/sports 6-7 days/week): RMR x 1.725

- Extra Activity (very hard exercise and a physical job or 2-a-day training) RMR x 1.9

Right now, you might fall into the sedentary or light activity category because you haven't started the *Strong Curves Program* yet and are not performing any other intense exercise. Nevertheless, I'd like you to calculate the calories needed based on the work you will take on in this program. I like to place my standard workout clients at the moderate activity level if they work a desk job. If I'm training athletes with desk jobs, I place them at the high activity level. Professional athletes during season usually fall in the extra activity level.

If we take our RMR calculation from above for a one hundred thirty-pound, five-foot six-inch, thirty-five year old woman, and decide she is moderately active, her daily caloric intake to maintain her weight would be as follows:

1,355 calories x 1.55 = 2,100 calories per day

I think it's hard to determine exact activity level using the Harrison Benedict formula, so if we decide she wants to maintain her body weight, we can go the simpler route and just multiply 130 pounds x 14 calories.

130 pounds x 14 calories = 1,820 calories per day

I find that the latter formula, though far more rudimentary, calculates caloric need surprisingly accurately because it's based on calories needed per day rather than an estimation of activity level, which can vary depending on how long you exercise and what type of exercise you perform.

Caloric Deficit for Fat Loss

Creating a caloric deficit can be as easy as reducing your daily caloric intake by a certain amount. For example, you might subtract five hundred calories from the calories you eat during a typical day prior to calculations. This doesn't always work, however, because your current caloric intake may be too high or too low. If we take our previous example and use this method, assuming the woman eats twenty-five hundred calories per day and reduces her caloric intake by five hundred calories, her intake would still be too high to create a sufficient deficit. For this reason, you may wish to create an even greater calculated caloric deficit. This can be done by multiplying your current body weight by eleven or twelve, as previously mentioned.

For example, let's say a woman who is five-foot six-inches tall and weighs one hundred fifty-five pounds. She would like to lose twenty pounds of fat mass. In order to eat the correct caloric deficit, she would calculate her daily calories as follows:

155 pounds x 11 calories = 1,705 calories per day

A Word of Caution About Hunger. As you get stronger and lose weight, your hunger will rise. You must fight the urge to eat more and struggle to stay disciplined to keep the weight moving in the right direction. The increased hunger is your body's way of telling you it's using fuel efficiently. Don't take this as a sign that you can splurge on your meals. Take this as a sign that you are getting closer to your goals. Know that your hunger will subside once your metabolism levels out. This may happen within a week or may take longer, but the hunger will go away naturally.

Calculating Macronutrients

Now that you know how many calories you need each day, it's time to figure out where those calories will come from. According to the Atwater Factor, proteins and carbohydrates contain four calories per gram, while fats contain nine calories per gram. These estimates were set a century ago based on rounding the caloric estimation of a large number of studied foods. These numbers are by no means absolute, but they provide a good starting point when it comes to setting your nutrition plan. If you want a formula for setting macronutrients, you can do the following:

Protein = consume .8-1 grams per pound of body weight

(Note that up to 1.5 grams can be used during hard dieting, and more protein should be consumed when losing weight as opposed to gaining or maintaining weight. Some women find that when consuming more than one gram of protein per pound of body weight, they experience constipation. If this occurs, make sure to supplement with fiber and eat plenty of fibrous vegetables.)

Fat = consume .3-.5 grams per pound of lean body mass

Carbohydrate = Subtract the sum of the protein and fat calories from your total daily caloric intake, and divide by 4 to get the number of grams.

If you take the example of our client who weighs one hundred thirty pounds and needs 1,820 calories per day to maintain her weight, her daily diet would look like this:

Total Calories = 1,820 calories/day
Protein = 130 pounds = 130 grams/day or 520 calories/day
Fat = 130(.5) = 65 grams/day or 585 calories/day
Carbohydrate = (Total calories minus protein calories minus fat calories) divided by 4

(1820-520-585) / 4 = 715/4 = 179 grams/day or 715 calories/day

She would, therefore, eat 130 grams of protein, 65 grams of fat, and 179 grams of carbohydrates per day.

You also must take into account how many calories per day you will burn. Calculating calories is never an exact science because on any given day, you will likely burn more or less than the previous day due to activity levels. That is why it's important to try to stick with these numbers but also give yourself some slack if you don't meet your exact needs every single day.

How Many Grams Are In What?

It's time to put together your meal plan by using these numbers. This is always the most confusing part of creating a nutrition plan, so here is a cheat sheet. These are estimations for common foods:

Protein Sources (protein in grams)
Chicken breast (4 oz)—30 grams
One chicken thigh—10 grams
One large egg—6 grams
Ground beef (4 oz)—26 grams
Steak (4 oz)—28 grams
Goat meat (4 oz)—29 grams
Lamb (4 oz)—30 grams
Most fillet fish (4 oz)—24 grams
Tuna (4 oz)—26 grams
Pork loin (4 oz)—29 grams
Ham (3 oz)—19 grams
Whole milk (1 cup)—8 grams
Cottage cheese (½ cup)—15 grams
Plain whole milk yogurt (1 cup)—8 grams
Tofu, firm (½ cup)—10 grams

Fat Sources (grams per serving)
1 tbs. olive oil—14 grams
1 tbs. coconut oil—14 grams
1 cup avocado—35 grams
2 tbs. peanut butter- 16 grams
2 tbs. almond butter—18 grams
1 ounce raw cashews—12 grams
1 tbs. butter—11 grams
1 large egg yolk—5 grams
1 ounce cheddar cheese- 9 grams
1 cup low fat cottage cheese- 2 grams
½ cup cottage cheese—5 grams
1 cup whole milk—8 grams
1 cup plain whole milk yogurt- 8 grams

Carbohydrate Sources (carbs in grams)
1 medium fresh apple- 21 grams
1 medium fresh banana- 26.7 grams
3 medium fresh apricots—11.8 grams
½ cup fresh blueberries- 10.2 grams
½ cup cantaloupe—22.3 grams
½ cup fresh cherries—12 grams
1 small fig—8 grams
½ medium grapefruit—17 grams
1 cup fresh grapes—15.8 grams
1 medium fresh mango—35.2 grams
1 medium orange—15.4 grams
1 medium fresh pear—25.1 grams
½ cup fresh watermelon—5.7 grams
½ cup beans (black, kidney, garbanzo, etc.) 17-19 grams
½ cup cooked lentils—20 grams
2 medium beets—16.3 grams
1 ounce Jicama—2.5 grams
1 small baked potato- 29.3 grams
1 medium yam—31.6 grams
½ cup pumpkin—10.1 grams
1 cup acorn squash- 14.6 grams
1 cup butternut squash—16.4 grams
1 cup cooked barley—41.6 grams
1 cup cooked pasta- 42.6 grams
1 cup cooked brown rice- 44.8 grams
1 cup cooked white rice—35.1 grams
1 cup cooked wild rice—35 grams
½ cup cooked rolled oats—27 grams
1 slice whole grain bread- 16 grams
½ cup cottage cheese—3 grams
1 cup whole milk—11 grams
1 cup plain whole milk yogurt- 12 grams

When setting up your diet, you must first determine how many times per day you will eat. Despite popular theory, eating five to six small meals a day should not be your standard rule. You don't need to constantly fuel the fire to make it burn. If you're more comfortable eating your regular three meals each day with a small snack, then do so. If you want to pack all of your calories into two sittings, that's fine too. Just make sure whatever you choose fits your comfort level and lifestyle. You can always figure this out by your appetite. If you have a hearty appetite, stick to three or four meals per day. If you eat like a bird, five or six meals might indeed work better for you. The important part is getting in those calories no matter when they fall into your schedule. My friend, Alan Aragon, has done a wonderful job dispelling this "stoke the fire myth" by citing multiple studies that show how more frequent daily meals do not result in increased metabolic rate.

You also want to time your meals around your workouts so that you have sufficient energy. This isn't to say that you absolutely must eat immediately before and after training. But it's good to have a meal in your system within two to three hours prior and one hour after you work out. If you train in the early morning in a fasted state (without eating), get in a good protein and carbohydrate source afterward to help with recovery.

Let's use our client example, who needs one hundred thirty grams of protein in her diet every day. If she wants to eat four meals per day, she might divide this up among her meals accordingly:

Meal 1: 3 whole eggs = 18 grams of protein

Meal 2: 6 oz. chicken breast, 1 cup whole milk = 53 grams of protein

Meal 3: ½ cup cottage cheese = 15 grams of protein

Meal 4: 6 oz. fish fillet, 1 cup plain yogurt = 44 grams of protein

Note that her meal plan is three grams over her daily goal. This is perfectly fine since her next day might be under. Calorie-counting is never an exact science. Just stay within close range, and it will work out. If you are going over or under your protein grams consistently, however, you should take a look at your food choices and see where you can make adjustments.

Next, let's formulate the fat component to her daily diet (goal—65 grams, actually 66 grams):

Meal 1: 3 egg yolks, 1 tsp. olive oil for cooking (3 tsp. in 1 tbs.) = 29 grams of fat

Meal 2: 1 cup whole milk = 8 grams of fat

Meal 3: 2 tbs. peanut butter, ½ cup cottage cheese = 21 grams of fat

Meal 4: 1 cup plain yogurt = 8 grams of fat

Her carbohydrate foods would look like this (goal - 164 grams, actually 171.2 grams):

Meal 1: 1 cup fresh cantaloupe = 44.6 grams of carbs

Meal 2: 1 medium yam, 1 cup whole milk = 47.4 grams of carbs

Meal 3: 1 medium banana, ½ cup cottage cheese = 29.7 grams of carbs

Meal 4: ½ cup cooked wild rice, ½ cup cooked lentils, 1 cup plain yogurt = 49.5 grams of carbs

To complete each meal, all you need is to add two to three cups of fibrous vegetables into the daily mix. A final meal plan would look like this:

Meal 1: 3 whole eggs, 1 tsp. olive oil for cooking, ½ cup mushrooms, 1 cup spinach, 1 cup fresh cantaloupe

Meal 2: 6 oz. chicken breast, 1 cup whole milk, 1 medium yam, 1 cup mixed greens with bell peppers, onions, and tomatoes

Meal 3: ½ cup cottage cheese, 1 medium banana sliced with 2 tbs. peanut butter

Meal 4: 6 oz. fish fillet, 1 cup yogurt, ½ cup cooked wild rice, ½ cup lentils

Each meal can be uniquely catered to your taste buds. This just gives you an example of what a daily menu should look like on the *Strong Curves Program*. When you want to fit in free meals and treats, try to stick with these whole foods for the first four weeks while on the *Strong Curves* plan. If your goal is weight loss, after the initial four weeks, fit in one free meal a week until you reach your target weight. From there, you can fit in two to three free meals a week. Free meals should consist of the same amount of calories as your regular meal, but can be whatever foods you want. Also, remember I said free meal, not free day.

If you are eating at maintenance when you start this plan, still avoid treats and free meals for the first four weeks until your body adjusts and you find the right balance of carbohydrates and fats. Once you have a pretty good handle on exactly what your body needs to run efficiently while reaching your goals, start introducing those free meals at your discretion. If you find yourself getting out of control at any time in your diet, go back to the original plan of treat-free eating.

Supplements for *Strong Curves*

I am not a strong proponent of sports supplements and do not recommend most of them to my clients. If asked, I will educate my clients on their choices but won't sway their opinion one way or another. While on the *Strong Curves Program*, I only recommend fish oil caps, vitamin D3, and a high quality multivitamin/ mineral. You may also take whey protein as a source of nutrition that is calculated into your macronutrients. Personally, I love whey protein as it helps me attain my daily protein goals without going overboard on calorie consumption. I also love the taste of it as long as I mix it with skim milk. However, I've found that most women do not like the taste and prefer real food over whey protein shakes. Some women even find that whey protein isn't easily digested.

I recommend that you take at least 1,200mg of quality fish oil per day if you cannot eat fresh fish twice per week.

I strongly suggest you take a high quality multivitamin/mineral once a day for insurance purposes, even if you eat a diet rich in fruits and vegetables. Our soil has been depleted throughout the years and does not contain as many vitamins and minerals as it once did.

If you avoid the sun, I recommend taking at least 800IU of vitamin D3 per day in addition to your multivitamin/mineral (and even more if you have a severe deficiency that needs to normalize).

Anything not mentioned in this book is not necessary to reach your goals. You can achieve an incredible physique without fat burners, BCAAs, glutamine, creatine, and all of the other high-priced products on the market. Research shows that some of them can indeed benefit performance, but for physique enhancement purposes, your money is best spent on quality food.

Keeping a Food Journal

Even if you're not big on documenting your progress, I recommend keeping a food journal for the first month while using the *Strong Curves Program*. Your nutrition directly relates to your strength and fat loss progress. If you aren't eating enough calories or enough of the right calories, you will feel it during training and see it on the scale. On days that you have high energy, take note of what you ate. The same rule applies for low energy days. The key to your success is becoming fully aware of how your body works.

Getting Everyone On Board

When you choose a fit lifestyle, you will face mixed reviews from friends and family. Most will be supportive, but others will offer advice and opinions that go against everything you are trying to accomplish. You can choose to confront or ignore them, but don't conform to their opinions. In time, they will see that your new lifestyle is doing wonders for your energy, physique, health, confidence, and attitude. Soon they will beg you for advice.

Your home kitchen may experience a big makeover on this program, so prepare your family members before you clean out their favorite treats from the pantry. Sit down together and discuss your weekly menu. Involve your partner and kids when you make the grocery list, and help them find healthy alternatives for their favorite snacks and meals.

One of the best things you can do for your children is invite them to the grocery store to help out. Give them the shopping list, and let them make some of the big decisions when buying groceries. Also involve them in meal preparation, especially when making lunch for school. The more involved your family becomes with your fit lifestyle, the more support you will receive from them.

What Digestive Health Has to Do With *Strong Curves*

While you'd rather not think about the inner workings of your digestion, digestive health is important if you want to meet your fitness and health goals. You were born with a completely sterile digestive tract and over time, microbes colonized it, making an incredibly diverse ecology in there. Certain elements in your diet and lifestyle may trigger an unhealthy balance, causing your digestion to go haywire. You may not like to associate certain symptoms with your digestion—symptoms like an inability to lose weight, add muscle, and even wake up feeling good. Nevertheless, your digestion plays an integral role in your overall well being.

I've met women who suffered gastric distress for years and learned to just accept that they were not going to feel well every day. Soon, they became in tune with how their eating affected their bodies and started eliminating potential food culprits. Once they found their trigger foods, they began healing within days. The majority of women who find foods that trigger health issues also find that once they eliminate those foods, they shed excess weight rapidly. Certain foods that irritate digestion or are allergens can cause you to store excess fat and water weight.

Experiment with your diet if you suffer from symptoms that disrupt your daily life. The first food you want to eliminate is refined sugar. Then, go for grains, including flours, wheat, barley, oats, and all sources of gluten. The next food to eliminate is dairy products. Make sure you eliminate food groups one at a time and track how you feel. If you don't see vast improvements after eliminating the first group move onto the next group of foods that may potentially trigger symptoms.

Once you find the food culprit and have it out of your system for two to three weeks, experiment by adding it back into one meal. Most people who have food intolerances will instantly notice the old symptoms come back. If this happens, make a conscious effort to keep that food out of your diet for good. You will be healthier and on the way to your fitness goal.

Digestion is one of the most overlooked aspects of building a beautiful physique and maintaining ideal weight. Your digestion is responsible for delivering nutrients to blood, organs, and tissue to maintain healthy body functions. Poor digestive health can be the number one indicator that your body is not receiving all of the nutrients it needs to sustain proper function.

You should become aware of how well your digestive system is functioning. Your muscles, physique, and entire body depend on it. If you suffer the symptoms of gas, bloating, constipation, diarrhea, stomach pains, or cramps, it's important that you learn to manage these issues since they directly relate to how your body absorbs nutrients. Don't ignore these symptoms; they can lead to larger problems in the future. Though the scope of this subject is too vast for the context of this book, I highly recommend that if these issues persist after eliminating potential food triggers, find a local nutrition expert who can help identify the root cause of the problem. Your mind and body will thank you. Whether you need to eliminate potential food irritants or not, you should also consider adding two important supplements to your daily diet.

Digestive Enzymes

Enzymes play a role in the entire digestive process, so if you suffer from any of the symptoms mentioned in the last section, you may benefit from a digestive enzyme supplement with each meal. If you have certain disorders such as a peptic ulcer, however, consult with your physician to find the best solution.

When selecting a digestive enzyme, you have three major choices. The first is Betaine HCl, which is a combination of a vitamin-like substance known as betaine and hydrochloric acid. This is sometimes prescribed to those who have too little hydrochloric acid in their stomachs or suffer from acid reflux. Another form of digestive enzymes is a multi-enzyme product, which supports the boost of enzymatic action throughout the course of digestion. The third is single enzymes that bond to certain proteins, sugars, or other macromolecules. These work well if you know that a single nutrient like dairy causes your gastric distress. It's best to consult with your holistic healthcare provider to find the right combination of digestive enzymes for your symptoms.

Healthy Intestinal Flora

In addition to digestive enzymes, you should also consider adding a quality probiotic to your daily regimen. There is plenty of scientific evidence that shows this is an opportunity to improve the beneficial bacteria (flora) in your gut. Eating a large base of plant foods is one way to improve good flora, but adding a probiotic is another. This renders almost immediate results by gently amending damaged intestinal colonies that may have suffered due to flora imbalances.

Rebalancing your gut flora will help to:

- Digest certain proteins and sugars for greater absorption.
- Speed up absorption of certain minerals, such as calcium, magnesium, and iron.
- Regulate appropriate fat storage.
- Prevent bloating, gas, and other digestive-related symptoms.
- Manufacture vitamin K and B vitamins.
- Use up nutrients that may otherwise become food for bacterial invaders.
- Secrete acids that bad bacteria find intolerable.
- Strengthen the intestinal lining to help block dangerous pathogens and allergens.
- Increase T-cells, producing natural antibiotics/antifungals to help stimulate the immune system.
- Metabolize and recycle hormones.

Eating a diet rich in fiber helps to feed healthy flora. Try to eat at least two cups of fibrous vegetables per day, and include fruits, legumes, seeds, and whole grains (if tolerated) in your daily diet. Also, fermented and cultured foods such as yogurt, kefir, miso, and sauerkraut will help keep bad bacteria at bay. Homemade pickles help, too. Limit refined sugars, alcohol, and refined flours, as bad bacteria love feeding on these foods.

Eight Simple Food Rules to Live By

If you read this entire chapter and cringed at the very thought of calculating calories and keeping tabs on macronutrients, you may just want to adhere to these eight simple rules adopted from Michael Pollan's *In Defense of Food* while progressing through the *Strong Curves Program.*

Many women are very strict with their nutrition when they first start training. They see excellent results and then get greedy. They might start eating a "low-carb brownie" each day or some other unhealthy food that's disguised as healthy. Common sense tells us that these foods should be avoided, as a healthy brownie is just too good to be true. In these cases, progress quickly comes to a halt, and the women fail to connect the dots.

Rule 1: Shop outside of the supermarket whenever possible.

Eating locally grown foods found at your farmer's market is the best thing you can do for your diet. Local farmers grow seasonal produce, feed livestock vegetarian diets, and allow their animals to roam free. Eating local ensures your food will always be fresh and in season, and your purchase will help sustain your local economy.

Rule 2: Eat less food, and stop eating before you feel full.

Eating at a caloric deficit has shown in numerous studies to slow the aging process in animals, and some researchers believe it is the single most prevalent link to cancer prevention. You don't always have to eat everything on your plate; it's better to leave some food behind.

Rule 3: Eat foods that will rot if you don't eat them.

The phrase "long shelf life" should be a dirty word in your household. Fungi and bacteria compete for your food in nature. The reason foods have a shelf life is that these little microbes won't go near them. So, if your food isn't good enough for fungi and bacteria, it shouldn't be good enough for you either.

Rule 4: Eat foods sweetened by nature.

If you have to add sugar to a food to make it sweet, don't eat it. Nature sweetens plenty of our foods for us, so make those your first choices when looking to satisfy your sugar cravings.

Rule 5: Eat foods that have been prepared by humans.

Whether you cook at home or go out for a meal, it's best to have your meal prepared by human hands than by a corporate factory. The same rule applies to corporate chain restaurants. Most of these restaurants add lots of salt, sugar, and other additives to their meals for flavor enhancement. Eat at a local restaurant known for serving high quality food, at a friend's house, or at home.

Rule 6: Put the right amount of food on your plate the first time.

Know how much you need to eat during a given meal, and place all of your food on your plate at one time. Then, don't go back for more. Often, when you go for a second helping, you tend to eat far more than originally anticipated. If your gut is telling you it's finished eating, stop.

Rule 7: You are what your food eats.

Eat animals that have consumed a healthy vegetarian diet. Grass-fed livestock or livestock fed a green diet are typically high in omega-3 fatty acids. Vegetarian-fed livestock contain more nutrients and live a much more humane life. The same rule applies to your produce. Eating local produce ensures that it has been grown in soil rich enough to support its growth and that it hasn't been sprayed with chemicals to speed up the ripening process.

Rule 8: Avoid foods that make health claims.

Apple farmers don't need to tell you to eat apples because they're good for you. If a food item needs to make up excuses as to why you should eat it, that's the first clue you shouldn't eat it. Always go with your gut instinct because you know what's good for you and what isn't. The same goes for foods that claim to be "light," "low fat," and/or "enriched." These are just polite ways of saying they are not nutritious.

Chapter 6:

Where'd You Get Those Moves?

As someone with a discerning eye for movement, I'm appalled at what I see in the commercial gyms these days. I don't expect every person who walks onto a gym floor to master movement patterns for squats and deadlifts (though this sure would be nice). What bothers me is when I see certified professionals forcing their clients to lift inappropriate amounts of weight with very poor form. I can't stress this enough: It's very important to develop proper movement patterns on the various fundamental motions such as squats, lunges, hip hinges, and bridges. You may find that you're limited in mobility, stability, and/or motor control and need to improve upon these qualities before loading up a pattern and adding resistance. You have to master your body weight before using a barbell. That's just all there is to it. Not only will doing the "right" exercises the "wrong" way fail to shape the glutes, but it will eventually end up causing pain or injury.

Evaluating Your Own Movement Patterns

Movement patterns are the foundation upon which strength is built, so good form is imperative to your success with *Strong Curves* and beyond. I run my clients through a battery of drills during their first session to evaluate their movement competency. Understanding how you move, where your weaknesses lie, and where to begin your training to build up weak areas and correct dysfunction will vastly improve your strength and form over time in addition to preventing serious injury. If you are not sure about your exercise form, I encourage you to find a Certified Functional Movement Screen (FMS) expert in your area to assess your mobility, stability, and motor control during fundamental movement patterns. You can do this by going to the FMS website: http://functionalmovement.com/.

Don't push yourself beyond limitations when you begin the *Strong Curves Program*. Regression with exercises may seem like you're working backward, but in reality, it will improve your strength and allow you to reach new personal records far faster by clueing in on your weaknesses and making corrections before using heavy loads.

With this assessment, you may find that you need to regress your squats to bodyweight or goblet squats until you improve your stability. If you have poor ankle dorsiflexion, you may need to stick with box squats until you bring up your mobility. Squatting may seem like a simple, natural movement, but many things have to happen for a proper squat to occur. The knees need to track over the toes, the spine needs to stay arched, the pelvis needs to keep its forward tilt, the body needs to stay centered over the feet, and the load needs to be distributed properly between the hips and knees. These criteria may be simple in a half-squat, but a deep squat is a different story.

In addition, many women struggle with proper plank and push-up form. I find that many of my female clients perform pushups incorrectly, and I often regress them by using an elevated bar while slowly moving it toward the ground over time until they're back in correct push-up form.

Krista was a former high school and collegiate athlete who arrived at my studio in Arizona after a couple of years out of her sport. She was in great shape but had one of the worst cases of valgus collapse I had ever encountered. I think of "valgus collapse" as a melting candle. Weak glutes and hip rotators fail to hold proper positioning during squatting tasks, and this causes the femurs to adduct and internally rotate, the opposite pelvis to drop (if performing single-leg squatting tasks), and the feet to pronate. Essentially, things "cave in" during the movement.

I filmed Krista during all of her exercises, and we reviewed them immediately after the set. This allowed her to see what she was doing and make rapid improvements. I showed her how her knees were caving in during squats and how she lacked symmetry during single-leg movements. She was accustomed to using a barbell, but I had her stick with a dumbbell and perform goblet squats and between-bench full squats. I placed my hands on the outside of her knees so that she focused on keeping them out throughout the movements. This greatly improved her motor control.

I also wrapped a band around her knees and had her perform band seated abductions, as well as x-band walks, side planks, and band rotary holds, to reinforce the "feel" of using the upper glutes. She did weekly bodyweight squats with the bands around her knees to improve the strength and stability of her hip abductors and external rotators through the squatting movement pattern. These strategies, in addition to all of the other lower body movements we employed, allowed her to make rapid improvements, and we were able to beat records and add loads each and every workout.

Krista cared a great deal about her physique, and prior to working with me, she had worked with several other trainers who failed to address her condition. She often left her trainers feeling frustrated due to lack of progress with her lower body lifts. With my corrective exercises, she was able to take her squat from ninety-five pounds to one hundred fifty-five pounds in eight weeks. She completely blew me away by bringing her deadlift up ninety pounds, to an incredible two hundred seventy-five pounds. By cleaning up her technique, we were able to make much greater strides. The moral of the story? Never sacrifice good form just to set a personal record!

The Aerobic Exercise Debate

Strong Curves doesn't have a set protocol for cardiovascular exercise. You will find that the work you do during the program greatly improves heart strength, endurance, and cardiovascular health without ever having to pound the pavement or jump on the cardio equipment at the gym. However, if you enjoy aerobic activity or believe your weight loss efforts could benefit from the fat-burning effects of cardio exercise, feel free to add this type of exercise into your weekly regimen. Two or three twenty to thirty minute sessions per week is all you need; don't go overboard.

Even when you add cardio sessions to your workout week, you still need to maintain proper nutrition. Extra exercise doesn't give you excuses to eat poorly. For example, a moderate thirty-minute elliptical workout for a woman weighing one hundred thirty pounds burns roughly two hundred ten calories. A Dunkin Donuts Blueberry Crumb donut contains five hundred calories. Not a fair trade off, is it?

Always prioritize your training around your goals. For example, sprinters should prioritize sprinting and perform their strength training after their sprint work. For your purposes, you will prioritize strength. The stronger you become, the greater your physique will look.

If you plan to add aerobic activity into your workout schedule, make sure the *Strong Curves Program* is prioritized over your cardio exercise (unless you are training for sport). This means that when you plan your schedule, you will perform your strength workouts first. If you want to add in twenty minutes of running to your strength program three times per week, you can either run after your strength workouts or on your days off from strength training. This ensures that you are using maximal effort with your strength programs, making aerobic activity your secondary priority for energy demands.

If you can only make it to the gym at night and only have time for a quick walk in the morning, however, don't skip your walk just to conform to this method. I want you to make the most of the *Strong Curves Program*, and I designed it to easily adapt to your needs.

Some of the other activities that women may wish to perform in addition to their *Strong Curves* workouts include:

Walking	Recreational Sports
Cardio equipment	Running hills
Complexes	Sled dragging
High-intensity interval circuits	Spin classes
	Step aerobics
Jumping rope	Swimming
Jogging	Tabatas
Pilates	Yoga
Plyometrics	Sprinting
Bike riding	

Cardio doesn't build shape, getting stronger does. And too much cardio will prevent you from getting stronger. I can't emphasize this enough. If you want rounder glutes, you'll need to build them up to be able to lift much heavier weight over time. The stronger the booty, the better the booty. Strength builds the shape while nutritional habits help reduce fat stores.

If you are new to training, I recommend adding light additional activity such as stationary walking on an inclined treadmill for fifteen to twenty minutes three times per week. If you are an advanced lifter, adding two fifteen-minute hill sprint workouts to your weekly schedule may benefit your stamina while not impairing your ability to recover from strength sessions.

Again, these additional activities are not required to be successful with *Strong Curves*, but cardiovascular and aerobic activities can benefit your program by allowing you to achieve your goals faster. Just don't overdo it! More is not better (yes, you will get constant subtle reminders of this).

It's important to pay attention to how your body feels each day. Wake up and assess any soreness or discomfort, and evaluate how your previous day's activities contributed to the discomfort. Is it from the newness of a particular movement, or is your body telling you to slow down and not overreach? If you are too tight or sore, you should make adjustments by decreasing the intensity or amount of activity. To improve recovery time and reduce risk of injury, dedicate at least one day per week to complete rest and recovery—even professional athletes take a day off. Assuming you stay the same weight, getting much stronger over time at hip thrusts, squats, and deadlifts will do far more toward developing *Strong Curves* than packing on miles of running without gaining strength.

Over-Training and Overreaching

Strength training is the most important aspect of training for physical purposes. It shapes and strengthens muscles while burning fat. Training for strength brings with it a number of health benefits, including improved bone density, cardiovascular health, and increased movement economy—just to name a few. But there is a fine line between beneficial exercise and too much exercise. One of the largest fitness myths is that in order to see great results, you must live in the gym and train for hours on end. This is the furthest thing from the truth. Round-the-clock training is not necessary or even ideal for muscle growth or body composition changes.

I can't tell you the number of times new clients have cried out in our first meeting, "I don't want to devote my life to working out!" This statement usually follows with, "I just don't have the time or energy to live in the gym." I can honestly tell you that unless you are directly speaking to a professional athlete whose livelihood depends on her ability to perform in peak condition, no one has time for this. Not you, not me, and not any of my clients. Yet, my clients are able to successfully accomplish the physiques they want by spending only a few hours per week in the gym or training at home, and you can, too.

I'm going to let you in on a little secret that many in the fitness industry don't want you to know. Most of my colleagues will tell you the truth because they truly care about your health, but the majority of the fitness industry sets you up for failure by making you believe that if you aren't devoting your entire free time to diet and exercise, you are never going to reach your goals. You will not achieve greater results by adding in more exercises, training for extra time, or working out seven days a week with *Strong Curves*. You will not achieve the body you want by adding in hours of cardio to your weekly strength-training plan in *Strong Curves* or by eating at a severe caloric deficit far below what is recommended in this book.

In fact, if you do any or all of these things, you will feel and look worse because your body will turn against itself. You have built-in survival mechanisms that are triggered when you are under great stress. Constantly over-training and under-eating sends out stress signals to your body around the clock. Eventually, your stress hormones will kick into overdrive and wreak havoc on your immune system. In turn, you will feel rundown, fatigued, irritable, and depressed rather than motivated and strong. If all of this is going on inside, imagine what you will look like on the outside.

One of the best things you can do is take my advice and never fall into this trap. Do not over-train, and do not under-nourish your body. Also, do not overeat because you feel all of this new exercise will compensate for the added calories. If you follow the *Strong Curves* plan to the letter, including both the nutrition and workout regimen, you will achieve your greatest physique to date. If you decide to manipulate your outcome by making changes to this plan that I strongly recommend against, don't send me an angry email when things start to go south.

You must stick with the "less is more" mindset, and remember these three phrases:

- Show up to train hard.
- Train smart, not long.
- Eat for nourishment.

Finding What's Right for Your Goals

When adding cardiovascular exercise to your *Strong Curves* plan, it's important to maintain structure. Though many new fitness fads claim that muscle confusion is the best method for fast results, I caution against this practice for several reasons. Think about the process of learning something new. As a kid, you didn't learn to ride your bike by getting on it every four weeks. After school every day, you reluctantly put your feet to the pedals as your dad thrust you out into the open road. You crashed, scraped a knee or two, and maybe even cried a little. But you consistently got back on that bike until you mastered it. Soon you were riding in a straight line down the road but couldn't figure out how to stop. Once you figured out how to stop, it was time to master turns.

After hours, days, or even months of consistently trying, you were riding your bike with the neighborhood kids like you were born to do it. The same goes for fitness training. Exercises may seem awkward, annoying, or even impossible at first. Some of these movements might make you feel downright silly or inadequate. I've felt that way several times with exercises that I've grown to enjoy over the years. The only way you're going to grow to enjoy the exercises in this book is to consistently incorporate them into your workouts and improve upon your form and strength with each session.

You might be familiar with and have already mastered some of the exercises. You may have heard of some of the exercises, but never had the guts or the inclination to test them out. Others may be completely new to you, but trust me when I say that all of them are worth adding to your program over time. In the *Strong Curves Program*, I encourage you to consistently use the same exercises during each individual phase. If there is an exercise in the program that you cannot use for whatever reason, choose a supplemental exercise offered in the Exercise Index, and stick with it throughout the duration of the phase.

This is important because of the adaptability of your neuromuscular system. You may not notice it, but it takes intricately detailed communication for your brain to tell your muscles what to do during an exercise. If you're new to the exercise, it makes the communication far more challenging for your brain. The more familiar your brain becomes with the movement, the more easily it can communicate with your muscles to create the correct movement patterns. The easier the communication, the more prepared you are for the lift. With each successive training session, your body will be better adapted to the lifts and ready to take on new challenges so that you can make steady strength gains over time. This process is known as "progressive overload." Essentially, you are pushing your muscles beyond adaptation with each session by adding weight or reps or by shortening the duration between sets.

For example, if your program requires that you perform squats during a given session, yet you don't do squats again for another four weeks, your brain has to recoordinate the movement. But if you perform squats in one session per week for four weeks, your coordination will greatly improve, which translates to a stronger squat. Remember that it takes thousands of repetitions in order for your brain to form a "motor engram," which is a memorized movement pattern.

After you complete *Strong Curves* phases one through three, you have the freedom to explore new techniques, tinker with exercises, and try different exercises listed in the Exercise Index. I offer a template that you can use for life, and I provide an extensive collection of exercises to choose from. Once you feel you are at a level where you are using excellent form in all of your big lifts (squats, deadlifts, lunges, hip thrusts, presses, and pulls), you have more opportunity to change your routine on a regular basis. As you advance, you may introduce more variety and will need to rotate exercises more frequently. But you will have mastered the movement patterns and will stay coordinated and strong with all movements due to the similarity of the various lower body exercises. For example, though squats, deadlifts, hip thrusts, and back extensions are all very different in terms of form, they all involve hip extension. As long as you perform movements that look like squats (double or single-leg), movements that look like deadlifts, and movements that look like bridges, you'll be fine. This is the "same but different" philosophy. For instance, a client might perform hip thrusts, full squats, and 45-degree hyperextensions one week, then barbell glute bridges, front squats, and sumo deadlifts the next week. This works because she is using the same global movement patterns, but they differ just enough to prevent boredom.

Follow these same guidelines when introducing aerobic activities to your weekly schedule. If you play soccer on Saturday and take a spin class on Tuesday, this works out to your advantage because you are consistently using the same movement patterns, increasing your coordination with each session. If you schedule Zumba classes on Monday, and kickboxing on Wednesday, but you take up jogging and skip these classes the following week, followed by taking up rock climbing instead the week after—well, you can see where this is going. Consistency is going to be key to your success. Without it, you will just flounder around with all of those new methods of exercise and never adapt well enough to become proficient at any of them. You may experience constant soreness because your body will not prepare properly for the activity. Over time you can vary your cardio each week, but try to stick to the same activities initially, and adapt gradually to avoid getting too sore.

Again, I advise you to really own your weekly schedule and make sure that you carefully plan how much you exercise. If you join a recreational volleyball league and practice twice a week for an hour, with an hour game on the weekends, make sure you incorporate this into your weekly schedule. In this case, you wouldn't want to strength train five days a week, completely neglecting your need for rest. Cut down to two or three strength training sessions per week until your body adapts or your season ends. Never fall into the trap of over-training because it's very hard to climb back out.

What to Do When Your Progress Comes To a Screeching Halt

If you are new to strength training, you will make great gains within the first several months. This happens to nearly everyone, and watching those numbers consistently go up on your lifts while your body fat percentage consistently goes down is great motivation. During your first couple of months, you will get accustomed to performing a couple more reps with the same weight or the same amount of reps with heavier weight than you did the week before. Over time, it becomes difficult to set personal records; simply getting one more rep or five additional pounds on an exercise can be challenging.

This happens to many long-term clients. I find that once they begin lifting at advanced levels, they couldn't care less how much more they lift because they have accomplished more than ninety-nine percent of the population.

But to ease you into these expectations, I will put things into perspective. If you could increase your strength by five pounds every week, you would increase your lifts by two hundred sixty pounds per year. Even if you only went up five pounds per month, this would equate to sixty pounds per year. This simply does not happen year in and year out. To think of it another way, if you could increase your reps by one per week, you would get fifty-two more reps on your exercises per year (at a constant weight). Even if it were just one rep per month, you would increase your reps twelve per year for that weight. So, if you squat one-hundred thirty-five pounds for one rep right now, in one year, you would be able to squat the same weight for thirteen reps. That will not always happen, especially after a couple of years of training.

After you have been training for six months or so, you will have reaped most of your beginner gains. You will then have to push hard to make incremental gains, which is perfectly fine. It's very important to understand that some experienced powerlifters train hard year round and see just moderate increases in strength. For example, one may see fifteen pounds added to her bench press, plus thirty pounds to her squats and deadlifts in twelve months. So, don't let strength plateaus discourage you because they happen to the best of us. They also mean that you are lifting near your threshold, which is quite an accomplishment.

Not only will your strength plateau once you reach an advanced level, but your weight will also taper off. In order to avoid frustration, understand that strength gains, weight loss, and body composition improvements are not linear over time. There will be times of great progress interspersed between times of stagnation. I have trained plenty of women who lost twenty-five pounds during their first month and only a total of five additional pounds over the next eleven months, for a total of thirty pounds net loss. Of course, these same women looked incredibly athletic and fit because they replaced fat mass with fat-free mass as they progressed through my program. Keep focused on changing your body composition rather than whether or not the scale is moving. I recommend taking a photo of yourself in a bikini each month from the same exact location, lighting, and camera position, as pictures often tell a different story than scales.

> **Kellie's Quick Tip:** *if your plateau lingers too long, check your diet and make sure you are eating enough calories and eating enough of the right calories. If your diet is slipping, your body will tell you by a decrease in your energy and performance levels.*

When plateaus happen, follow these suggestions in order to continually progress:

- Hone in on your diet (eating the right amount and the right types of food). Although your strength has stagnated, your physique will head in the right direction.

- Focus on new strength goals such as higher rep ranges or new exercises. For example, set out to perform one hundred non-stop walking lunges or a set of twenty-rep deadlifts with one hundred thirty-five pounds.

- Deload for a week, which involves intentionally pulling back on the intensity of your workout and adding an easy week. This will provide added recuperation, allowing strength levels to rebound. In this situation, perform your workouts at around fifty to eighty percent of your usual intensity. Mentally, it isn't easy to stop a set far short of failure—for example, a set of bench presses with eighty-five pounds for five reps when you're used to doing that weight for ten reps. But training like this for an entire week can spark new gains by allowing for optimal restoration and hormonal homeostasis. Some women do very well with deloading while others do not. There are many ways to tweak a deload, such as simply performing one or two sets rather than three or four sets, thereby keeping intensity up but reducing volume. The important thing is to never stop trying and to not give up and feel defeated.

Modifying Exercises To Fit Your Needs

If you train in a busy gym or a gym that has limited equipment available, you may not be able to perform the *Strong Curves Program* exactly as it is prescribed. Don't let this discourage you, as I have provided ample supplemental exercises to keep you on track and focused. I encourage you to jot down at least one supplemental exercise in all of the big lift categories (your first four exercises of your workout) so that if anything prevents you from performing those lifts, you have options readily available.

For instance, if you arrive at your gym and the squat racks are filled with a line behind them, supplement the exercise with goblet squats or Bulgarian split squats instead of box squats. If you don't have a certain piece of equipment, such as a 45-degree hyperextension, supplement that exercise with Swiss ball reverse hyperextensions and really squeeze the lockout portion for a three-second pause to increase its difficulty. If you always show up at the gym prepared for any changes, you will feel confident with your workouts.

Also, use this practice for exercises that you are not physically able to perform. If you have physical limitations that prevent you from performing certain exercises, flip to the Exercise Index to find one that works for your level and ability. Remember to write this down in your workout journal to get a good understanding of the exercise before you head to the gym. When in doubt, take the *Strong Curves* book with you for additional support and information. The more prepared you are, the more successful you will be.

Strong Curves for Expecting Mothers

Exercise is one of the most beneficial practices you can implement during pregnancy for both you and your baby. Planning your exercise program while expecting can be daunting, though. Knowing what exercises to use is important for the health and safety of your changing body and growing baby. *Strong Curves* offers numerous exercises that you can add to your daily activity throughout your pregnancy. Of course, it's important to consult with your physician and obtain medical clearance prior to engaging in any exercise program. If no contraindications exist, adding three days of resistance training per week to your schedule will greatly contribute to a healthy pregnancy and labor.

Benefits of Strength Training During Pregnancy

While an interpretation of the research is a little fuzzy because many studies do not delineate between aerobic and anaerobic activity, it's pretty clear that adding strength training to your activity schedule during pregnancy will improve your overall health and aid in post-partum recovery. The following are benefits you may experience from using a modified *Strong Curves Program* during each term of your pregnancy:

- Weight management: Studies indicate that women experience a majority of weight gain during the childbearing years (ages twenty-five to thirty-four), but excess weight gain can be controlled by regular strength training sessions during pregnancy. Researchers found that women who maintain regular strength training programs during pregnancy gain twenty percent less weight on average than those who neglect exercise.

- Decreased incidents of pregnancy complications and disorders: Resistance training during pregnancy has been shown to decrease your risk of complications, including low back pain, gestational diabetes, preeclampsia, and depression.

- Improved fetal development: Not long ago, women were advised to avoid strength training during pregnancy for fear of poor fetal development. Luckily, these myths have been debunked, and exercise has actually been found to have positive effects on the development of your baby.

- Labor ease: Resistance training during pregnancy has shown to have positive effects on the ease of your labor. Studies have found that women who use resistance training during pregnancy have shorter durations of active labor and lower incidents of operative delivery.

- Miscarriage concerns: It should be mentioned that women largely fear that strength training may increase the risk of miscarriage during pregnancy, but studies have shown that women who strength train are at no greater risk of miscarriage than those who do not.

Strong Curves Guidelines for Pregnancy

Safety is always the primary concern when implementing exercise routines while pregnant. When pregnant, you should always seek to maintain a reasonable level of fitness rather than maximize it. Aim to stay healthy, but don't lift too heavy or attempt to set personal records at this time (unless you're unfit and new to training). Once you have your baby and get clearance from your doctor to return to the gym, you can start going for those big numbers again, but there is no reason to do so while pregnant.

This isn't to say you can't exercise vigorously during this time, but you always have to keep safety in the forefront. Your joints are looser than normal and after your first trimester, your balance shifts quite a bit. These changes take some getting used to when you're pregnant.

When training with resistance while pregnant, it greatly benefits you to focus on strengthening the entire body, including the core, and to receive plenty of rest in between workouts. The *Strong Curves* plan is structured to give you the option of training three days a week with rest days built in between each session. If you're brand new to strength training, I recommend performing just one set per exercise during your first few workouts. If you're more adept at strength training, you may perform up to three sets per exercise for each workout.

As mentioned previously, your joints are a little more lax during pregnancy, so you will benefit from higher repetitions of ten or more per set. This is best achieved using intensity less than seventy percent of your one-repetition maximum. During your first trimester, you may experience symptoms, including nausea, vomiting, fatigue, headaches, and dizziness. It's important to adjust your fitness plan accordingly so as not to provoke these symptoms.

During the third trimester, some restrictions must be implemented to accommodate the changes in your body. Just listen to your body, and adjust accordingly based on your body's "biofeedback." If something doesn't feel right, don't do it; there are plenty of exercises available, so stick to the ones that are comfortable. Avoid exercises that require lying on your back because this position tends to block venous return to your uterus. You may also omit exercises that require excessive forward flexion at the hips and/or waist. Doing these movements may result in increased stress on your low back, dizziness or heartburn. However, I feel that a set of bodyweight hip thrusts or sumo squats during the workouts should not be feared, as women have reported positive feedback from these exercises while pregnant.

Strong Curves Workouts During Pregnancy

During your first trimester, you may use the *Strong Curves* Booty-ful Beginnings Program in a modified form. As previously mentioned, I recommend reducing your sets to one per exercise if you're new to strength training. Substitute bodyweight hip thrusts for barbell hip thrusts during weeks nine to twelve for workout A.

During your second and third trimester, switch to the *Strong Curves* Best Butt Bodyweight Program, or substitute exercises in the *Strong Curves* Booty-ful Beginnings Program by using the Exercise Index. I recommend sticking with beginner level exercises and working on higher repetitions as opposed to heavier weight and lower repetitions. Of course, if you ever feel discomfort or experience adverse symptoms, stop the exercise immediately.

Chapter 7:

Ladies, Meet Your *Strong Curves Programs*

I've provided three separate workouts in this book based on your individual fitness level. In addition, the Exercise Index provides multiple supplemental exercises to use as substitutions in the pre-formulated workouts or to use when designing your own programs. Whether you use the *Strong Curves* for Beginners, Advanced, Body-weight, or Glutes Only, you will follow the same basic template. I designed it after years of research, EMG testing, and field-testing with clients and athletes. I learned that most women achieve the greatest results when following this format regardless of their overall goals. This is a template you can use for life as the foundation for all of your workouts going forward. Once you work through a twelve-week *Strong Curves Program* or two, you can start designing your own workouts based on this template. In the Exercise Index, I provide a blank template for you to fill in on your own. I encourage you to work through at least one of the programs before branching out on your own, even if you are well versed in program design already.

Before I dive into the exact structure of the template, I need to establish a few structural rules so that you understand how and why the program works the way it does. Again, the template is only the foundation of the *Strong Curves* method. How you use it will determine your success with the program.

How Often and When To Sculpt Those Curves

Four training days per week is optimal, performing workout A twice per week and workout B and C once per week:

Day one: Workout A
Day two: Workout B
Day three: Active rest
Day four: Workout A
Day five: Workout C
Day six: Active rest
Day seven: Rest

However, you might find that you achieve the best results training three days per week, or even five days per week. Perhaps your schedule only allows for two workouts per week, but a good rule is to train between two

and five days a week on this program. Of course, I'd rather see you use the program once per week than not at all. But I don't think you invested your hard earned money in this book just to train once a week.

I also advise you not to strength-train six or seven days per week because you might see a decline in your results. If you plan to only strength-train twice a week, make sure you do other activities during the week when your schedule allows for them. I've trained hundreds of women over the course of my career. Each had her own agenda and lifestyle that I catered her workouts around, and they all saw tremendous results when they stuck to the plan I gave them. You have the same option with this program, but you need to fit your workouts in around your schedule and not skip them if you get too busy. If you have time to watch television, play computer games, read a novel, or hang out with friends, you have time to work out. This isn't to say that you shouldn't have a life. But you must make workouts your priority.

Take It Easy, Pleas-y

What if you embarked on an entirely new career? If you had been a pharmacist for years and suddenly became a kindergarten teacher, what would your reaction be if you walked into the classroom having never taken one education course? You would feel completely frazzled, and the kids would run amok the entire day. That's how your muscles would feel if you jumped into a new workout program that was completely different from anything you had done in the past.

Humans live in excess. Whether it's material goods, rich foods, or a strenuous lifestyle, we tend to over-stimulate our lives on many levels. When it comes to training, lack of adequate physical preparation leads to unbearable soreness, frustration, and possible injury. I have to hold my tongue when I overhear someone talk about how sore she is from her workout the night before. I'm talking sore to the point that she can't walk up the stairs or sit down. This is not progress. When a workout renders you immobile, how do you plan to bring your best effort the next day?

I want you to succeed, and you will do so by gradually introducing this program into your life. This will allow your body to adapt to new stressors while quickly building up capacity for the workload. That is the primary reason why I wrote the programs in this book using progressive overload.

If you are completely new to strength training, do one set of each exercise with moderate intensity on your first day, and call it a day. There is nothing wrong with starting out light and not training full force. This gives you a chance to see how your body reacts to the new movements so that you can gauge how hard to push yourself during the following workout. What is important is that you get much stronger over time, and strength gains do not require excessive pain in the days following a workout.

When I start training a new client, my goal is to build them up to be incredibly strong and fit women over the course of several months while using perfect form the entire way through. I have seen women make unbelievable strength gains without ever feeling too sore along the way. Of course, a reasonable amount of soreness is inevitable and in the nature of training. I will be the first to admit that I look forward to a bit of soreness after a new program just to remind me that I'm working my muscles. High frequency training greatly reduces soreness, and you will find that after the first week of training, you will feel much better. But, again, too much soreness can and will work against you, so don't chase it.

Become the Master Manipulator... of Intensity

On days when you feel drained, rundown, or achy, it's best to assess how you feel after your warm-up routine. Sometimes the warm-up helps your muscles feel better so that you can have a productive training session, maybe even setting some new records. Other times, you will feel beat-up even after a good warm-up. If this is the case, manipulate your training to avoid making things worse. Don't fall for the "no pain, no gain" message. That may work in the armed forces, but not when building *Strong Curves*.

As you get stronger, you will push your body to new heights. You may set records every week for two straight months, but eventually your body will require a break. Remember that you can't linearly increase your strength every week for a matter of years. Strength gains fluctuate, and your strength will increase rapidly at times, while it will stagnate at other times. Your energy levels are influenced by a number of factors, including the previous day's workout, sleep patterns, nutrition, stress levels, hormones, and immune system health.

Listen to your body and make appropriate adjustments. If your lower back feels tight, avoid deadlifts or good mornings. Perhaps you opt for single-leg hip thrusts, walking lunges, high rep back extensions, and/or band seated abductions. If your adductors are sore and feel like they're going to pull, don't do any single-leg exercises or deep squats. Perhaps you opt for barbell glute bridges, high box squats, rack pulls, and/or band standing abductions.

If you feel drained all over, reduce the intensity of your training that day. Stay far away from failure, and focus on using excellent form. Often, you come back a couple of days later with rebounded strength, executing strong lifts and maybe even seeing some increased strength. The most important aspect of this program is to gain strength over time. This will not happen if you're constantly injured, overly sore, or beat down and drained. So, train smart, and listen to your body.

Working It All Out

Rather than digging into why I'm against women doing body part splits for the sake of body transformation, let's look at why full body training is your best bet:

• Greater training frequency for each muscle group: With full body workouts, you hit all of your major muscle groups multiple times per week. The more you stimulate your muscles, the more they will grow. It's imperative that you hit your glutes several times a week for optimum transformation. I will have you activating and firing your glutes pretty much every time you move by the end of this program.

• Greater calorie expenditure: Due to the large amount of muscle mass that is taxed in each training session, full body workouts burn more calories per session. This means you can avoid starvation diets, skip the cardio sessions if you want, and gain muscle without gaining fat. Heck, you will probably lose fat while you're at it.

• Greater hormone stimulation: When you work a large amount of muscle at once, you increase the plasma anabolic hormone concentrations for a short period of time. While this occurs to a greater extent in men than it does in women, this brief increase may improve long-term muscle growth.

Principle of Prioritization

You will perform the largest glute stimulators first, which are the bridging/quadruped movements. Give these exercises your fullest attention, as these big lifts allow for the most improvement in glute strength. In fact, you may find that during the barbell glute bridge, your glutes contract so forcefully and create so much tension that they cramp up. If you get to this point, know that it's a good thing, as there is no doubt that you're activating your glutes to their utmost potential. Just make sure that you stop the set prior to cramping as you don't want to sustain an injury. You'll figure this out as you progress, so don't worry about it too much for now.

I can already hear you question me: "But, Bret, shouldn't I do squats and deadlifts first?" While it's true that pre-exhausting your glutes prior to squats or deadlifts may negatively impact your strength levels on those lifts, remember that this program is based on aesthetics (physique-related) goals, not on powerlifting strength. Some trainees find that with their squats or deadlifts, they have to drop down in weight around ten percent after they have hip-thrusted or glute-bridged, while others find that heavy bridging first does not impact their strength much. Don't sweat this; you're trying to build your best booty imaginable. So, doing your bridges first is the wisest strategy. Regardless, if you want to demonstrate your squat or deadlift strength at some point, you can simply perform one of them first in the workout and potentially set a PR (personal record). If you see strength decreases on squats and deadlifts following heavy bridging, it's perfectly fine to use slightly less weight on the squats and deadlifts. Many tend to overdo it on these lifts anyway (well, usually the "many" are men, not women).

So, the gauntlet has been thrown down—heavy bridging comes first. I promise you will grow to love this practice, especially when your glutes start responding favorably to the new style of training.

That brings up another important point. Why on earth would a woman only train her glutes one day per week? I can say with certainty based on all the success my clients have had that hitting the glutes multiple times per week is far superior than training them only once per week. The glutes need frequent stimulation to grow best. After using this program, you will look back at your old routine and realize it didn't work well to stimulate glute growth.

This program seeks to achieve optimal stimulation and variety in order to prevent old habits from creeping back in—the ones where you get stuck in a routine and can't get out. But you aren't going to aim for variety just for variety's sake. The movement patterns will follow a certain format, but the exercises will vary. From session to session, you will alternate between high reps and low reps, as well as bilateral and unilateral variations. For example, one day you might perform low rep squats and deadlifts. Maybe the following day, you will perform high rep lunges and single-leg back extensions. These are the similar movement patterns (squat/lunge motions and hip hinge motions) that stress different ranges of motion. You will perform integrative and targeted movements and will tinker around with different stances, widths, foot flares, elevations, ranges of motions, positions of loading, and types of equipment. But you will always be thrustin', squattin', lungin', and pullin'. For upper body, you'll do vertical pressing some days and horizontal pressing on other days. Then, you'll do vertical pulling some days and horizontal pulling on other days.

The Template for *Strong Curves* Full Body Workouts

Here is the template that you'll perform each day you train:

1. **Glute dominant exercise:**
   2-4 sets of 5-20 reps (page 193)

2. **Horizontal pull or vertical pull exercise:**
   2-4 sets of 5-20 reps (pages 264 and 280)

3. **Quad dominant exercise:**
   2-4 sets of 5-20 reps (page 209)

4. **Horizontal press or vertical press exercise:**
   2-4 sets of 5-20 reps (pages 272 and 287)

5. **Hip dominant, straight-leg hip dominant or hamstring dominant exercise:**
   2-4 sets of 5-20 reps (pages 231, 248, 259)

6. **Glute accessory exercise:**
   1-2 sets of 10-30 reps (page 204)

7. **Linear core exercise:**
   1-2 sets of 10-20 reps or 30-60 seconds (page 292)

8. **Lateral or rotary core exercise:**
   1-2 sets of 10-20 reps or 30-60 seconds (page 300)

The Template for *Strong Curves* Glutes-Only Workouts

This template is perfectly fine, and many women prefer it to full body training because they aren't interested in developing any upper body muscle mass.

1. **Glute dominant exercise:**
   2-4 sets of 5-20 reps (page 193)

2. **Quad dominant exercise:**
   2-4 sets of 5-20 reps (page 209)

3. **Hip dominant, straight-leg hip dominant or hamstring dominant exercise:**
   2-4 sets of 5-20 reps (pages 231, 248, 259)

4. **Glute accessory exercise:**
   1-2 sets of 10-30 reps (page 204)

Become the Glute Firing Squad

Yes, I'm bringing up this topic again, but it's so important to your success that I figured it was about time to give you a reminder. Throughout the entire workout, you're going to focus on getting maximum glute activation for every lower body exercise performed. Chances are, you won't feel your glutes working too hard when you first start this program. You will probably feel the low back, hamstrings, and quads taking over during exercises, but you're not going to let them. You're going to concentrate on the glutes and force them to contribute as much as they can to each action. The more you focus on squeezing your glutes into action, the more nervous system impulses you will send to those muscle fibers. After several training sessions, you will have that "ah-ha" moment when you start to feel those muscles kick into action. Your muscle contractions will feel more forceful, and other muscles will work much less to compensate for your weak booty.

Within two months of beginning this program, you will feel your glutes firing very hard during all types of glute exercises, including squats, deadlifts, back extensions, lunges, good mornings, and hip thrusts. Mark my words: You will feel the glutes squeezing together to erect your torso during back extensions, good mornings, and deadlifts. You will feel the glutes power you up during squats and lunges. Your glutes will burn intensely during barbell glute bridges and hip thrusts, which is the perfect sign that the exercises are working. I want you thinking about glutes all the time during training or any other activity you do during the day. Having glutes on your mind may sound crazy, but it makes a huge difference. Soon, you won't be able to walk your dog without squeezing your glutes with each step. It will become automatic. The more you squeeze, the better your glutes will look, and the more confident you will feel.

The Equipment: Below is a list of equipment used for this book. Most of it was purchased from www.Elitefts. com or www.PerformBetter.com. Rather than go into the equipment that I own and used at my studio, Lifts, I'd like to describe how I'd do it now. If I had to construct a garage gym from scratch on limited discretionary income, here's what I'd buy first:

Round One

Matting

Olympic bar (Pendlay Bar)

Squat stands

Bumper plates

Airex pad or Hampton thick bar pad (for hip thrust and barbell glute bridge padding)

Aerobics step and eight risers (for optimal hip thrust height and the ability to do single-leg hip thrusts)

Elastic bands

Heavy kettlebell (for swings)

TRX unit

Adjustable bench

Stability ball

Iron gym

Chalk bin and chalk (dramatically improves grip strength)

Round Two

Power rack/platform with monkey chin bar, dip handles, step-up attachment, and box squat box

Dual cable column with lat pulldown and attachments including rope handle, single handles, and d-handle

Texas power bar

Plates

Dumbbells and dumbbell rack

Cook bar

Trap bar

Ab wheel

Deadlift lever (makes unloading the plates much easier)

Round Three

Competition bench press bench

Incline press bench

Seated military press bench

Glute/ham developer

45-degree hyper

Reverse hyper

Landmine unit

Don't panic if you don't have access to all of this equipment. Whether you train at home using just your body weight, or you're fortunate enough to go to a well-equipped gym, *Strong Curves* will work for you. This is just to prepare you for what lies ahead and what options are possible within these programs.

Over the years, I've grown tired of training at commercial gyms. If you have extra space in your house and money to spare, I highly recommend that you consider constructing a home gym over time. It could be a gradual process. Having optimal booty-building training equipment, being able to play your own music and train whenever you want, and not having to wait for someone to finish using a piece of equipment are all invaluable advantages.

Method to My Madness (Yes, It Has a Purpose)

When you see the template, it might appear very simple, but know that much time and effort has gone into the planning of this program. It contains the right amount of pushing and pulling, backside and front-side, upper body and lower body, core and periphery, horizontal and vertical, and any other type of symmetry you can think of. This is very important for good posture and pain/injury prevention, which will allow you to train productively over the long haul.

This template ensures that you will not become quad-dominant, which happens when the focus is on movements that favor the muscles around the knee joints and leads to an imbalanced quad/posterior chain strength ratio. In other words, this happens when your front lower half becomes stronger than your back lower half. It's common for some women because they choose exercises that work the legs more than the glutes. This includes leg extension machines, leg press machines, hack squat machines, and any other leg exercise ending in "machine" that has you seated for the majority of your workout. You will notice this program has none of those exercises in it and for good reason. The exercises I chose are far superior for the glutes and will render far greater results. In fact, I think hip dominant exercises that require lots of glute work are so important that the *Strong Curves Programs* require you to perform twice the amount of hip dominant hip extension work (hip thrusts and Romanian deadlifts) than quad dominant hip extension work (squats and lunges).

For upper body work, make sure you balance out vertical and horizontal pressing and pulling throughout the week. If you stick to the program and train four days per week, perform horizontal presses and pulls twice per week and vertical presses and pulls twice per week. But if you train an odd number of times per week, skew your training toward more horizontal work. If you train three days per week, choose horizontal pulls and presses twice per week and vertical presses and pulls once per week. If you train five days per week, choose horizontal pulls and presses three times per week and vertical pulls and presses twice per week. This will ensure balanced shoulder joint strength and stability. I have all of this built into the program, so use this as a reference when you finish a few of the programs in the book and are ready to design your own.

You are probably scratching your head right now, wondering why I'm telling you all of this. Yes, I'm giving away all of my secrets so that you can successfully design your own programs once you work through the ones provided for you. I didn't spend the past several years of my life up to my eyeballs in research so that I could hoard all of my knowledge for my own personal use. I want you to become proficient at designing and creating your own workouts so that you can walk into any gym with confidence. I think trainers rob their clients of power when they become a crutch for their clients' success. I want you to feel empowered and completely capable of taking your strength to the next level with a little guidance from me.

Wanna Get Away?

Vacation doesn't always have to mean a break from exercise. Your hotel may have a gym facility, you could enjoy a hike, or you could factor in some other activity while spending time away from your busy life. Sometimes, however, you do need to take a little time away from exercise. This is perfectly fine, and you might even make strength gains while you rest. To prepare for this break in training, engage in "planned overreach-

ing." To do this, you increase the volume (number of sets and reps), as well as the intensity (how hard you push yourself), of your workouts leading up to your vacation. You will experience fatigue, but the extra days of recovery while on vacation will have you amped up for your return to the workouts. Just add in an extra set or two, perform an extra exercise or two, or push your sets a bit harder than usual. Then, enjoy the time off and know that your glutes are growing while you're relaxing and having fun.

If you still want to train while away on vacation, take this book with you, and perform sessions from the Twelve-week Best Butt Bodyweight Program. You can either start with week one or begin the week you left off with your current program. For example, if you're on week five, you can start at week five with the Best Butt Bodyweight program.

Stick With It, but Create Change Along the Way

As time goes on and you learn more about your body, make adjustments to the template. We're all unique in terms of physiology and anatomy, so our programs should differ slightly. The workouts I provide in this book are a starting point for you, but I want you to learn how to adjust your program based on how you respond and adapt to the exercises. You might find that you prefer to do more or less sets of certain categories of exercises or that you prefer higher or lower rep ranges of certain exercises. You may respond better, too, when you switch the order of exercises. Don't be afraid to experiment in order to figure out what suits you best once you work through at least one program in this book, but do not stray too far from my original format because it is important to follow a tried and true method.

Moreover, you need to enjoy your training and like your program. Mindset and psychology play a huge role in your success. When you know an exercise might be optimal, but you curl up in a ball at the very thought of doing it, you must learn to compromise. Make a bargain with yourself. If you don't like an exercise, allow yourself to do only one set if you beat your previous personal record for that exercise. For example, if dumbbell walking lunges are tough for you, try to add a few more reps to your record from the previous week. If you do, then you're finished with that exercise for the day. It's far more important to do the exercise correctly and with proper intensity than to stomp your way through it half-heartedly.

On a personal note, I cannot stand high rep squatting or deadlifting. These methods might be the best hypertrophy movements ever invented, but the mere thought of doing them makes me cringe. I barter with myself by sticking with heavier weight and lower rep sets with these two movements. Then, I do higher reps on exercises that I enjoy such as hip thrusts, back extensions, and high step-ups. I don't enjoy performing multiple sets of single-leg work, and if I was told to do four sets of walking lunges, single-leg RDL's, or single-leg hip thrusts, I would probably do the same thing I did with my dirty laundry as a kid—tuck it away somewhere so that I didn't have to see it. But I know they're necessary for my program, so I do single sets of each. Since I'm only doing one set, I push the intensity hard, knowing that I will not have to go another round.

Growing Stronger Everyday

Right now, you might be a novice at strength training. You may not be able to perform a single lunge or bodyweight squat, which is perfectly fine. It just means that your glutes have plenty of room for improvement. Any number of the women whose physiques you ad-

> **Train for Life:** This book was written with a long-term vision in mind. It isn't meant to be a routine that you follow for only a month; it's a way of training for life. For now, this book provides methods found to benefit women most. I will continue researching and experimenting and will undoubtedly learn more about training, and I'll update my methods as my research advances.
>
> I have included some very advanced exercises in this book because while you might not be strong enough right now to perform these movements, you will continue to gain strength if you stick to the template and push yourself. Most strength training books omit highly advanced variations or exercises that require unique equipment because they don't apply to most readers. In the interest of giving you a program that you can use for life, however, I wanted to give you ideal methods for maximal booty-building. Over the years, you may find yourself joining a better gym, building your own gym, and/or reaching strength levels far greater than you ever imagined. Promise that you will email me when you make these gains because I want to give you a virtual high-five!

mire all started in the same place as you, and their results certainly didn't happen overnight. Forget instant gratification because it doesn't exist. Commit to this program for the long haul, and know that you will be fit for life. It just takes time.

Many of my clients start out with just body weight for exercises like squats, lunges, glute bridges, and forty-five-degree hyperextensions. Within a few months, these same clients are using a barbell plus additional weight for squats and hip thrusts, heavy dumbbells for lunges and back extensions, and performing much more difficult exercises.

Every six months, you will feel substantially stronger than you were six months prior. As I mentioned earlier, however, you will not see linear improvements. For your first six months, you'll see huge gains in strength, and these gains will taper somewhat. For example, I'm at a point where a ten-pound increase in hip thrust, squat, or deadlift strength is difficult. But as a beginner, my strength increased about ten pounds each week. Depending on how long you have been strength training, you may see measurable strength increases across the board every week or minor gains every month or so. When I say strength training, I mean lifting a considerable amount of weight. If you have only attended aerobics classes at your gym or have been lifting the same ten-pound weights for the past ten years, you will make serious strength gains on this program right away if you push yourself.

Paired Supersets Make You a Superhero

Paired supersets involve pairing up non-competing exercises such as a lower body and upper body exercise to increase the amount of work done in a fixed amount of time. It also reduces rest time, which fires up your metabolism to burn more fat. In each of the twelve-week programs, I denote paired supersets in your training logs as A1 and A2 or B1 and B2. This means that you perform one set from exercise A1, and immediately follow it with one set from exercise A2. Once you complete both sets, rest for sixty to one-hundred twenty seconds, and repeat until all sets are completed.

Sometimes gyms are crowded, and claiming two pieces of equipment might be a bit selfish. So, it isn't always realistic to perform paired supersets in gyms. In this case, opt to perform straight sets, and work your way through all of the sets of each exercise before moving on to the next one. Bear in mind that you need to do the same amount of sets for your lower body and upper body exercises for this to work. I have it set up in each twelve-week program to work this way, so keep that in mind when you decide to design your own *Strong Curves* workouts. You will only be able to do this for the first two paired sets of exercises. Doing so with the rest of the workout will compromise your strength, and your glutes won't reap the full benefit of the program. Don't worry; this will all make sense once you read the programs.

Taking a Break Between Sets

Rest up to two minutes between sets for exercises that require using multiple large muscle groups like squats and deadlifts. Rest about thirty seconds between sets for muscles that are single-joint movements or require less energy like seated band abductions or bodyweight reverse hypers. When performing paired supersets, rest one to two minutes in between sets. You can either wear a watch or read a wall clock. These numbers don't have to be exact, but it's a good practice to time your rest periods so that you don't rest too long or neglect adequate recovery time.

I Just Want a Nice Butt!

I've had several clients who prefer training their lower half only. If this is your desired training regimen, you will like the glutes-only program in this book. I created a Gorgeous Glutes Program for lower body-only training that offers twelve weeks of non-stop glute action. You will notice that no paired supersets are performed with these workouts because the exercises compete with each other, interfering with strength. If you choose this program, please stick to this idea, and don't attempt to pair supersets.

> **Kellie's Quick Tip:** *Even when performing just the Beautiful Glutes Program, you will get a significant upper body workout from the compound movements without the added muscle size. This will help to create symmetry with your curves.*

Having trained hundreds of women throughout my life, I'm not foolish enough to think that most women will opt for this plan. In my experience, women enjoy performing upper body exercises, and they're exhilarated when they're finally able to complete a bodyweight push-up or chin-up with proper form and range of motion.

But I want it to be known that I believe this is the best option for most women. When I owned my studio, I would ask my female clients to choose their ideal body from a bunch of pictures of female physiques. Most of them pointed to the photos of Jessica Biel from her July 2007 photo shoot for GQ Magazine. (I can't blame them; she looks absolutely incredible in those pictures). They'd say, "Yes! Can you make me look like that? This is exactly what I want to look like."

When a woman gets lean, her upper body and abdominals appear muscular and toned. In fact, a woman's arms can be very small and still look impressive with low body fat. So, the secret to a nice upper body is to simply get lean through diet and training, and the best type of training to reduce body fat levels is done at a high intensity.

If you've ever performed high rep barbell hip thrusts, heavy barbell squats or deadlifts, walking lunges with dumbbells, or back extensions while holding a dumbbell underneath your chin, you know how metabolically taxing these exercises are and how much they elevate your heart rate. Therefore, glute exercises are not only the secret to building the perfect booty, but the secret to making the upper body and core look amazing as well. Heavy resistance training can tax the metabolism more than any other form of training.

Of course, I can't get all of my clients to look like Jessica Biel, but I know that the closest they'll get to looking like her in her 2007 pictures is by adhering to the *Strong Curves Program*, and the Beautiful Glutes program is the most efficient route. I realize that Jessica has an incredible shape everywhere, including the legs, butt, arms, back, and shoulders. Just mark my words, if you become incredibly strong at the glute exercises in this program while getting down to your ideal body weight, your entire body will look fantastic. Your booty will be shapelier, your legs will be firm, your upper body will be lean, and your core will look much better. Nevertheless, most women will undoubtedly wish to perform upper body and core movements, which is certainly fine.

Stop the "Six-Pack Abs" Insanity

Abdominal training should not be in your vocabulary, and you should definitely never take a half-hour abdominal class at your gym multiple times per week. While you may feel inclined to train your abs so that they're toned with little belly fat, these classes are not the correct way to make those improvements. Remember that strength training not only increases your muscle strength but also how large your muscles grow. The more you train your abdominal muscles, the larger they will get.

You are actually adding size to your waist, but not targeting belly fat. Belly fat decreases when you reduce your caloric intake and burn more calories than you take in. Your body doesn't automatically trigger a fat-burning mechanism in certain regions when you begin training those muscles. Fat burning is part of your overall metabolic process, and for women, it often begins from the top down. So, your belly will likely be one of the first regions on your body to burn fat, but it won't happen from doing abdominal exercises in excess. This "spot reduction" myth has been debunked in research. You can't train a certain body part and expect it to accelerate fat loss in that particular region.

Strong Curves builds in core exercises to each workout, and you will find them at the end of every training session. You will perform two core exercises, each targeting different regions of your core. This is all you need to sculpt a nice, curvy waist. Anything more than this, and you may start adding size rather than reducing. Plus, your core will get stimulated from heavy compound exercises, so you don't need to hammer them relentlessly with endless sets of abdominal exercises. Do you really want to significantly increase the muscularity of your rectus abdominis and obliques? Think about it.

> **Kellie's Confession:** *I have a very short waist, and for many years, I did abdominal exercises every day. In middle and high school, I performed two hundred to three hundred crunches five days per week. I learned over the years that this was actually taking away from that coveted X-frame, so I cut back to no more than two abdominal exercises per week. It has made a huge difference in the contour of my waist.*

Overworking your abs will give you a boxy, boyish figure regardless of the length of your torso. Once you build a strong foundation in the first twelve-week program, your core will grow strong with compound and bodyweight exercises. You can supplement direct abdominal exercises for other exercises that improve core strength. For example, band hip rotations work the obliques, but they hit the glutes very hard when you learn how to do them properly.

The Not So Welcome Pleasure of Exercise

My first regular female client used to squirm around when she performed certain exercises. I'd hound her, telling her she needed to stay tight. One day, she mustered up the courage to inform me that the reason she squirmed was because she was experiencing orgasms while she exercised. I had never heard about this at the time, but I was very understanding. She explained that she did not want it to happen because it was uncomfortable and inopportune.

Recent research suggests that about fifteen percent of women experience orgasms when they exercise, although I'm pretty certain this figure is overestimated. The scientific name is exercise-induced orgasm or EIO, but the fitness industry has coined the phenomenon a "coregasm." This is nothing new. In fact, sexologist Albert Kinsley first wrote about the phenomenon in 1953. About fifty-one percent of the time, this happens during exercises that involve the lower abdominals, such as when using the Captain's Chair to perform leg raises or during reverse crunches or other abdominal exercises. And it usually happens after fifteen reps or so.

Women who experience this phenomenon are not thinking sexual thoughts while exercising, and they're self-conscious and usually embarrassed by it. If you experience this sensation while exercising, don't feel ashamed. You could try stopping the set prematurely if you feel the sensation coming on, or you could save "problematic" exercises for home. You could also choose to simply roll with it since other people won't know what's going on.

In Search of the Secret Form of Exercise

You will run into a lot of marketing masterminds in the fitness industry—gurus, if you will. These are the trainers who hold "big secrets" they are willing to give up for large sums of money. With regard to glute training, there is a science behind building a better butt. These marketing whizzes disguised as trainers come up with a myriad of magical exercises promised to instantly perk up your posterior.

But these trainers don't get the science behind gluteal hypertrophy, and they lack the testimonials to prove otherwise. Over the years, I've heard it all. Pilates and yoga "develop long lean muscles." Thankfully this won't happen. If you could lengthen muscles significantly, they would eventually fail to stabilize joints. Plus, many forms of exercise don't allow for progressive overload. Cardio kickboxing and spin might make the glutes burn, but endurance athletes don't have the glutes that power athletes have, so this is not ideal for glute development. Sprinting and plyometrics are good forms of exercise for the glutes, but they don't quite activate the glutes to their fullest potential. They also don't take advantage of a couple of key mechanisms of hypertrophy. Kettlebells provide an efficient glute workout, but barbells out perform them in terms of gluteal muscle activation. The list goes on and on.

Bodybuilders are the masters of muscle development and attaining low levels of body fat. If something works, they figure it out. While all of these forms of exercise can improve the glutes of a sedentary individual and are way better than doing nothing, they are not superior to plain and simple resistance training. Performing bodyweight, dumbbell, barbell, band, and kettlebell movements through a complete range of eccentric and concentric motion in a variety of rep ranges makes full use of the three primary mechanisms of hypertrophy mentioned earlier: muscle damage, metabolic stress, and mechanical tension.

So, focus on getting stronger at the best glute exercises while using perfect form and activating the glutes, and you can't go wrong for booty sculpting.

> **Glute Fun Fact:**
> A simple bodyweight squat typically activates sixty percent MVC for the quads and only ten percent MVC for the glutes in women. This is why most women feel squats only in their quads.

With regard to fat loss, your body can only produce certain results based on your level of training. It's important to understand that most beginners can only expend about five to ten calories per minute while training. More advanced exercisers can get to fifteen per minute and possibly even twenty per minute for very brief intervals. But in this case, the duration of the workout wouldn't be that great. So, an intermediate exerciser would typically burn around six hundred calories during an hour-long workout. As you can see, this is not very impressive. That's where nutrition comes to the rescue.

Sure, high intensity interval training creates an "after burn" effect in which your body continues to burn calories long after you hang up those running shoes, but so does weight training. In fact, heavy, intense resistance training can be costlier than interval sprinting in terms of caloric expenditure. Based on my experience, it's much easier to remove daily calories than to perform high amounts of cardio day in and day out. The upside (well, there are a lot of upsides to not being a slave to the treadmill) is that this gives you more free time and gives your muscles more time to recover and grow stronger. Better recovery and stronger muscles equal great training sessions every week. I hope you can see that resistance training is the way to go for optimal physique enhancement purposes.

Cellulite Facts

Cellulite is present in about ninety-eight percent of post-pubertal women, is most often found in the buttocks and thighs, and can affect individuals regardless of their body mass index (BMI). It's an architectural disorder characterized by dimples in the skin and is caused by the herniation of subcutaneous fat within fibrous connective tissue. Currently, there is no definitive explanation for cellulite's presentation and prevalence.

There is a considerable genetic component to cellulite, and it's much more common in women than in men. Caucasian women get cellulite more than Asian women, and excessively high carbohydrate diets can provoke hyperinsulinemia (excess insulin levels) and promote lipogenesis (fat formation). Sedentary lifestyles impede blood flow, causing alterations in cellulite prone areas. Pregnancy often exacerbates cellulite via increased prolactin and insulin secretion, which leads to lipogenesis and fluid retention. Sometimes, weight loss can improve cellulite severity, but not always. While many proposed treatments exist, ranging from topical creams to invasive procedures, no single treatment is completely effective.

The way I see it, since ninety-eight percent of women have cellulite, you shouldn't feel like you're in the minority if you have it. *The Strong Curves Program* helps to shrink fat cells and build sexy shape underneath, so nobody will notice some minor cellulite when there's an amazing booty and thighs to admire. Do what you can through proper exercise, nutrition, and lifestyle choices, and don't worry if you are left with a little cellulite.

Points to Ponder Before You Get Glute-ified

There are two things you need to always keep in mind with regard to diet and exercise:

1. Sculpting the perfect body takes time.
2. It's your body forever, so take care of it.

You can find many diet manipulations that will provide instant and drastic results, but they won't support long-term health and longevity. Many athletes go to dietary extremes to prepare for competition. These extremes slip into the mainstream arena and get inside the average woman's head. Sure, fighters can lose thirteen pounds overnight to meet weigh-in requirements, and bodybuilders can cut water within a couple of days to show as many muscle striations as possible on stage. But how will these practices benefit you? Normally, they won't, and unless done under careful supervision, they can cause serious damage to your body. Besides, these methods hardly provide lasting solutions.

If you're seeking long-term results that will improve your health and physique over time, stay away from drastic measures. If you're looking for a "quick fix," close this book and return it to the store. When you go into the *Strong Curves Program*, results will take time, as they would with any good program.

Of course, you will see incredible changes within the first several weeks of this program. But unlike most fad diets, that is not the end result. In fact, I hope you never reach the end result and keep striving for greater strength, leaner muscles, and new feats of courage and perseverance every single month for years to come. Some of my most cherished emails and letters come from clients I haven't trained in years. They decided to send me an update to let me know they are still using my methods two, four, and even six years later. They are still achieving great results, hitting new personal records, and feeling and looking years younger than their peers.

My goal is to get you stronger, especially with your glutes. I also want you to learn to use your muscles properly, nourish your body with the right nutrients, and improve your body composition. All of these goals go hand-in-hand, and you will not achieve one if the other two aren't in line. Your body will not change if you aren't eating right or lifting with proper form.

Weighing in on a Weighty Topic

I'm a huge proponent of weekly weigh-ins with my clients because I feel it keeps them honest. My clients know they have to step on that scale at the first session of every week (usually right after a weekend), and that number will tell me their secrets. But I advise you to use your scale at your own discretion. Your weight will fluctuate depending upon many factors, including the time of day, your level of hydration, how many carbohydrates you've recently consumed, and where you are in your menstrual cycle. It will also fluctuate if you've gained or loss any tissue (including fat and muscle).

At home, weighing yourself weekly will keep your head in check. If you threw away the scale and solely relied on how your clothes fit, you could set yourself up for failure. For instance, if your jeans become tight in the thighs, you might think you aren't achieving results. The last thing I want is for this book to end up in your wastebasket. Your jeans may get tighter because you are adding muscle to your glutes and thighs, but you may have lost a few pounds in the process. The scale might tell you, "Hey, you've lost three pounds. Great job!" So, don't underestimate the power of the scale.

Also, if you avoid the scale altogether, it will be much harder to calculate your calories. Remember that calories are based on bodyweight and goals. For example, Jessica Biel is 5'8" tall and weighs about one hundred-fifteen pounds. If your ultimate goal is to have a physique like Jessica, you will likely want to know how your body measures up to hers. At this point, weight loss may be your goal so that you can build that ideal body. Once you reach your ideal weight, your ultimate goal will require eating at maintenance while working on changing body composition (increasing muscle while shedding fat). How will you know what maintenance is for you if you don't know your own body weight? Use your scale with caution, and don't go overboard weighing yourself every time you eat. But try to weigh yourself at the beginning or end of every week. Also, remember that you may gain a few pounds while on this program, especially right off the bat, but it will be fat-free mass if you follow the plan exactly.

One more note on body composition: If you're trying to reach your ideal weight, chances are you will get there within a period of months depending on how far away you are from your goal. Still, that's only fifty percent of the battle. The other fifty percent will take you years to achieve, but that's the fun of strength training. Transforming and attaining a pleasing physique are hard work, and most people simply don't have the guts and determination to realize their full potential. That's why it's so impressive and admirable to others.

The key is to remain consistent. It's important to realize that muscle takes up about twenty percent less space than fat, so it's quite possible to lose volume (size) while staying the same weight. This happened all the time when I owned my studio. Women bragged that they had to go clothes shopping because their clothes no longer fit, but their weight on the scale hadn't changed.

So, it's important to note that your scale won't tell the whole picture. Take measurements around your waist, hips, thighs, and buttocks at least once a month to note the changes. After a while, the scale may stop moving, but you will likely still see incredible changes in your measurements.

Ultimately, a variety of feedback will let you know how you're progressing, so it's important to pay attention to your body weight, measurements, how your clothes fit, how you look in the mirror, your strength on the big lifts, and how you feel.

Chapter 8:

Become the Ultimate Workout Tracker

A training log is one thing that sets a competent lifter apart from someone who randomly shows up at the gym. Tracking your workouts ensures that you are making appropriate progress with this program. It also keeps you motivated and striving toward bigger goals. The *Strong Curves Program* focuses on progressive overload, where you increase the weight or number of reps for each exercise in your workout over the course of four weeks. Though I would like to think you have the memory of an elephant, it's still better to write everything down than to simply go by what you remember from your previous workout.

You will find a blank workout template at the end of each twelve-week program that allows you to fill in the information from your training sessions. You can photocopy these and bring them with you to the gym, or write down the workouts in a notebook. You don't need to spend gobs of money on a fancy workout journal; a simple notebook works just fine. You will be even more successful if you track both your nutrition and workouts in the same place, so set up your notebook accordingly.

In your training log, jot down the date, and consider writing down your current weight (using the same scale each day). Underneath the date, write the names of your exercises and the loads (weights) and number of repetitions performed for each set. This is set up for you in

the workouts provided if you choose to photocopy those pages.

When you begin a new workout week, look back to determine your previous record for a certain exercise. If you did sixteen bodyweight back extensions during your last performance, aim for eighteen in your next session. You will not go up in strength each week, but you can still strive for continuous gains by increasing your number of reps or using more weight on specific exercises. I encourage you to jot down notes about the workout such as whether you went too heavy or too light or some things to remember about technique for the next time. See below for an example of a training log entry for a single workout. Note that "BW" stands for bodyweight.

Date: _11/15/2011_   Weight: _135_

Exercise	Set 1	Set 2	Set 3
A1: Bodyweight hip thrust 3 sets, 10-20 reps	Weight **BW** Reps **13**	Weight **BW** Reps **12**	Weight **BW** Reps **10**
A2: Seated row 3 sets, 8-12 reps	Weight **40lbs** Reps **10**	Weight **40lbs** Reps **9**	Weight **40lbs** Reps **8**
B1: Goblet squat 3 sets, 10-20 reps	Weight **20lbs too light** Reps **20**	Weight **25lbs** Reps **18**	Weight **25lbs** Reps **16**
B2: Barbell bench press 3 sets, 8-12 reps	Weight **Bar (45lbs)** Reps **8**	Weight **Bar (45lbs)** Reps **8**	Weight **Bar (45lbs)** Reps **8**
Barbell Romanian deadlift 3 sets, 10-20 reps	Weight **70lbs** Reps **15**	Weight **70lbs** Reps **15**	Weight **70lbs back rounded** Reps **15**
Side lying abduction 1 set, 15-30 reps (each)	Reps left **20** Reps right **20**		
RKC Plank 1 set, 20-60 seconds	Seconds **35**		
Side plank 1 set, 20-60 seconds (each)	Seconds left **30** Seconds right **30**		
Notes:	*Felt much stronger this week*	*Ate 3 hrs prior to training*	*Need to work on deadlift form*

Setting Personal Strength Goals

Strength is highly dependent on natural and genetic phenomena such as your natural body shape (somatotype), proportions of body segment lengths (anthropometry), tendon insertion points, muscle fiber type composition (type II fibers are stronger than type I), and natural hormonal levels. You will be great at some lifts, while others will make you cower in the corner.

Be inspired by what you see others accomplish, but keep things in perspective when setting your own strength goals. Don't label yourself a failure if you can't muster up the strength for unassisted chin-ups, and don't throw in the towel if you can't get past five bodyweight lunges on each side. You will accomplish these tasks, but it takes time to get there. You have to start somewhere, and you are likely beginning right where many powerful women stood not so long ago.

The CDC report for 2003 to 2006 shows that sixty-four percent of women over the age of twenty in the U.S. have a body-mass index over twenty-five and are considered overweight or obese. This number can be skewed for those who carry a good amount of muscle, but I conclude that this isn't the case for the majority within this statistic. As for the remaining thirty-six percent of the female population who are of normal weight, probably only one-third of them perform proper resistance training. This means about ten percent of women are competing with you for strength. I would venture to guess that if you can perform a chin-up, you are in the 95th-pecentile in terms of upper body pulling strength among women. In other words, if you took a random sample of one hundred women, it's unlikely that more than five could perform a full-range, unassisted chin-up starting from a dead hang. If you aren't there yet, know that working toward that goal puts you at a much higher level than the majority of women.

Some women base their perception of female strength on what they see advanced lifters doing in the gym. If you feel that way, I encourage you to review the real life breakdown on the chart that follows. At one point several years ago, I had more than thirty female clients, and I managed to train them all by myself week in and week out. While my strong female colleagues probably think that this chart is a bit "easy," I believe it to be accurate if you consider the entire female resistance training population.

Female Strength Chart

Exercise	Beginner	Intermediate	Advanced	Elite
Back squat	BW x 10	45 x 10	95-135 x 10	135-225 x 10
Dumbbell walking lunge	BW x 10	20 x 10	30-40 x 10	40-60 x 10
Push up	zero	1-8 reps	8-20 reps	20-40 reps
Bench press	zero	45 x 10	65-85 x 10	85-135 x 10
Dumbbell Bench press	20 x 10	20 x 10	25-35 x 10	35-50 x 10
Incline press	zero	45 x 10	65-85 x 10	85-115 x 10
Dumbbell Incline press	15 x 10	20 x 10	25-35 x 10	35-50 x 10
Military press	zero	45 x 5	45-65 x 10	65-95 x 10
Dumbbell Military press	10 x 10	15 x 10	20-25 x 10	25-35 x 10
Deadlift	45 x 10	65 x 10	95-185 x 10	185-275 x 10
Hip thrust	BW x 20	45-95 x 10	95-185 x 10	185-275 x 10
Dumbbell 45-degree hyper	BW x 20	10-20 x 10	20-50 x 10	50-100 x 10
Chin up	zero	1-3 Eccentric reps	1-8 reps	8-15 reps
One-arm row	20 x 10	25 x 10	30-40 x 10	40-60 x 10

As mentioned previously, anthropometry plays a huge role in the display of strength. It is not uncommon for a tall woman with long femurs to front squat just the barbell but deadlift well over one hundred thirty-five pounds. Most women can hip thrust more than they can squat, and they can deadlift more than they can hip thrust. A woman with a slender upper body and shapely legs may never be able to do a chin-up no matter how lean and strong she gets. Bodyweight reverse hyperextensions are an excellent exercise for her, as her ratio of lower body weight to upper body weight makes it quite challenging. Conversely, a woman with this body type can perform bodyweight 45-degree hyperextensions very easily and needs to hold onto a dumbbell to make it challenging.

Another huge factor with real strength is whether you take exercises through a full range of motion. This is the only legitimate measure of strength for those movements. Some women partial squat ninety-five pounds for ten reps but cannot do a single rep to parallel or deeper with the same weight. On the same subject, some women perform three partial range chin-ups but cannot do a single rep when attempting to start from a dead hang and stop at the top of the sternum. I have seen women claim to dumbbell military press a ton of weight, but it is a whole different story when forced to use a complete range of motion by starting at shoulder level and progressing to lockout while maintaining a tall stance with a strong spine that doesn't arch back.

Typically, women who have trained in the past do not show up at my gym with the ability to perform barbell full squats. If you're a beginner, start off with bodyweight exercises, ensuring proper levels of mobility, stability, and motor control—and use basic progression. Build a foundation by gaining flexibility, getting your glutes to activate properly, and learning how to stabilize your core. In addition, build your scapular muscles so you can perform exercises with proper form. Progress gradually when it comes to range of motion, repetition, resistance, and exercise variation before you take on more challenging lifts. For example, perform goblet squats—a good intermediate exercise that bridges the gap between bodyweight and barbell squats. Barbell glute bridges come before barbell hip thrusts, and rack pulls come before deadlifts.

Dumbbells for the upper body are often necessary to bridge the gap between bodyweight and barbells. Use bands for assistance with chin-ups. Elevate the angle on inverted rows and push-ups to make them easier. All of this is set up for you in the twelve-week *Strong Curves Programs*, but I want you to keep this information in mind as you progress beyond those twelve weeks.

> **Kellie's Notes:** *Exude pride if you are at the "advanced" or "elite" stage in any of the exercises listed above, as that comes only from hard and consistent work over time. Notice that the elite range on the chart is very broad. If you are in the elite category, set a goal to get on the upper end of different exercises. Hopefully, this chart will help you keep your strength in proper perspective. I'm very strong with my lower body exercises, but my upper body exercises put me in the advanced category, rather than the elite. I just keep striving to make greater gains.*

Progress is as Progress Does

If you start with the twelve-week Booty-ful Beginnings Program for beginners, it's fine to move on to the twelve-week Gluteal Goddess Program for advanced lifters next. You may find some of the lifts challenging beyond your current strength, however. If this is the case, I encourage you to find supplemental exercises in the Exercise Index to perform in place of those that are too challenging for your level. Just keep those lifts you couldn't do as future goals.

This book provides a chart that will help you track your progress. Each exercise offers a place for you to write your lifts at your low rep maximum record, medium rep maximum record, and high rep maximum record. Fill in how much weight you lift for a single rep, yet fail on the second rep in the first section. In the second section, fill in how much weight you lift for ten consecutive reps, failing on the eleventh rep. In the last section, attempt the lift at bodyweight, and see how many reps you can accomplish.

I recommend working on these records in small increments once you have become accustomed to your *Strong Curves* workouts. Give yourself a few sessions in the routine before you attempt to set personal records. Use these records as a means to gauge your progress and as fuel to push yourself even harder. You will be amazed at how far you come from the time you make your first attempt to an attempt two months down the road.

Note that some of these exercises are not written in your program. You can save these sheets for when you do implement them into your workout because attempting them only once and not consistently will not give you accurate, recordable gains. As you will see in our example, not every single slot has to be completed, as some exercises don't lend themselves well to low reps. Knowing your records on all of the lifts in various rep ranges allows you to succeed by giving you many more opportunities to set personal records and achieve progressive overload.

Advanced Chart

Exercise	Low Rep Record (example 1RM)	Medium Rep Record (example 10RM)	High Rep Record (example max bodyweight reps)
Dumbbell between bench squat			
Goblet squat			
Barbell front squat			
Barbell full squat			
Barbell Zercher squat			
Barbell low box squat (10-inch height)			
Barbell med box squat (12-inch height)			
Barbell conventional deadlift			
Barbell sumo deadlift			
Barbell American deadlift			
Barbell good morning			
Barbell glute bridge			
Barbell hip thrust			
Dumbbell back extension			
Dumbbell 45-degree hyper			
Barbell Bulgarian split squat			
Dumbbell Bulgarian split squat			
Barbell walking lunge			
Dumbbell walking lunge			
Dumbbell high step up (30-inch height)			
Bodyweight pistol squat			
Dumbbell single-leg RDL			
Bodyweight single-leg hip thrust			
Bodyweight prisoner single-leg back ext.			

Example: **Krista**

Exercise	Low Rep Record (example 1RM)	Medium Rep Record (example 10RM)	High Rep Record (example max bodyweight reps)
Dumbbell between bench squat		70 x 10	
Goblet squat			50 x 20
Barbell front squat	135 x 1	95 x 10	65 x 30
Barbell full squat	155 x 1	115 x 10	95 x 20
Barbell Zercher squat	155 x 1	115 x 10	
Barbell low box squat (10-inch height)	115 x 1	95 x 10	
Barbell med box squat (12-inch height)	155 x 1	115 x 10	
Barbell conventional deadlift	255 x 1	205 x 5	135 x 30
Barbell sumo deadlift	275 x 1	225 x 5	135 x 40
Barbell American deadlift			95 x 25
Barbell good morning		95 x 10	65 x 30
Barbell glute bridge		225 x 10	135 x 40
Barbell hip thrust	185 x 5	135 x 20	95 x 40
Dumbbell back extension		60 x 10	Bw x 200
Dumbbell 45-degree hyper		70 x 10	Bw x 200
Barbell Bulgarian split squat		45 x 10	Bw x 70
Dumbbell Bulgarian split squat		25 x 10	
Barbell walking lunge		65 x 10	Bw x 100
Dumbbell walking lunge		30 x 15	
Dumbbell high step up (30-inch height)		10 x 8	Bw x 15
Bodyweight pistol squat	Bw x 3		
Dumbbell single-leg RDL		30 x 10	
Bodyweight single-leg hip thrust			Bw x 25
Bodyweight prisoner single-leg back ext.			Bw x 25

Beginner Chart

Exercise	Maximum Reps
Bodyweight low box squat (13-inch height)	
Bodyweight hip thrust	
Barbell Romanian deadlift (45-lb bar)	
Bodyweight low step up (13-inch height)	
Bodyweight 45-degree hyper	
Bodyweight walking lunge	
Bodyweight single-leg glute bridge	

Example: Katherine

Exercise	Maximum Reps
Bodyweight low box squat (13-inch height)	Bw x 16
Bodyweight hip thrust	Bw x 18
Barbell Romanian deadlift (45-lb bar)	45 x 20
Bodyweight low step up (13-inch height)	Bw x 12
Bodyweight 45-degree hyper	Bw x 20
Bodyweight walking lunge	Bw x 10
Bodyweight single-leg glute bridge	Bw x 8

Chapter 9:

The *Strong Curves* Warm-Up

I've learned over the years that warming up means something different to everyone. Women are typically far more flexible than men, so stretching isn't always a necessary component to their warm-up (plus, strength training is just as effective for increasing flexibility as stretching). Those who are better conditioned might not need to warm-up as much before lifting but might need a longer warm-up when sprinting or performing sports activities. Others cannot do a single lift without first doing a long warm-up.

I designed warm-ups for each of your workouts so that you feel comfortable going into your routine. If you are new to strength training or this type of training, I recommend sticking with these warm-up routines. If you have your own method of warming up to workout, you may use that in place of what is provided in this book. However, warming-up using these routines for at least the first four weeks of your *Strong Curves Program* will help ensure that your muscles are properly primed for the workload you are about to take on. It's probably far different from anything else you've done in the past, and the last thing I want is for you to suffer injury during your first weeks of *Strong Curves*.

Most workout programs follow a standard warm-up that looks something like this: ten minutes on the stationary bike at a moderate pace, five minutes of static stretching, and a specific warm-up set (or two) for the first exercise of the workout. The largest problem with this warm-up routine is that it doesn't address all of your needs prior to training. The warm-up has many purposes, including increasing tissue temperature, priming the nervous system, and getting your blood flowing.

But the *Strong Curve* warm-up extends beyond this standard by addressing common problems due to our professions and lifestyles. What happens when you sit at your desk for a full workday? You neglect to take your joints through a full range of motion, your muscles shut down because they decide you don't need them to work, and some muscles get shortened.

For the *Strong Curves Program*, I want you to do a dynamic warm-up because it will address your preliminary needs (increased temperature and blood flow), while doing an even better job at priming your nervous system and joints for your workout. Before you begin the first exercise in each workout, you will do the ten to fifteen-minute warm-up shown below.

Warm-Up for Workouts A and C

Foam roller/medicine ball
- erectors, IT band, quads, hamstrings, adductors, glutes, calves, lats

p. 178
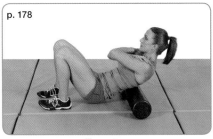
Erector

p. 176
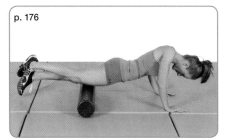
Quads

p. 177
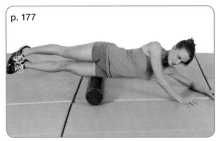
IT bands

p. 176
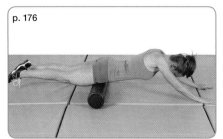
Hip flexors

p. 176
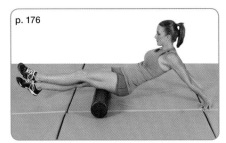
Hamstring

p. 177
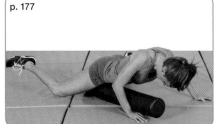
Adductors

p. 174
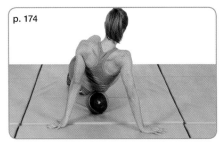
Glutes

p. 175
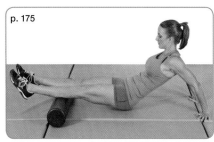
Calves

p. 178
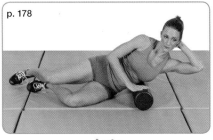
Lats

Static stretches
- foot elevated hamstring, psoas, adductors

p. 179
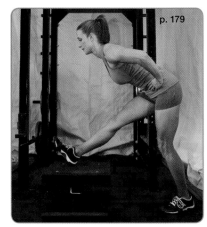
Foot elevated hamstring

p. 184
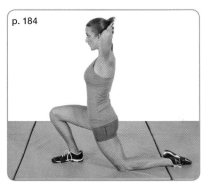
Psoas

p. 181
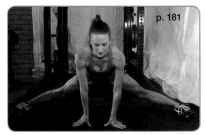
Adductors

p. 181
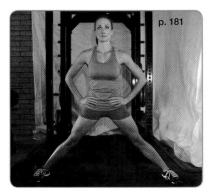
Adductors

Activation

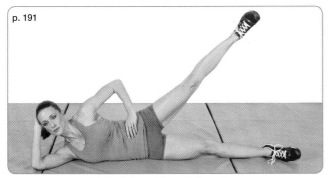
p. 191
Side lying hip abduction

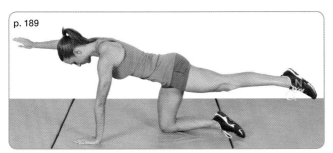
p. 189
Bird dog

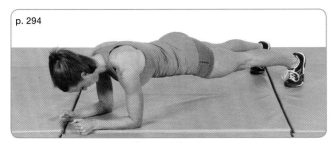
p. 294
Front plank

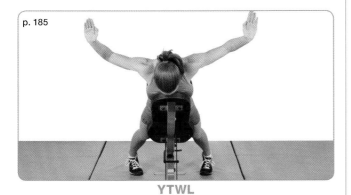
p. 185
YTWL

Mobility

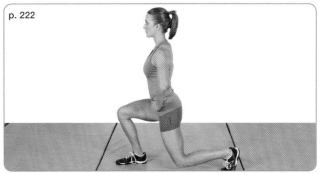
p. 222
Walking lunge

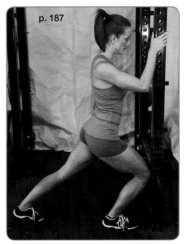
p. 187
Wall ankle mobility

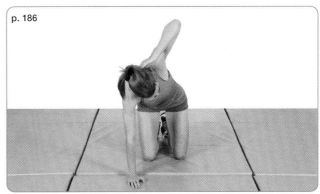
p. 186
Quadruped thoracic extension/rotation

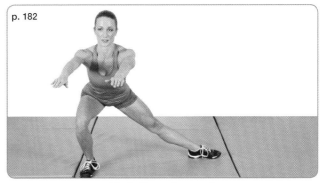
p. 182
Rotational squat

The stick or tiger tail

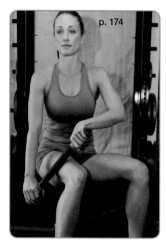

IT band

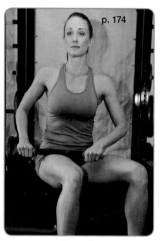

Quads

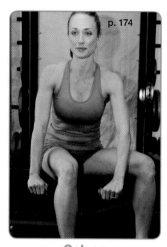

Calves

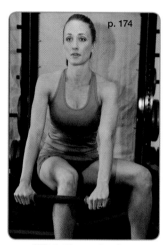

Tibialis anterior

Med ball and tennis ball SMR

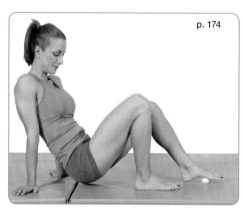

Plantar fascia

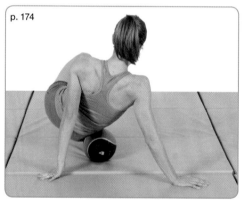

Upper glutes

Static stretches

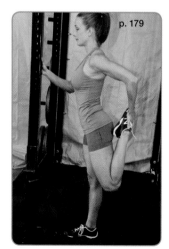

Rectus femoris

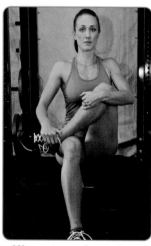

Hip external rotators

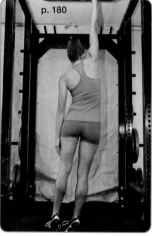

Lats

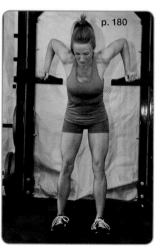

Pecs

Activation	Mobility

Activation

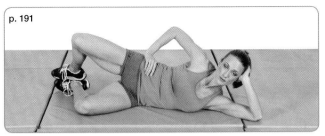

p. 191

Side lying clam

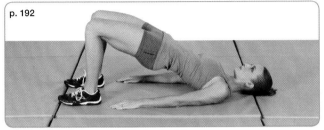

p. 192

Glute bridge

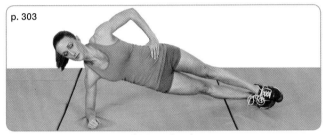

p. 303

Side plank

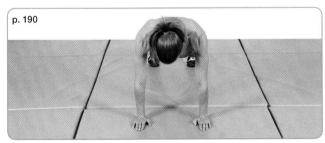

p. 190

Push-up plus

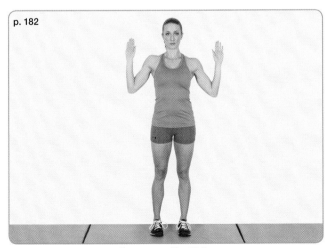

p. 182

Scap wall slide

Mobility

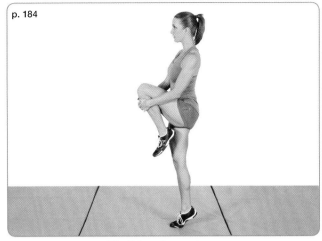

p. 184

Walking knee hug

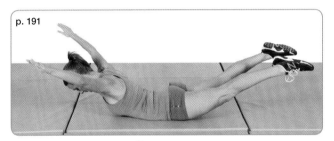

p. 191

Superman

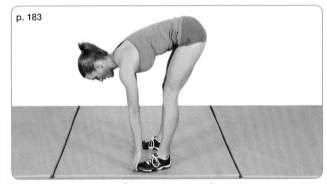

p. 183

Squat to stand

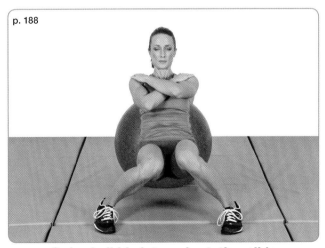

p. 188

Swiss ball hip internal rotation slide

When to Perform Cardio

In an ideal world, you would perform your cardio session on your days off from strength training. A perfect schedule would look like this:

Monday: Workout A
Tuesday: Workout B
Wednesday: Cardio or HIIT session A
Thursday: Workout C
Friday: Workout A
Saturday: Cardio or HIIT session B
Sunday: Off

Let's say you prefer to strength train three times per week rather than four times per week. Here is a recommended schedule:

Monday: Workout A
Tuesday: Cardio or HIIT session A
Wednesday: Workout B
Thursday: Cardio or HIIT session B
Friday: Workout C
Saturday: Cardio or HIIT session C
Sunday: Off

Either you looked at that and nodded in agreement, or you rolled your eyes, saying, "Yeah, right, Bret. Like I have time for this." If you don't live in this ideal world, don't panic. This program was designed to fit your lifestyle, and I know you have other things going on that may deter you from training six days per week. The most important part of this program is the strength training workouts. However, a good cardio workout or two during your week could improve how quickly you burn fat.

In this program, you need to perform your cardio workouts after your strength training sessions, never before. Cardio workouts should not be a part of your warm-up. You need to save your energy reserves for strength training to reap the maximum benefits of this program. If you train at night, do your cardio sessions the next morning. If you train in the morning, do your cardio sessions that evening or the next day. The exception is low-intensity cardio. You can go for a brisk walk the morning of your strength session or in the evening before it.

I recommend performing up to two high intensity cardio sessions each week along with your strength workouts. This could be hill sprints, HIIT, tabatas, a kickboxing class, or any form of exercise that causes a rise and fall in your heart rate. I believe that this can be beneficial in terms of health and self-confidence; just don't overdo it.

These activities don't shape the glutes like heavy resistance training, though. Improving your performance during resistance training is your best bet with regard to perking up those glutes. Becoming more efficient at HIIT can make you a bit leaner and improve the glutes if that's the only exercise you perform, but it isn't superior to a proper combination of optimal nutrition and progressive strength training. So, don't feel compelled to perform cardio or HIIT if you'd rather not. On the other hand, don't avoid cardio or HIIT if you enjoy it and it makes you feel better. The program you enjoy is likely to deliver superior results.

Chapter 10:

Strong Curves Twelve-Week Booty-ful Beginnings Program for Beginners

If you are completely new to strength training, haven't worked out in a while, or feel that you have stopped making progress with your current training plan, this is the right starting place for you. In fact, unless you have used a majority of the exercises in this book for a good amount of time, I recommend you start here.

Once you dive into the Twelve-week Booty-ful Beginnings Program for beginners, you can assess whether or not you're ready for a greater challenge with the Twelve-week Gluteal Goddess Program for advanced lifters. I think you will be surprised at how challenging the *Strong Curves* beginners program is—even for experienced lifters. Many of the exercises used in this program are probably new to you or are presented in a new way. You may currently work each muscle group only once per week, or you may have not previously targeted your glutes the way you will in this program. If you aren't sure where to start, give this program a try for a week and evaluate how you feel. If you walk away from your workouts feeling like you just breezed through the park, step up your challenge with the advanced program. But if you leave feeling a bit winded and sore, stick with this program for the remaining eleven weeks. You will greatly benefit from doing so because this program teaches you proper form and technique.

One of the largest challenges of this Twelve-week program is mastering quality movement patterns. As mentioned in Chapter Four, it isn't just moving, but how you move that matters. Anyone can throw a significant amount of weight on a bar and lift it. The integrity of your muscle development and strength progress relies heavily on mastering your motor competency. This means executing each individual lift with excellent form. I need you to make one promise to me while working through any program in this book. Promise me that if you feel your form is breaking down or that you aren't moving as well in your lifts as you did during your first repetition that you will set the weight back down and rest.

I cannot stress enough how important this is for your progress. Once your form starts to crumble, you usually decrease your range of motion, overcompensate with single muscle groups rather than moving synergistically, leak energy and cave in at various joints, and risk injury. Over the next twelve weeks, I want you to focus on understanding how your muscles work during each movement. Pay attention to how they feel. Squeeze your muscles during concentric movements (shortening of the muscle to develop tension). Stretch them during eccentric movements (active lengthening of the muscle). You should feel tension in your muscles all the way up in a lift and all the way back down.

I also want you to focus on activating your glutes with every exercise. At first, this may seem impossible to do. Just keep at it, and you will start to feel them working during your hip dominant movements. Once they kick in during glute exercises, you will begin to feel them working during other lower body exercises. Your overall goal is to work your glutes every time you move. That's right—every single time you perform a compound lower body movement, your glutes should be activated. I know for Kellie and many of my other advanced lifters, her glutes turn on during every lift automatically. She even activates them during bench presses, pull-ups, military presses, barbell curls, rope tricep extensions, and any exercises where she is not seated. I want you to accomplish this as well. Just remember that it will take time and a great amount of adjustment when you begin this workout.

In this twelve-week program, I've given you guidelines as to how many repetitions you should aim for during each exercise set. This is just a goal to keep in mind while lifting. I would rather you achieve five high quality reps with great form than squeeze out twenty mediocre reps with only a few high quality ones in the beginning of your set. Also, note that if you can bang out a set of twenty reps without even creasing your brow a tiny bit, you probably need to ramp up the amount of weight that you use. The only way you will progress toward the physique you want is to challenge yourself every time you train and consistently set records each month. I cannot tell you how many times I have trained a female client for the first time and gotten her to achieve thirty repetitions or so with a weight she had previously done for just ten reps. I achieved this only by motivating and encouraging her to push the set as hard as possible (without letting form break down, of course).

Before you start, figure out how much weight you are going to use for each set by finding your ten-rep max (10RM). Do so by selecting a weight you think you can lift ten times with perfect form. This means that the weight is heavy enough that your form would break down on the eleventh rep. If you only make it to five reps, the weight is too heavy. If you maintain perfect form after ten reps, then the weight is too light. Think of it like Goldilocks finding the perfect porridge. Once you do, write down the weight in your fitness journal, and get to work. This will be different for some of the exercises. For example, the activation exercises in this program aim to stimulate dormant muscles so that you can incorporate them into all of your movements. Believe me, they will present a great challenge to your muscles and tax your metabolic system. So, don't even think about adding weight to these exercises. Just get those glutes working properly, and you will feel the burn immediately. In fact, I want you to feel like running for the ice bath right after each set.

Twelve-Week Booty-ful Beginnings Program for Beginners

- The goal of these sessions is to master quality movement patterns. Think quality and not quantity. It's better to do five great repetitions than twenty average ones.

- You're establishing movement patterns that will eventually become automatic, so make sure you take full advantage of this critical period to gain an understanding of proper form.

- Don't get caught up with the suggested rep ranges. If you can only get six quality repetitions, stop there. The set ends when you can no longer perform perfect repetitions. And if your form is perfect, and you can do more repetitions, feel free to do more.

- When performing single-arm or single-leg (unilateral) exercises, always begin with the weaker limb first, and match the number of repetitions with the stronger limb. Over time, your strength will converge, and there won't be much of an imbalance.

Date: _____   Weight: _____

Equipment needed for weeks 1-4:

- *Exercise mat*
- *Flat bench*
- *Dumbbells*
- *Exercise box (may use flat bench or multiple aerobics steps if box is not available)*
- *Cable lat pulldown machine (see Exercise Index for substitute exercises if training from home or if machine is not available)*
- *45-degree back extension apparatus (see Exercise Index for substitute exercises if training from home or if apparatus is not available)*

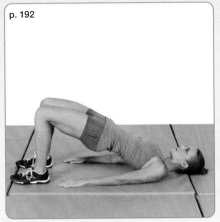
p. 192
A1: Bodyweight glute bridge
—3 sets of 10-20 reps

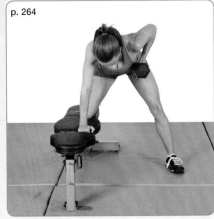
p. 264
A2: One-arm row
—3 sets of 8-12 reps (each side)

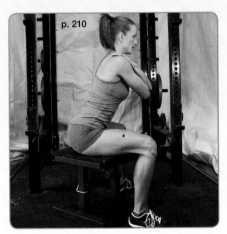
p. 210
B1: Bodyweight box squat
—3 sets of 10-20 reps

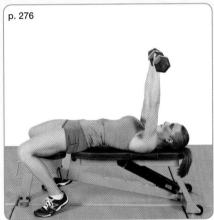
p. 276
B2: Dumbbell bench press
—3 sets of 8-12 reps

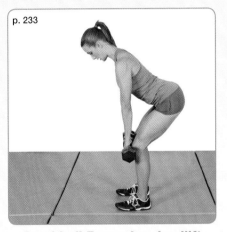
p. 233
Dumbbell Romanian deadlift
—3 sets of 10-20 reps

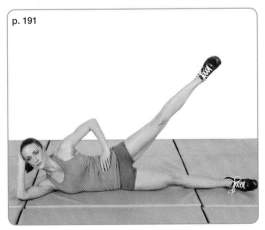
p. 191
Side lying abduction
—1 set of 15-30 reps (each side)

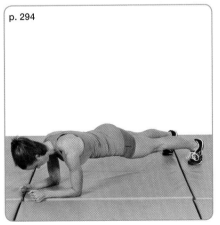
p. 294
Front plank
—1 set of 20-120 seconds

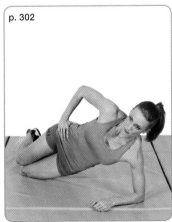
p. 302
Side plank from knees
—1 set of 20-60 seconds (each side)

Date: _____   Weight: _____

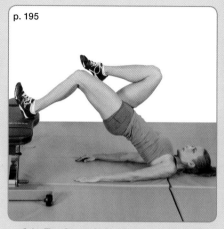

A1: Bodyweight foot elevated single-leg glute bridge
—3 sets of 10-20 reps (each side)

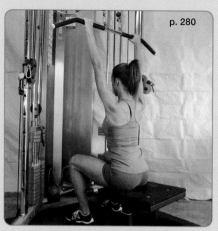

A2: Front lat pulldown
—3 sets of 8-12 reps

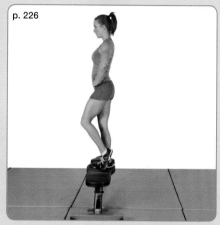

B1: Bodyweight step up
—3 sets of 10-20 reps (each side)

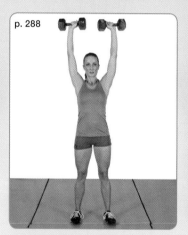

B2: Dumbbell standing overhead press
—3 sets of 8-12 reps

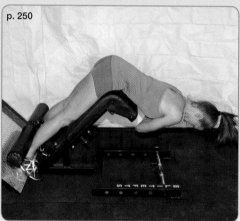

Bodyweight 45-degree hyper extension
—3 sets of 10-20 reps

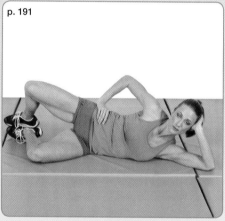

Side lying clam
—1 set of 15-30 reps (each side)

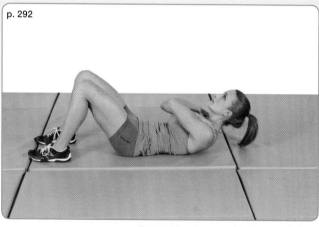

Crunch
—1 set of 15-30 reps

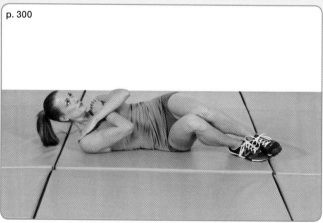

Side crunch
—1 set of 15-30 reps (each side)

Date: _____   Weight: _____

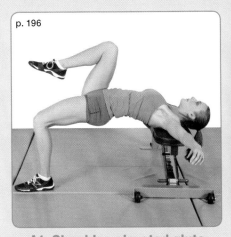

A1: Shoulder-elevated glute march
—3 sets of 60 seconds (alternating legs in "marching fashion")

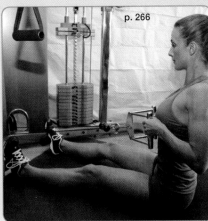

A2: Cable Column
—3 sets of 8-12 reps

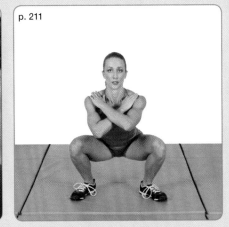

B1: Bodyweight squat
—3 sets of 10-20 reps

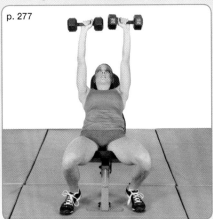

B2: Dumbbell incline press
—3 sets of 8-12 reps

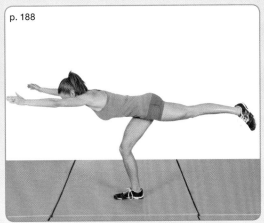

Reaching single-leg Romanian deadlift
—3 sets of 10-20 reps (each side)

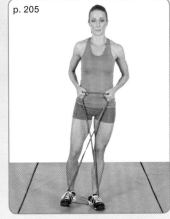

X-band walk (light tension)
—1 set of 10-20 steps (each side)

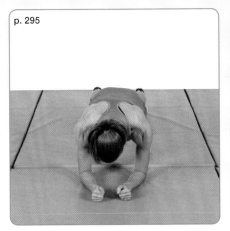

RKC plank
—1 set of 10-30 seconds

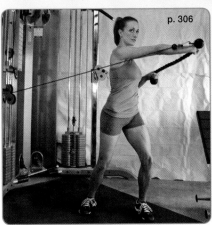

Rope horizontal chop
—1 set of 10 reps (each side)

Date: _____   Weight: _____

Equipment needed for weeks 5-8:

- *Exercise mat*
- *Seated cable row machine*
- *Chin-up bar*
- *Exercise box (may use flat bench or multiple aerobics steps if box is not available)*
- *Flat barbell bench*
- *Barbell (may need plate weights and clips, too)*
- *Dumbbells*
- *Table or support mechanism for bodyweight reverse hyperextensions*
- *Swiss ball*
- *Kettlebell*

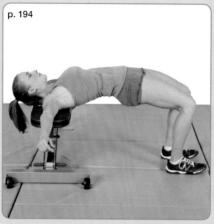

p. 194

A1: Bodyweight hip thrust
—3 sets of 10-20 reps

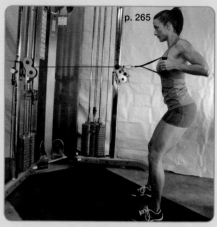

p. 265

A2: Standing single-arm cable row
—3 sets of 8-12 reps

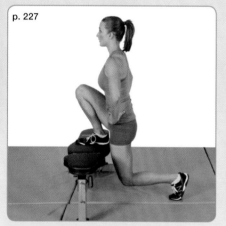

p. 227

B1: Bodyweight step up/ reverse lunge combo
—3 sets of 10-20 reps

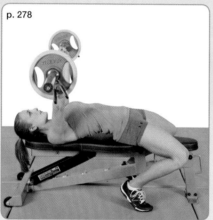

p. 278

B2: Barbell bench press
—3 sets of 8-12 reps

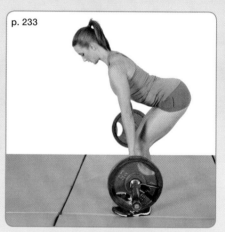

p. 233

Barbell Romanian deadlift
—3 sets of 10-20 reps

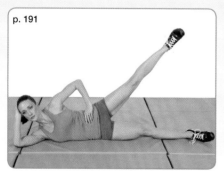

p. 191

Side lying abduction
—1 set of 15-30 reps (each side)

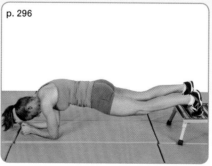

p. 296

Feet-elevated RKC plank
—1 set of 20-60 seconds

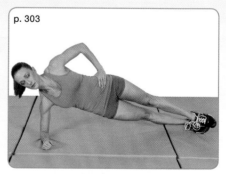

p. 303

Side plank
—1 set of 20-60 seconds (each side)

Date: _____　　　　　　　　Weight: _____

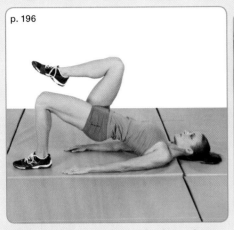

A1: Bodyweight single-leg glute bridge
—3 sets of 10-20 reps (each side)

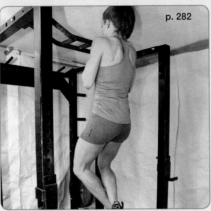

A2: Negative chin-up (or underhand grip pulldown)
—3 sets of 3 reps

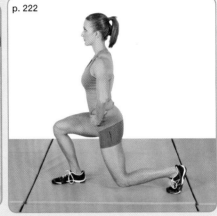

B1: Bodyweight walking lunge
—3 sets of 10-20 reps (20-40 steps total)

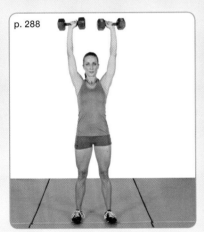

B2: Dumbbell standing overhead press
—3 sets of 8-12 reps

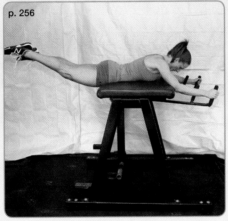

Bodyweight reverse hyper
—3 sets of 10-20 reps

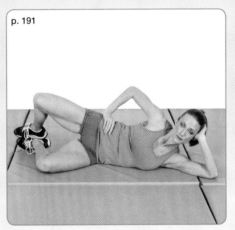

Side lying clam
—1 set of 15-30 reps (each side)

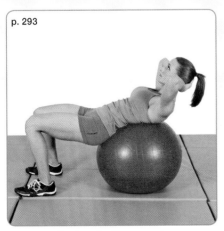

Swiss ball crunch
—1 set of 15-30 reps

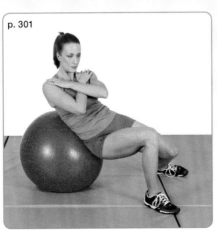

Swiss ball side crunch
—1 set of 15-30 reps

Date: _____   Weight: _____

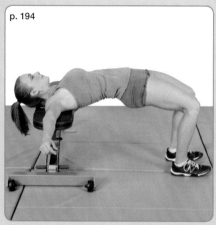

A1: Bodyweight hip thrust (pause rep method)—3 sets of 10-20 reps (3 second pause at top)

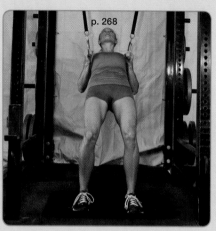

A2: Modified inverted row —3 sets of 8-12 reps

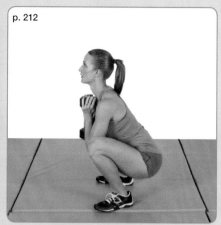

B1: Goblet squat —3 sets of 10-20 reps

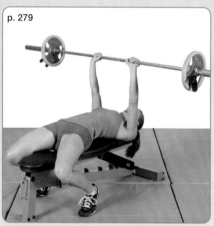

B2: Barbell close grip bench press —3 sets of 8-12 reps

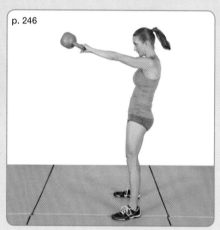

Russian kettlebell swing —3 sets of 10-20 reps

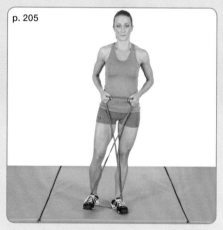

X-band walk (moderate tension) —1 set of 15-30 steps (each side)

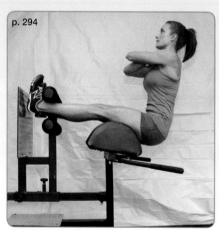

Straight-leg sit-up —1 set of 15-30 reps

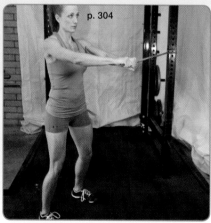

Band anti-rotation hold —1 set of 10-20 seconds (each side)

Date: _____   Weight: _____

Equipment needed for weeks 9-12:
- *Exercise mat*
- *Barbell*
- *Weight plates*
- *Barbell clips*
- *Hampton thick bar pad*
- *Dumbbells*
- *Exercise box (may use flat bench or multiple aerobics steps if box is not available)*
- *Swiss ball*
- *Cable column*
- *Chin-up bar*
- *Squat rack*
- *Flat bench*
- *Band*

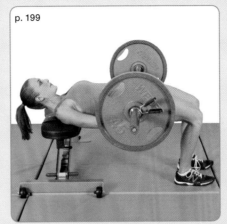

p. 199

A1: Barbell hip thrust
—3 sets of 10-20 reps

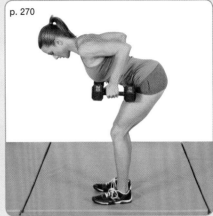

p. 270

A2: Dumbbell bent over row
—3 sets of 8-12 reps

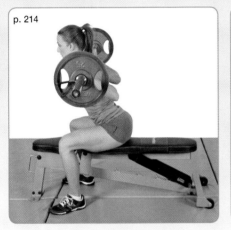

p. 214

B1: Barbell box squat
—3 sets of 10-20 reps

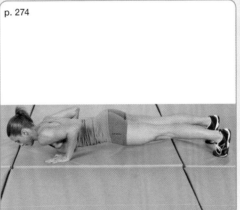

p. 274

B2: Push-up
—3 sets of 3-10 reps

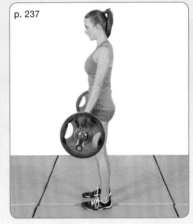

p. 237

Barbell American deadlift
—3 sets of 10-20 reps

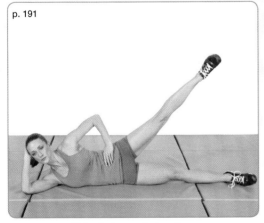

p. 191

Side lying abduction
—set of 15-30 reps (each side)

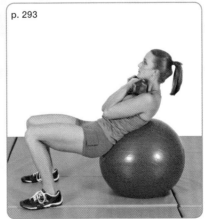

p. 293

Dumbbell Swiss ball crunch
—1 set of 15-30 reps (each side)

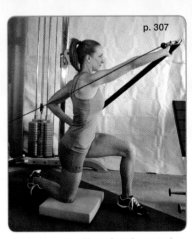

p. 307

Half-kneeling horizontal chop
—1 set of 10-15 reps (each side)

Date: _____   Weight: _____

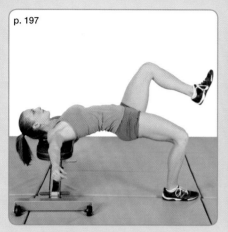

A1: Shoulders-elevated single leg hip thrust
—3 sets of 10-20 reps (each side)

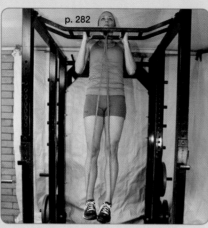

A2: Band-assisted parallel grip pull-up
—3 sets of 1-5 reps

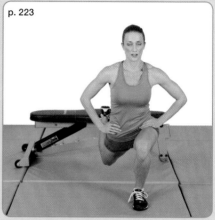

B1: Bodyweight Bulgarian split squat
—3 sets of 10-20 reps

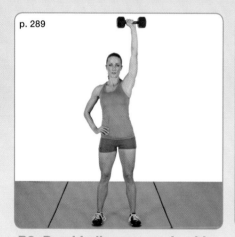

B2: Dumbbell one-arm shoulder press
—3 sets of 8-12 reps

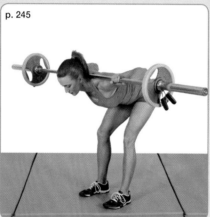

Barbell good morning
—3 sets of 10-20 reps

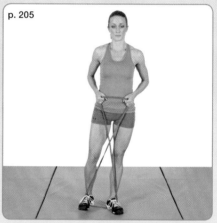

X-band walk (moderate tension)
—1 set of 15-30 steps (each side)

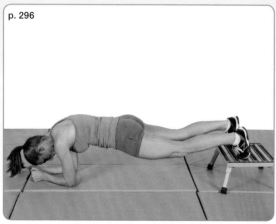

Feet-elevated RKC plank
—1 set of 60-120 sec

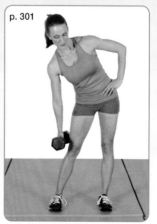

Dumbbell side bend
—1 set of 15-30 reps (each side)

Date:_____   Weight:_____

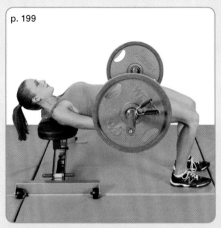

A1: Barbell hip thrust (pause rep method)—3 sets of 8-15 (3 second pause at top)

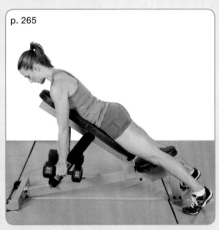

A2: Dumbbell chest supported row—3 sets of 8-10 reps

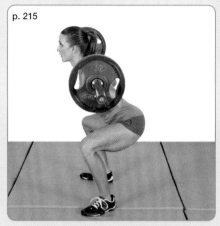

B1: Barbell parallel squat—3 sets of 10-20 reps

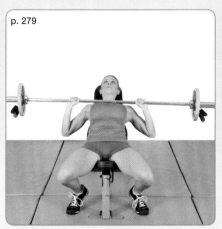

B2: Barbell incline press—3 sets of 3-10 reps

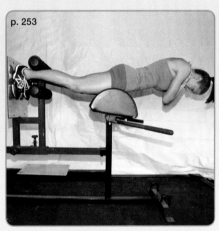

Bodyweight back extension—3 sets of 10-30 reps

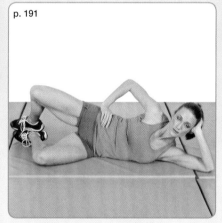

Side lying clam—1 set of 15-30 reps (each side)

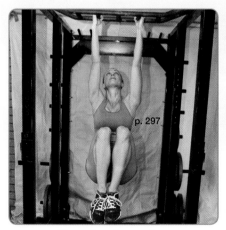

Hanging leg raise—1 set of 10-20 reps

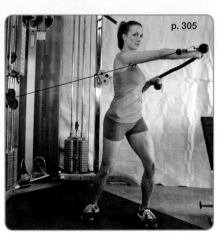

Rope horizontal chop 1 set of 10-15 reps (each side)

Name: _____ Date: _____ Weight: _____

Exercise	Set 1	Set 2	Set 3
A1: Bodyweight glute bridge 3 sets, 10-20 reps	Weight Reps	Weight Reps	Weight Reps
A2: One arm dumbbell row 3 sets, 8-12 reps (each)	Weight Reps	Weight Reps	Weight Reps
B1: Bodyweight box squat 3 sets, 10-20 reps	Weight Reps	Weight Reps	Weight Reps
B2: Dumbbell bench press 3 sets, 8-12 reps	Weight Reps	Weight Reps	Weight Reps
Dumbbell Romanian deadlift 3 sets, 10-20 reps	Weight Reps	Weight Reps	Weight Reps
Side lying abduction 1 set, 15-30 reps (each)	Weight Reps		
Front plank 1 set, 20-120 seconds	Seconds		
Side plank from knees 1 set, 20-60 seconds	Seconds		
Notes:			

Note: Perform one set of A1 then immediately follow it with one set of A2. Rest 30-90 seconds, and repeat until all sets are completed. Do the same for B1 and B2.

Booty-ful Beginnings Workout B: Weeks 1-4 Training Log

Name:_____ Date:_____ Weight:_____

Exercise	Set 1	Set 2	Set 3
A1: Bodyweight foot elevated single-leg glute bridge 3 sets, 10-20 reps	Weight Reps	Weight Reps	Weight Reps
A2: Front lat pulldown 3 sets, 8-12 reps (each)	Weight Reps	Weight Reps	Weight Reps
B1: Bodyweight step up 3 sets, 10-20 reps (each)	Reps left Reps right	Reps left Reps right	Reps left Reps right
B2: Dumbbell military press 3 sets, 8-12 reps	Weight Reps	Weight Reps	Weight Reps
Bodyweight 45-degree back ext. 3 sets, 10-20 reps	Weight Reps	Weight Reps	Weight Reps
Side lying clam 1 set, 15-30 reps (each)	Reps left Reps right		
Crunch 1 set, 15-30 reps	Reps		
Side crunch 1 set, 15-30 (each)	Reps left Reps right		
Notes:			

Note: Perform one set of A1, and immediately follow it with one set of A2. Rest 30-90 seconds, and repeat until all sets are completed. Do the same for B1 and B2.

Name: _____   Date: _____   Weight: _____

Exercise	Set 1	Set 2	Set 3
A1: Glute march 3 sets, 60 sec	Weight Reps	Weight Reps	Weight Reps
A2: Seated row 3 sets, 8-12 reps	Weight Reps	Weight Reps	Weight Reps
B1: Bodyweight parallel squat 3 sets, 10-20 reps	Reps left Reps right	Reps left Reps right	Reps left Reps right
B2: Dumbbell incline press 3 sets, 8-12 reps	Weight Reps	Weight Reps	Weight Reps
Bodyweight single-leg RDL 3 sets, 10-20 reps (each side)	Weight Reps	Weight Reps	Weight Reps
X-band walk (light tension) 1 set, 10-20 steps (each side)	Reps left Reps right		
RKC plank 1 set, 10-30 sec	Reps		
Rope horizontal chop 1 set, 10 reps (each side)	Reps left Reps right		
Notes:			

Note: Perform one set of A1, and immediately follow it with one set of A2. Rest 30-90 seconds, and repeat until all sets are completed. Do the same for B1 and B2.

Name: _____   Date: _____   Weight: _____

Exercise	Set 1	Set 2	Set 3
A1: Bodyweight hip thrust 3 sets, 10-20 reps	Weight Reps	Weight Reps	Weight Reps
A2: Standing single-arm cable row 3 sets, 8-12 reps	Weight Reps	Weight Reps	Weight Reps
B1: Goblet squat 3 sets, 10-20 reps	Weight Reps	Weight Reps	Weight Reps
B2: Barbell bench press 3 sets, 8-12 reps	Weight Reps	Weight Reps	Weight Reps
Barbell Romanian deadlift 3 sets, 10-20 reps	Weight Reps	Weight Reps	Weight Reps
Side lying abduction 1 set, 15-30 reps (each)	Reps left Reps right		
Feet elevated plank 1 set, 20-60 seconds	Seconds		
Side plank 1 set, 20-60 seconds (each)	Seconds left Seconds right		
Notes:			

Note: Perform one set of A1, and immediately follow it with one set of A2. Rest 30-90 seconds, and repeat until all sets are completed. Do the same for B1 and B2.

Name: _____ Date: _____ Weight: _____

Exercise	Set 1	Set 2	Set 3
A1: Bodyweight single-leg glute bridge 3 sets, 10-20 reps (each)	Weight Reps	Weight Reps	Weight Reps
A2: Negative chin-up 3 sets, 3 reps	Weight Reps	Weight Reps	Weight Reps
B1: Bodyweight walking lunge 3 sets, 20-40 total steps	Weight Reps	Weight Reps	Weight Reps
B2: Dumbbell military press 3 sets, 8-12 reps	Weight Reps	Weight Reps	Weight Reps
Bodyweight reverse hyperextension 3 sets, 10-20 reps	Weight Reps	Weight Reps	Weight Reps
Side lying clam 1 set, 15-30 reps (each)	Reps left Reps right		
Swiss ball crunch 1 set, 15-30 reps	Reps		
Swiss ball side crunch 1 set, 15-30 reps (each)	Reps left Reps right		
Notes:			

Note: Perform one set of A1, and immediately follow it with one set of A2. Rest 30-90 seconds, and repeat until all sets are completed. Do the same for B1 and B2.

Name: _____ Date: _____ Weight: _____

Exercise	Set 1	Set 2	Set 3
A1: Bodyweight hip thrust (pause rep method) 3 sets, 10-20 reps (3 sec pause at top)	Weight Reps	Weight Reps	Weight Reps
A2: Modified inverted row 3 sets, 8-12 reps	Weight Reps	Weight Reps	Weight Reps
B1: Goblet squat 3 sets, 10-20 reps	Weight Reps	Weight Reps	Weight Reps
B2: Close grip barbell bench press 3 sets, 8-12 reps	Weight Reps	Weight Reps	Weight Reps
Russian kettlebell swing 3 sets, 10-20 reps	Weight Reps	Weight Reps	Weight Reps
X-band walk (moderate tension) 1 set, 15-30 reps (each)	Reps left Reps right		
Straight-leg sit-up 1 set, 15-30 reps	Seconds		
Band rotary hold 1 set, 10-20 seconds (each)	Seconds left Seconds right		
Notes:			

Note: Perform one set of A1, and immediately follow it with one set of A2. Rest 30-90 seconds, and repeat until all sets are completed. Do the same for B1 and B2.

Name: _____ Date: _____ Weight: _____

Exercise	Set 1	Set 2	Set 3
A1: Barbell hip thrust 3 sets, 10-20 reps	Weight Reps	Weight Reps	Weight Reps
A2: Dumbbell bent over row 3 sets, 8-12 reps	Weight Reps	Weight Reps	Weight Reps
B1: Barbell box squat 3 sets, 10-20 reps	Weight Reps	Weight Reps	Weight Reps
B2: Push-up 3 sets, 3-10 reps	Weight Reps	Weight Reps	Weight Reps
Barbell American deadlift 3 sets, 10-20 reps	Weight Reps	Weight Reps	Weight Reps
Side lying abduction 1 set, 15-30 reps (each)	Reps left Reps right		
Dumbbell Swiss ball crunch 1 set, 15-30 reps	Reps		
Half-kneeling cable anti-rotation press 1 set, 10-15 reps (each)	Reps left Reps right		
Notes:			

Note: Perform one set of A1, and immediately follow it with one set of A2. Rest 30-90 seconds, and repeat until all sets are completed. Do the same for B1 and B2.

Name: _____   Date: _____   Weight: _____

Exercise	Set 1	Set 2	Set 3
A1: Bodyweight single-leg hip thrust 3 sets, 10-20 reps (each)	Weight Reps	Weight Reps	Weight Reps
A2: Chin-up (band assisted) 3 sets, 1-5 reps	Weight Reps	Weight Reps	Weight Reps
B1: Bodyweight Bulgarian split squat 3 sets, 10-20 reps (each)	Weight Reps	Weight Reps	Weight Reps
B2: Barbell military press 3 sets, 8-12 reps	Weight Reps	Weight Reps	Weight Reps
Good morning 3 sets, 10-20 reps	Weight Reps	Weight Reps	Weight Reps
X-band walk 1 set, 15-30 reps (each)	Reps left Reps right		
Feet elevated plank 1 set, 60-120 sec	Reps		
Dumbbell side bend 1 set, 15-30 reps (each)	Reps left Reps right		
Notes:			

Note: Perform one set of A1, and immediately follow it with one set of A2. Rest 30-90 seconds, and repeat until all sets are completed. Do the same for B1 and B2.

Name: _____ Date: _____ Weight: _____

Exercise	Set 1	Set 2	Set 3
A1: Barbell hip thrust (pause rep method) 3 sets, 8-15 reps (3 sec pause at top)	Weight Reps	Weight Reps	Weight Reps
A2: Dumbbell chest supported row 3 sets, 8-12 reps	Weight Reps	Weight Reps	Weight Reps
B1: Barbell parallel squat 3 sets, 10-20 reps	Weight Reps	Weight Reps	Weight Reps
B2: Barbell incline press 3 sets, 8-12 reps	Weight Reps	Weight Reps	Weight Reps
Bodyweight back extension 3 sets, 10-30 reps	Weight Reps	Weight Reps	Weight Reps
Side lying clam 1 set, 15-30 reps (each)	Reps left Reps right		
Hanging leg raise 1 set, 10-20 reps	Reps		
Rope horizontal chop 1 set, 10-15 reps (each)	Reps left Reps right		
Notes:			

Note: Perform one set of A1, and immediately follow it with one set of A2. Rest 30-90 seconds and repeat until all sets are completed. Do the same for B1 and B2.

Chapter 11:

Strong Curves Twelve-Week Gluteal Goddess Program for Advanced Lifters

You really need a quality base of strength and good understanding of strength training before diving into the Twelve-Week Gluteal Goddess Program for Advanced Lifters.

I recommend this program for women who have accomplished most of the following:

1. 50 non-stop bodyweight hip thrusts
2. 1 bodyweight chin-up from a dead hang
3. 5 bodyweight full-range push-ups (without sagging at the hips)
4. 20 non-stop bodyweight Bulgarian split squats
5. 30 non-stop bodyweight back extensions
6. 10 deadlifts with 135 pounds

"Progressive overload" is the gradual increase of intensity with training over a period of time. It's likely the best way to improve strength, build quality lean mass, and gain greater endurance because each week you force your body out of its comfort zone. Progressive overload incrementally increases the stress you put on your muscles each week, forcing them to re-adapt. Notice that I said incremental changes. You want these changes to be just right. Otherwise, the effects will not be positive. Too little change in your intensity, and your muscles won't need to adapt. If your workouts are the same one year from now as they are today, your muscles probably won't be any shapelier, and you won't look much different (unless you dropped significant body fat). Too much change in your intensity, and you'll end up allowing your form to suffer, which won't end pretty. You'll be incredibly sore each week and will probably end up on the injured list.

Remember, tension is the key to increased muscular shape. You must do more over time so that you place more tension on the muscles. Think how much tension is required of the glutes when you perform a two hundred twenty-five-pound hip thrust compared to a bodyweight glute bridge. That's the key to great glutes!

The best way to overload your neuromuscular system is to add more weight to your lifts each week. I want you to attempt this for at least one major lift during your session. Though it would be ideal for you to go up in weight with every exercise, the more proficient you become at training and the stronger you are, the less likely this will happen. Elite male lifters sometimes take well over a year to add only twenty pounds of weight to the bigger lifts like squats, deadlifts, and bench presses. If you can't muster another lift with any more weight, either increase how many reps you do per set or decrease the amount of rest you allow between your sets.

Just to recap, here is what progressive overload looks like:

- Increase the weight for each lift each week by five to ten pounds while performing the same number of reps,
- Increase the amount of reps for each lift each week by one to two while using the same amount of weight, or
- Decrease the amount of rest you take between sets by about thirty seconds while using the same amount of weight and the same number of reps.

Remember, the first option is always the best, but this will not happen each week. Listen to what your body tells you, and do your best. But don't ever let your form suffer just to try to beat a personal record. There will be plenty of weeks when you don't beat a personal record for certain lifts. There will even be weeks when you feel weak and don't set any personal records on any set of any exercise. But there are plenty of opportunities to set personal records throughout the week, and initially, this is very doable.

I want you to focus on progressive overload and setting records for the last three weeks during Phase I, II, and III. I recommend a deload week at the end of Phase III, as your muscles will be ready for a break. For deloading, you can simply go back to the first week of Phase I, using the same weight that you used during that week, or stick to the advice I provided earlier and reduce the intensity by twenty to fifty percent (or just perform one set per exercise). There are plenty of ways to deload, but the point is to provide only the bare minimum of stimulation necessary for the body to hold onto gains, while allowing for optimal recovery and preparation for upcoming weeks of hard work.

At the end of this chapter, you will find a set of templates to copy and use in the gym. Here's an example of a month-long progression for the box squat exercise. Let's say that during week one you're able to perform three sets of five box squats with a sixty-five-pound barbell. The next week, you might aim for three sets of six box squats with sixty-five pounds. Or, you could go for eight reps the first set, then five reps on the second and third sets. Finally, you could add five pounds and jump up to seventy pounds of total weight, attempting to achieve three sets of five reps again. Let's assume that you chose this route and went with seventy pounds but were only able to achieve five reps during set one and two. Then, during set three you only performed three reps. During week three, you might stick with seventy pounds and try to complete the three sets of five reps. During week four, you might choose to deload and go with sixty pounds for three sets of five reps, attempting to use picture-perfect form. These small jumps add up over time and make a huge difference in the long-run.

Remember, when you don't write down the volume and intensity of your workouts, you must rely on memory, which might not always be accurate. You already have plenty on your mind, so make your workouts simple by using the templates offered in this chapter.

Twelve-Week Gluteal Goddess Program for Advanced Lifters

- The goal of these sessions is to progressively add weight or repetitions without compromising good form.

- Up the repetitions until you've reached a certain number, then add load. For example, stick with 65 pounds until you can do it for 12 reps, then increase to 70 or 75 pounds and stick with that until you can do it for 12 reps, etc.

Date:_____ Weight:_____

Equipment needed for workout A weeks 1-4:

- Exercise mat
- Barbell with weight plates and rack
- Hampton pad
- Flat bench
- Set of dumbbells
- Band
- Chin-up bar
- Dumbbells
- Back extension (if not available, see Exercise Index for substitute exercises)
- Band
- Cable machine with ankle cuff
- Light kettlebell

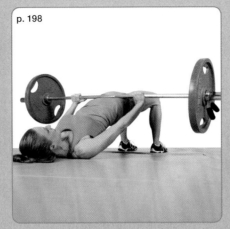

p. 198

A1: Barbell glute bridge
—3 sets of 20 reps

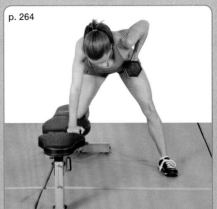

p. 264

A2: One-arm row
—3 sets of 8 reps (each side)

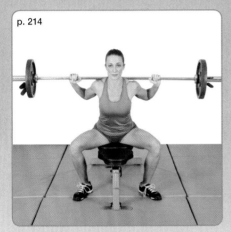

p. 214

B1: Barbell box squat
—3 sets of 5 reps

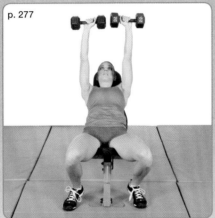

p. 277

B2: Dumbbell incline press
—3 sets of 8 reps

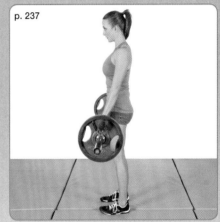

p. 237

Barbell American deadlift
—3 sets of 5 reps

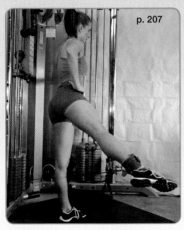

p. 207

Cable standing abduction
—1 set of 20 reps (each side)

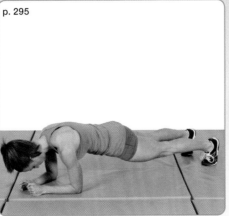

p. 295

RKC Plank
—1 set of 60 seconds

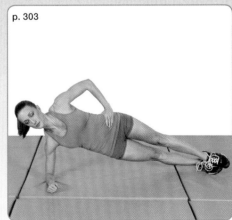

p. 303

Side plank
—1 set of 60 seconds (each side)

Date:_____   Weight:_____

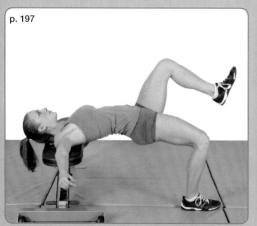

p. 197

A1: Bodyweight shoulder elevated single-leg hip thrust
—3 sets of 8-20 reps (each side)

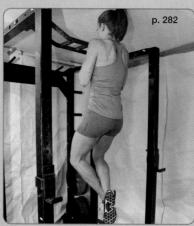

p. 282

A2: Chin-up
—3 sets of 5 reps

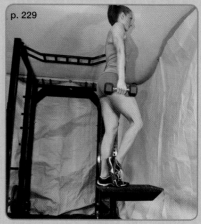

p. 229

B1: Dumbbell high step up
—3 sets of 10 reps (each side)

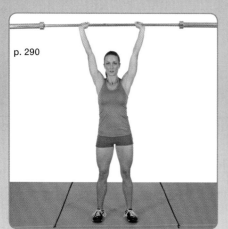

p. 290

B2: Barbell military press
—3 sets of 8 reps

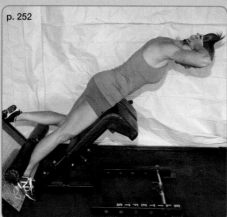

p. 252

Prisoner single-leg 45-degree hyperextension
—2 sets of 12 reps

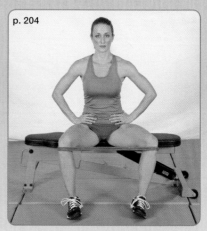

p. 204

Band seated abduction
—1 set of 20 reps

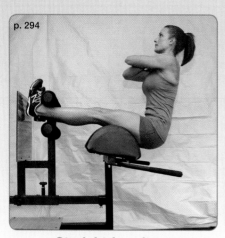

p. 294

Straight-leg sit-up
—1 set of 20 reps

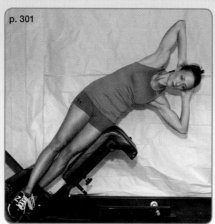

p. 301

45-degree side bend
—1 set of 20 reps

Date:_____   Weight:_____

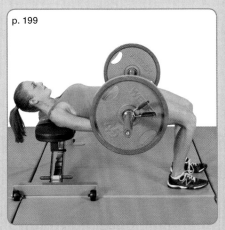

p. 199

A1: Barbell hip thrust
—3 sets of 20 reps

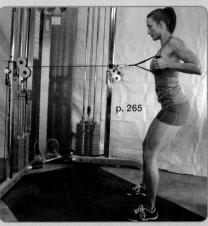

p. 265

A2: Standing single-arm cable row
—3 sets of 8 reps (each side)

p. 212

B1: Dumbbell goblet squat
—3 sets of 5 reps

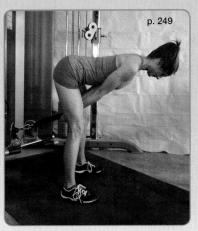

p. 276

p. 249

B2: Dumbbell one-arm bench press
—3 sets of 8 reps

Cable straight-leg pull-through
—3 sets of 8-12 reps

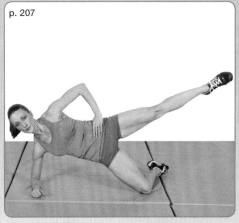

p. 207

Side lying hip raise
—1 set of 10 reps (each side)

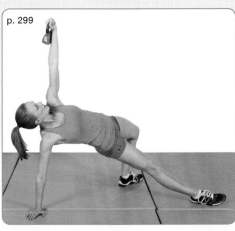

p. 299

Turkish get up
—1 set of 5 reps (each side)

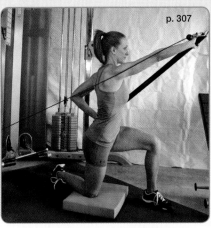

p. 307

Bar half-kneeling horizontal chop
—1 set of 8-12 reps (each side)

Date:_____

Weight:_____

Equipment needed for workout A weeks 5-8:

- Exercise mat
- Barbell with weight plates
- Hampton pad
- Barbell with weights and rack
- Dumbbells
- Ab wheel
- Two flat benches or a flat bench and box (to elevate feet)
- Chin-up bar
- Dumbbells
- Back extension (if not available, see substitute exercises)
- Band
- Cable machine

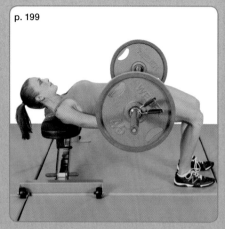

p. 199

A1: Barbell hip thrust
—3 sets of 3-8 reps

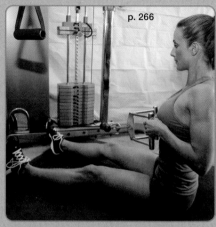

p. 266

A2: Seated cable row
—3 sets of 8 reps

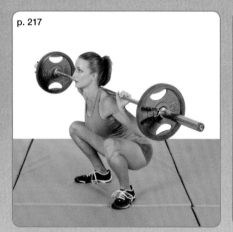

p. 217

B1: Barbell full squat
—3 sets of 5 reps

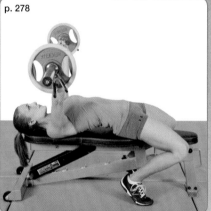

p. 278

B2: Barbell bench press
—3 sets 3-8 reps

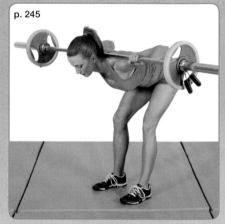

p. 245

Barbell good morning
—3 sets of 8-12 reps

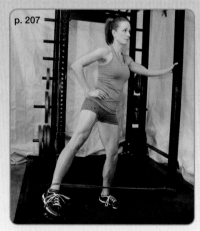

p. 207

Band standing abduction
—1 set of 10-30 reps (each side)

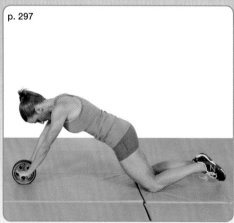

p. 297

Ab wheel rollout from knees
—1 set of 8-20 reps

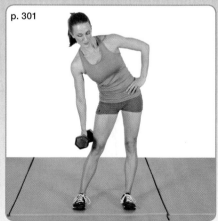

p. 301

Dumbbell side bend
—1 set of 10-20 reps (each side)

Date:_____   Weight:_____

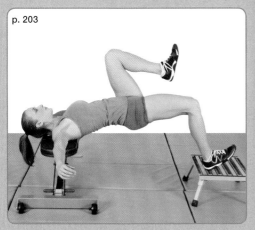

A1: Bodyweight single-leg hip thrust (shoulders and foot elevated)
—3 sets of 8-20 reps

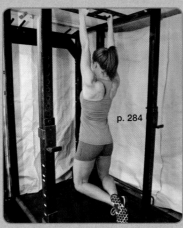

A2: Bodyweight parallel grip pull-up
—3 sets of 3-8 reps

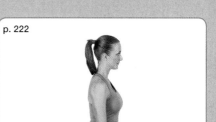

B1: Dumbbell walking lunge
—3 sets of 10 reps (20 total steps)

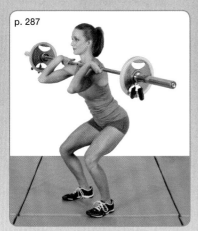

B2: Barbell push press
—3 sets 6 reps

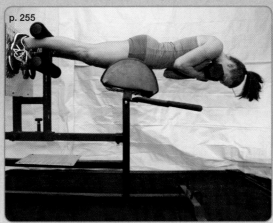

Dumbbell back extension
—2 sets of 20 reps

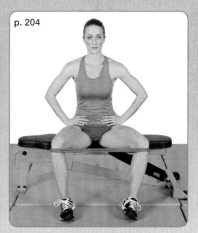

Band seated abduction
—1 set of 10-30 reps

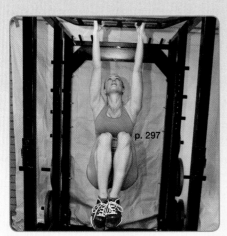

Hanging leg raise
—1 set of 8-20 reps

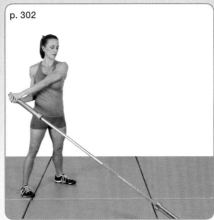

Landmine
—1 set of 8-12 reps (each side)

Date:_____   Weight:_____

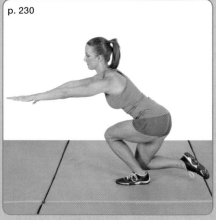

p. 199

**A1: Barbell hip thrust
(isohold method)**
—3 sets of 30-60 seconds

p. 281

A2: D-handle lat pulldown
—3 sets of 8 reps

p. 230

B1: Skater squat
—3 sets of 8 reps

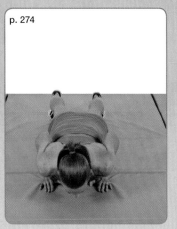

p. 274

B2: Close-width push-up
—3 sets 5-15 reps

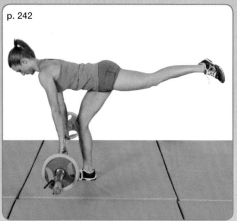

p. 242

Barbell single-leg Romanian deadlift
—3 sets of 8-12 reps

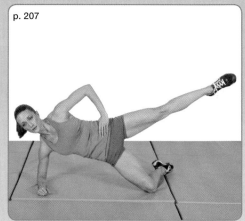

p. 207

Side lying hip raise
—1 set of 10-30 reps

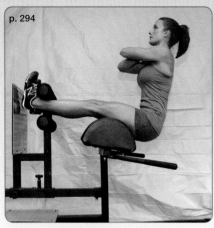

p. 294

Straight-leg sit-up
—1 set of 10-20 reps

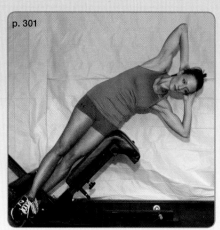

p. 301

45-degree side bend
—1 set of 10-20 reps (each side)

Date:_____

Weight:_____

Equipment needed for workout A weeks 9-12:

- Barbell with weight plates
- Hampton bar pad
- Band
- Dumbbell
- Swiss ball
- Chin-up bar
- Incline bench rack
- Smith machine or rack with secure barbell
- Flat bench
- Valslides or Gliders (two towels on smooth floor will work)
- Cable machine
- Airex pad or exercise mat
- Pull-up bar
- Back extension

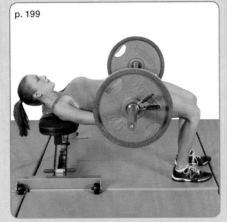

p. 199

A1: Barbell hip thrust (rest pause method)—3 sets of 10 reps (6 in a row, then 1, then 1, then 1)

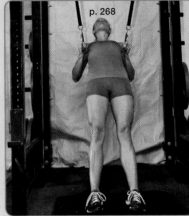

p. 268

A2: Bodyweight inverted row—3 sets of 6-12 reps

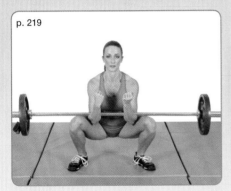

p. 219

B1: Barbell Zercher squat—3 sets of 5-10 reps

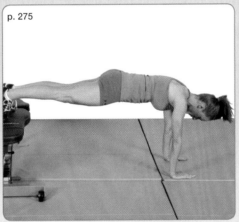

p. 275

B2: Feet elevated push-up—3 sets of 5-20 reps

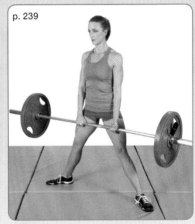

p. 239

Barbell Sumo deadlift—3 sets of 6-12 reps

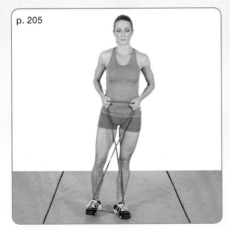

p. 205

X-band walk—1 set of 20 reps (20 to the right, 20 to the left)

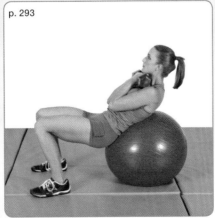

p. 293

Dumbbell Swiss ball crunch—1 set of 20 reps

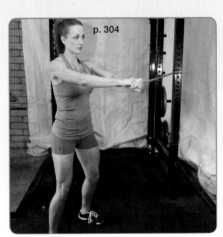

p. 304

Band anti-rotation hold—1 set of 15 seconds (each side)

Date:_____   Weight:_____

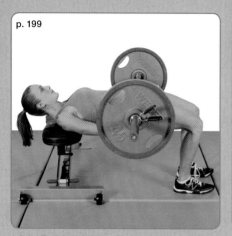

A1: Barbell hip thrust (constant tension method)
3 sets of 20-30 reps (no stopping)

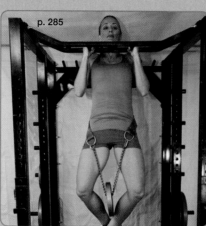

A2: Weighted parallel pull-up
—3 sets of 1-3 reps

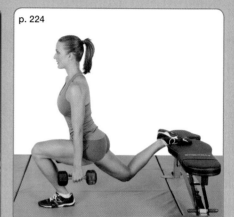

B1: Deficit dumbbell Bulgarian split squat
—3 sets of 10 reps (each side)

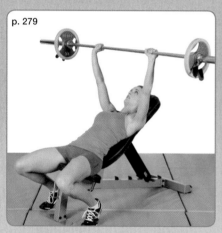

B2: Barbell incline press
—3 sets of 6-10 reps

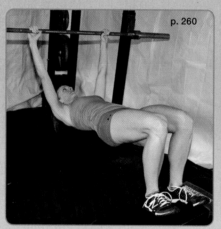

Gliding leg curl
—2 sets of 6-15 reps

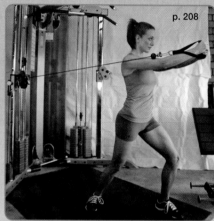

Cable hip rotation
—1 set of 8-15 reps

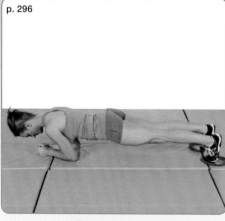

Body saw
—1 set of 8-15 reps

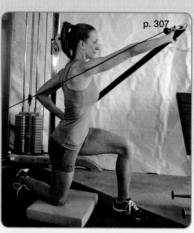

Bar half-kneeling horizontal chop
—1 set of 8-12 reps (each side)

Date:_____   Weight:_____

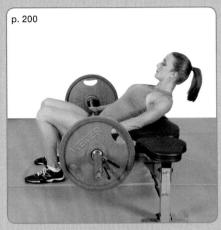

A1: American hip thrust
—3 sets of 5 heavy reps

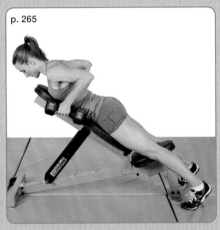

A2: Dumbbell chest supported row
—3 sets of 6-12 reps

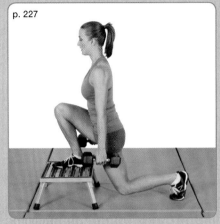

B1: Dumbbell step up/reverse lunge combo
—3 sets of 8-15 reps (each side)

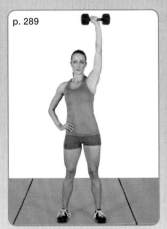

B2: One-arm shoulder press
—3 sets of 8-15 reps

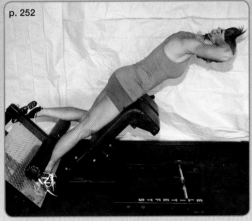

Prisoner single-leg back extension
—3 sets of 8-15 reps (each side)

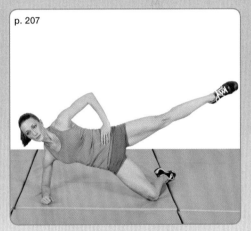

Side lying hip raise
—1 set of 10-30 reps (both sides)

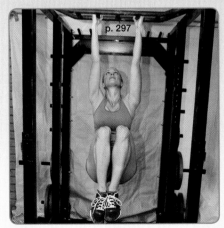

Hanging leg raise
—1 set of 8-20 reps

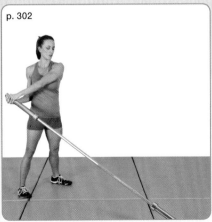

Landmine
—1 set of 8-12 reps (each side)

Name: _____ Date: _____ Weight: _____

Exercise	Set 1	Set 2	Set 3
A1: Barbell glute bridge 3 sets, 20 reps	Weight Reps	Weight Reps	Weight Reps
A2: One-arm dumbbell row 3 sets, 8 reps (each)	Weight Reps	Weight Reps	Weight Reps
B1: Barbell box squat 3 sets, 5 reps	Weight Reps	Weight Reps	Weight Reps
B2: Dumbbell incline bench press 3 sets, 8 reps	Weight Reps	Weight Reps	Weight Reps
Barbell American deadlift 3 sets, 5 reps	Weight Reps	Weight Reps	Weight Reps
Cable standing abduction 1 set, 20 reps (each)	Weight Reps		
RKC plank 1 set, 60 seconds	Seconds		
Side plank 1 set, 60 seconds	Seconds		
Notes:			

Note: Perform one set of A1, and immediately follow it with one set of A2. Rest 30-90 seconds and repeat until all sets are completed. Do the same for B1 and B2.

Name:_____ Date:_____ Weight:_____

Exercise	Set 1	Set 2	Set 3
A1: Bodyweight shoulder elevated single-leg hip thrust 3 sets, 8-20 reps (each)	Weight Reps	Weight Reps	Weight Reps
A2: Chin-up 3 sets, 5 reps	Weight Reps	Weight Reps	Weight Reps
B1: Dumbbell high step up 3 sets, 10 reps (each)	Reps left Reps right	Reps left Reps right	Reps left Reps right
B2: Barbell military press 3 sets, 8 reps	Weight Reps	Weight Reps	Weight Reps
Prisoner single-leg 45 back extension 2 sets, 12 reps (each)	Weight Reps	Weight Reps	
Banded seat abduction 1 set, 20 reps	Reps left Reps right		
Straight-leg sit-up 1 set, 20 reps	Seconds		
45-degree side bend 1 set, 20 reps (each)	Seconds		
Notes:			

Note: Perform one set of A1, and immediately follow it with one set of A2. Rest 30-90 seconds and repeat until all sets are completed. Do the same for B1 and B2.

Name:_____ Date:_____ Weight:_____

Exercise	Set 1	Set 2	Set 3
A1: Barbell American hip thrust 3 sets, 20 reps	Weight Reps	Weight Reps	Weight Reps
A2: Standing single-arm cable row 3 sets, 8 reps each side	Weight Reps	Weight Reps	Weight Reps
B1: Goblet full squat 3 sets, 5 reps	Weight Reps	Weight Reps	Weight Reps
B2: Single-arm dumbbell bench press 3 sets, 8 reps	Weight Reps	Weight Reps	Weight Reps
Cable straight-leg pull-through 3 sets, 8-12 reps	Weight Reps	Weight Reps	Weight Reps
Side lying hip raise 1 set, 10 reps (each)	Weight Reps		
Turkish get up 1 set, 5 reps (each)	Seconds		
Half-kneeling cable anti-rotation press 1 set, 8-12 reps (each)	Seconds		
Notes:			

Note: Perform one set of A1, and immediately follow it with one set of A2. Rest 30-90 seconds and repeat until all sets are completed. Do the same for B1 and B2.

Name:_____ Date:_____ Weight:_____

Exercise	Set 1	Set 2	Set 3
A1: Barbell hip thrust 3 sets, 3-8 reps	Weight Reps	Weight Reps	Weight Reps
A2: Seated row 3 sets, 8 reps	Weight Reps	Weight Reps	Weight Reps
B1: Barbell full squat 3 sets, 5 reps	Reps left Reps right	Reps left Reps right	Reps left Reps right
B2: Barbell bench press 3 sets, 3-8 reps	Weight Reps	Weight Reps	Weight Reps
Barbell good morning 3 sets, 8-12 reps	Weight Reps	Weight Reps	Weight Reps
Band standing abduction 1 set, 10-30 reps (each)	Weight Reps		
Ab wheel rollout from knees 1 set,8-20 reps	Reps		
Dumbbell side bend 1 set, 10-20 reps	Reps		
Notes:			

Note: Perform one set of A1, and immediately follow it with one set of A2. Rest 30-90 seconds and repeat until all sets are completed. Do the same for B1 and B2.

Name:_____ Date:_____ Weight:_____

Exercise	Set 1	Set 2	Set 3
A1: Bodyweight single-leg hip thrust (shoulder and foot elevated) 3 sets, 8-20 reps (each)	Weight Reps	Weight Reps	Weight Reps
A2: Bodyweight neutral grip pull-up 3 sets, 3-8 reps	Weight Reps	Weight Reps	Weight Reps
B1: Dumbbell walking lunge 3 sets, 10 steps (20 total steps)	Weight Reps	Weight Reps	Weight Reps
B2: Barbell push press 3 sets, 6 reps	Weight Reps	Weight Reps	Weight Reps
Dumbbell back extension 2 sets, 20 reps	Weight Reps	Weight Reps	
Banded seat abduction 1 set, 10-30 reps	Weight Reps		
Hanging leg raise 1 set, 8-20 reps	Reps		
Landmine 1 set, 8-12 reps	Reps		
Notes:			

Note: Perform one set of A1, and immediately follow it with one set of A2. Rest 30-90 seconds and repeat until all sets are completed. Do the same for B1 and B2.

Name:_____ Date:_____ Weight:_____

Exercise	Set 1	Set 2	Set 3
A1: Barbell hip thrust (isohold method) 3 sets, 30-60 sec	Weight Reps	Weight Reps	Weight Reps
A2: D-handle lat pulldown 3 sets, 8 reps	Weight Reps	Weight Reps	Weight Reps
B1: Skater squat 3 sets, 8 reps (each)	Reps left Reps right	Reps left Reps right	Reps left Reps right
B2: Narrow base push-up 3 sets, 5-15 reps	Weight Reps	Weight Reps	Weight Reps
Barbell single-leg RDL 3 sets, 8-12 reps (each)	Weight Reps	Weight Reps	Weight Reps
Side lying hip raise 1 set, 10-30 reps (each)	Weight Reps		
Straight-leg sit-up 1 set, 10-20 reps	Reps		
45-dgree side bend 1 set, 10-20 reps (each)	Reps		
Notes:			

Note: Perform one set of A1, and immediately follow it with one set of A2. Rest 30-90 seconds and repeat until all sets are completed. Do the same for B1 and B2.

Name:_____ Date:_____ Weight:_____

Exercise	Set 1	Set 2	Set 3
A1: Barbell hip thrust (rest/pause method) 3 sets, 6 reps, 1 rep, 1 rep, 1 rep	Weight Reps	Weight Reps	Weight Reps
A2: Bodyweight inverted row 3 sets 6-12 reps	Weight Reps	Weight Reps	Weight Reps
B1: Barbell Zercher squat 3 sets, 5-10 reps	Weight Reps	Weight Reps	Weight Reps
B2: Feet elevated push-up 3 sets, 5-20 reps	Weight Reps	Weight Reps	Weight Reps
Barbell sumo deadlift 3 sets, 6-12 reps	Weight Reps	Weight Reps	Weight Reps
X-band walk (heavy tension) 1 set, 20 reps (each)	Weight Reps		
Dumbbell Swiss ball crunch 1 set, 20 reps	Reps		
Band rotary hold 1 set, 15 seconds (each)	Seconds		
Notes:			

Note: Perform one set of A1, and immediately follow it with one set of A2. Rest 30-90 seconds and repeat until all sets are completed. Do the same for B1 and B2.

Name:_____ Date:_____ Weight:_____

Exercise	Set 1	Set 2	Set 3
A1: Barbell hip thrust (constant tension method) 3 sets, 20-30 reps (non-stop)	Weight Reps	Weight Reps	Weight Reps
A2: Weighted parallel pull-up 3 sets, 1-3 reps	Weight Reps	Weight Reps	Weight Reps
B1: Dumbbell Bulgarian split squat 3 sets, 10 reps (each)	Reps left Reps right	Reps left Reps right	Reps left Reps right
B2: Barbell incline press 3 sets, 6-10 reps	Weight Reps	Weight Reps	Weight Reps
Gliding leg curls 2 sets, 6-15 reps	Weight Reps	Weight Reps	
Banded hip rotation 1 set, 8-15 reps (each)	Weight Reps		
Body saw 1 set, 8-15 reps	Reps		
Half-kneeling cable anti-rotation press 1 set, 8-12 reps (each)	Reps		
Notes:			

Note: Perform one set of A1, and immediately follow it with one set of A2. Rest 30-90 seconds and repeat until all sets are completed. Do the same for B1 and B2.

Name:_____ Date:_____ Weight:_____

Exercise	Set 1	Set 2	Set 3
A1: American hip thrust 3 sets, 5 heavy reps	Weight Reps	Weight Reps	Weight Reps
A2: Dumbbell chest supported row 3 sets, 6-12 reps	Weight Reps	Weight Reps	Weight Reps
B1: Dumbbell step up/reverse lunge combo 3 sets, 8-15 reps (each)	Weight Reps	Weight Reps	Weight Reps
B2: Single-arm dumbbell military press 3 sets, 8-12 reps (each)	Weight Reps	Weight Reps	Weight Reps
Prisoner single-leg back extension 3 sets, 8-15 reps (each)	Weight Reps	Weight Reps	Weight Reps
Side lying hip raise 1 set, 10-30 reps (each)	Weight Reps		
Hanging leg raise 1 set, 8-20 reps	Reps		
Landmine 1 set, 8-12 reps (each)	Reps		
Notes:			

Note: Perform one set of A1, and immediately follow it with one set of A2. Rest 30-90 seconds and repeat until all sets are completed. Do the same for B1 and B2.

Chapter 12:

Twelve-Week Best Butt Bodyweight Program (At-Home)

You may not go to a gym, or you may have days when you can't make it there. The *Strong Curves* Twelve-week Best Butt Bodyweight Program is perfect for beginners, someone who prefers training at home, or for those days when the gym is not an option. If you are working through another *Strong Curves Program* in this book, these workouts are also good substitutes if you miss the gym one day. Just select a workout from the same phase and day that you are on.

In order to perform the program designed for this twelve-week phase, you will need to purchase a few small items that store easily in your closet and will not take up much room. There is no need to go out and purchase tons of home gym equipment because you can train efficiently using your own body weight and just a few tools.

The equipment you need at home for this workout include:

- Exercise mat
- Swiss ball
- Valslides (may substitute a towel if you have a smooth floor)
- Chin-up bar (Iron Gym works well)
- PVC pipe or some other dowel (a broomstick could work)

You will also need several surfaces to use for elevation. Be creative by using coffee tables, chairs, a bed railing, walls, and any other surface with the right elevation. I also encourage you to purchase a Jungle Gym XT by Lifeline USA. It's an industrial suspension system that allows you to perform many exercises shown in this book. The Twelve-Week Bodyweight Program specifies several workouts that use inverted rows. While you can perform these using other utilities, the Jungle Gym XT would greatly benefit your progression with this exercise.

Just as I mentioned in the Twelve-week Booty-ful Beginnings program, I want you to master quality movement patterns because how you move matters more than anything else in this program. It's easy to do a significant amount of repetitions with this program, but if you are performing them incorrectly or with poor movement patterns, you aren't making proper gains. Your first and last repetition must look similar. If you start to break down, take a rest. Also, if you aren't feeling the right muscles working, regress until you can work the right way.

In the Exercise Index, I demonstrated some of the most common mistakes when performing popular exercises and how to correct those mistakes, but know that these corrections take time. You won't figure out how to do the exercises overnight, and that's why I chose specific progression patterns for this program.

I need you to make another promise to me while working through any program in this book: Pay attention to how your muscles feel during every exercise. If they don't feel like they are working hard, you're performing the exercise incorrectly. Bodyweight workouts are highly underrated. Beginners benefit more from this workout than from using weights in a gym. Many bodyweight exercises use a high percentage of the body's weight for loading. As a matter of fact, they put more loading on the muscles than typical barbell or dumbbell exercises with beginners. For example, a beginner might use very light dumbbells for incline press, one-arm rows, or Romanian deadlifts. By sticking with variations of push-ups, inverted rows, and hip thrusts, the loading on the pecs, lats, scapula retractors, and hip extensors is higher with the bodyweight movements than with the dumbbell movements. By really challenging yourself during the next twelve weeks, you will build the most incredible physique without ever having lifted a single weight.

Date:_____   Weight:_____

Twelve-Week Best Butt Bodyweight Program at Home
- *Goal is to first master the movement patterns.*
- *Once coordinated and feeling the correct muscles doing the job, increase in repetitions, and learn to make the movement more challenging.*

Equipment needed for workout A weeks 1-4:
- *Exercise mat*
- *Jungle Gym XT or two chairs*
- *Table or other raised surface*
- *Swiss ball*
- *Chin-up bar*

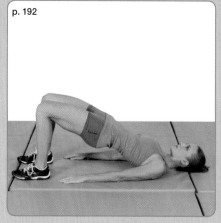
p. 192

A1: Bodyweight glute bridge
—3 sets of 10-20 reps

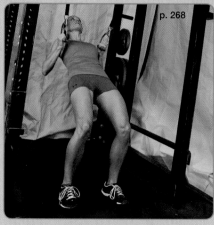
p. 268

A2: Bodyweight modified inverted row
—3 sets of 8-12 reps)

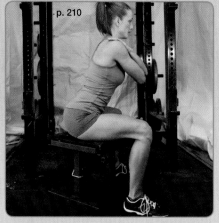
p. 210

B1: Bodyweight box squat
—3 sets of 10-20 reps

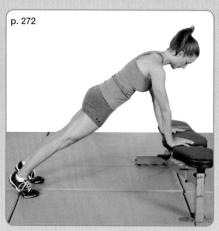
p. 272

B2: Torso-elevated push-up
—3 sets of 8-12 reps

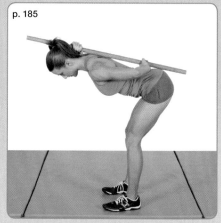
p. 185

Bodyweight hip hinge with dowel
—3 sets of 10-20 reps

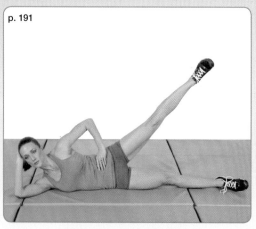
p. 191

Side lying abduction
—1 set of 10-30 reps (each side)

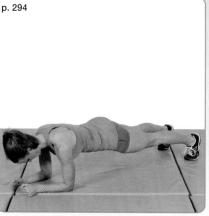
p. 294

Front plank
—1 set 30-120 seconds

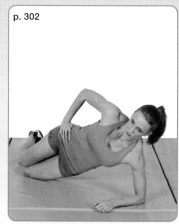
p. 302

Kneeling side plank
—1 set of 20-60 seconds (each side)

Date:_____ Weight:_____

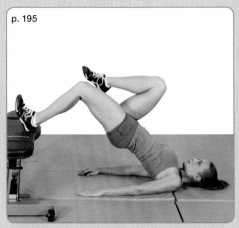

A1: : Bodyweight foot elevated single-leg glute bridge
—3 sets of 10-20 reps (each side)

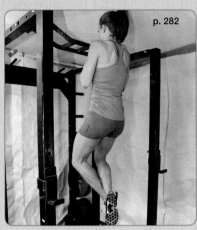

A2: Bodyweight chin-up (negative)
—3 sets of 1-3 reps

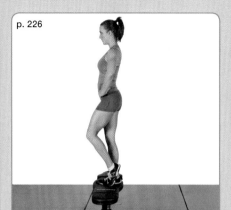

B1: Bodyweight step up
—3 sets of 10-20 reps (each side)

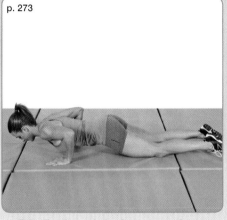

B2: Bodyweight knee push-up
—3 sets of 5-15 reps

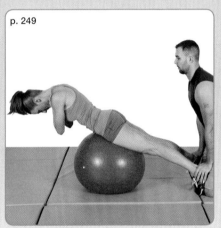

Bodyweight Swiss ball 45-degree back extension
—3 sets of 10-20 reps

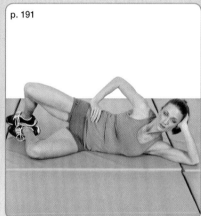

Side lying clam
—1 set of 20-30 reps (each side)

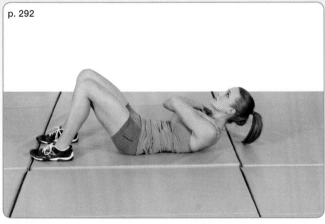

Crunch
—1 set of 20-30 reps

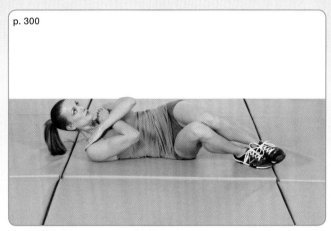

Side crunch
—1 set of 20-30 reps (each side)

Date:_____   Weight:_____

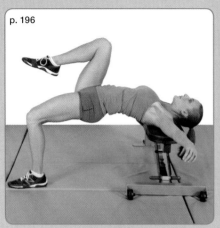

A1: Shoulders-elevated glute march
—3 sets of 30-60 second (alternating legs in marching fashion)

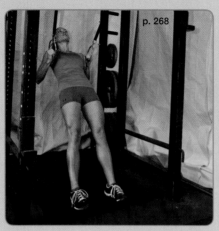

A2: Bodyweight inverted row
—3 sets of 8-12 reps

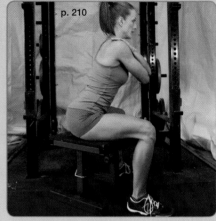

B1: Bodyweight box squat
—3 sets of 10-20 reps (each side)

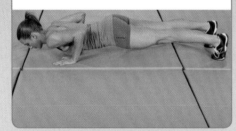

B2: Bodyweight negative push-up
—3 sets of 3-5 reps

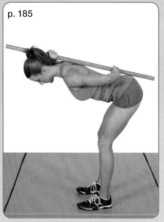

Bodyweight hip hinge with dowel
—3 sets of 10-20 reps

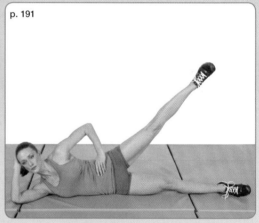

Side lying abduction
—1 set of 10-30 reps (each side)

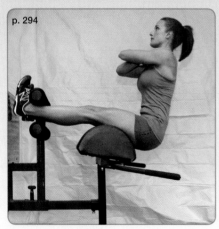

Straight-leg sit-up
—1 set of 15-30 reps

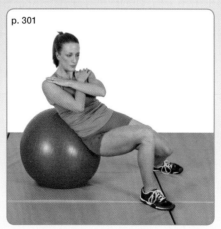

Swiss ball side crunch
—1 set of 15-30 reps (each side)

Date:_____

Weight:_____

Equipment needed for weeks 5-8:

- *Exercise mat*
- *Jungle Gym XT or two chairs*
- *Table or other raised surface*
- *Swiss ball*
- *Chin-up bar*

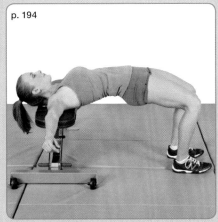

p. 194

A1: Bodyweight hip thrust
—3 sets of 10-30 reps

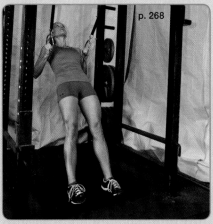

p. 268

**A2: Bodyweight inverted row
(less torso angle than previous
month)**—3 sets of 8-12 reps

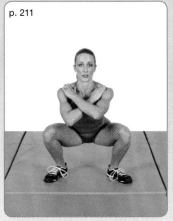

p. 211

B1: Bodyweight squat
—3 sets of 10-30 reps

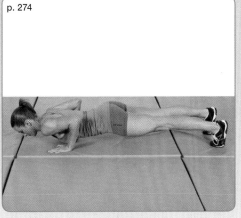

p. 274

**B2: Bodyweight push-up
(strict singles)**
—3 sets of 1 rep

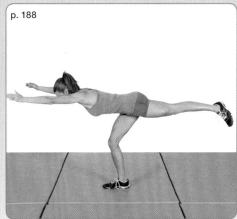

p. 188

Reaching single-leg RDL
—3 sets of 10-20 reps (each side)

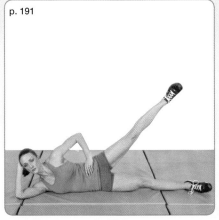

p. 191

Side lying abduction
—1 set of 20-30 reps (each side)

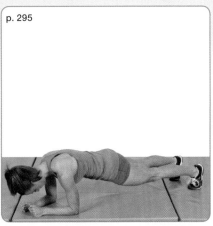

p. 295

RKC plank
—1 set of 20-60 seconds

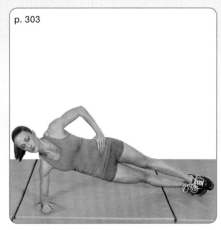

p. 303

Side plank
—1 set of 20-60 seconds (each side)

Date:_____   Weight:_____

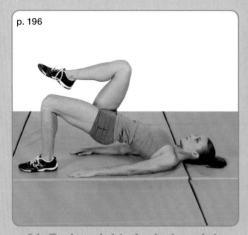

p. 196

A1: Bodyweight single-leg glute bridge
—3 sets of 10-20 reps (each side)

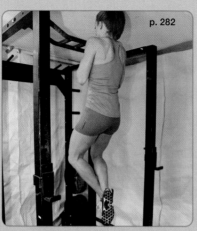

p. 282

A2: Bodyweight chin-up (single reps)
—3 sets of 1 rep

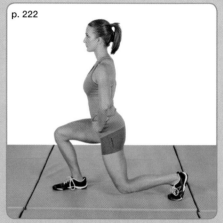

p. 222

B1: Bodyweight walking lunge
—3 sets of 10-20 reps (20-40 total steps)

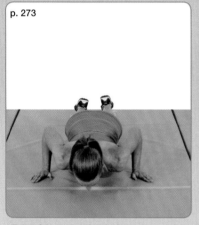

p. 273

B2: Close-width knee push-up
—3 sets of 6-20 reps

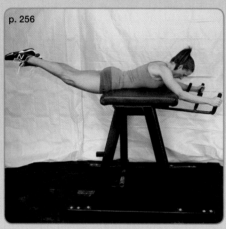

p. 256

Bodyweight reverse hyper
—3 sets of 10-30 reps

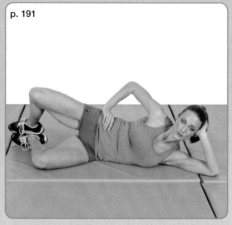

p. 191

Side lying clam
—1 set of 10-30 reps (each side)

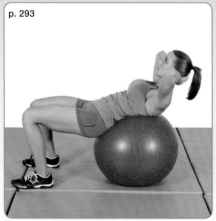

p. 293

Swiss ball crunch
—1 set of 10-30 reps

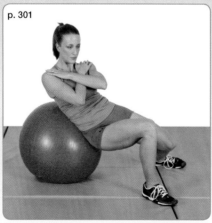

p. 301

Swiss ball side crunch
—1 set of 10-30 reps (each side)

Weeks 5-8: Workout C (perform on day five of workout week)

Date:_____   Weight:_____

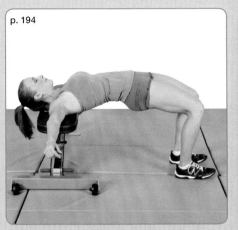

A1: Bodyweight hip thrust
—3 sets of 10-30 reps

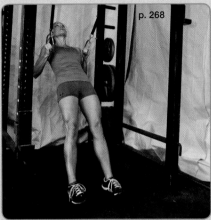

A2: Bodyweight inverted row (steep torso angle)
—3 sets of 8-12 reps

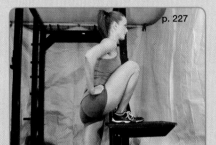

B1: Bodyweight high step up
—3 sets of 10-20 reps (each side)

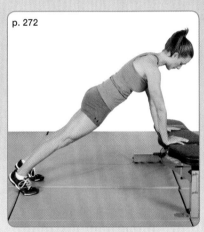

B2: Bodyweight torso elevated push-up
—3 sets of 8-12 reps

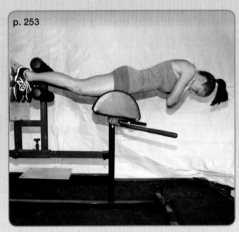

Bodyweight back extension
—3 sets of 20-30 reps

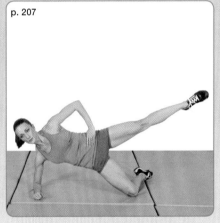

Side lying hip raise
—1 set of 10-20 reps (each side)

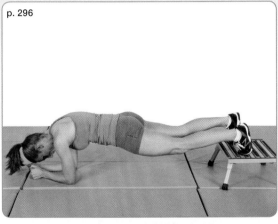

Feet elevated RKC plank
—1 set of 60-120 seconds

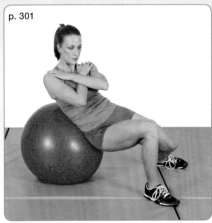

Swiss ball side crunch
—1 set of 10-20 reps (each side)

Date:_____   Weight:_____

Equipment needed for weeks 9-12:

- *Exercise mat*
- *Table or other raised surface*
- *Jungle Gym XT or two chairs*
- *Swiss ball*
- *Chin-up bar*
- *Valslides, Gliders or towel on a smooth surface*

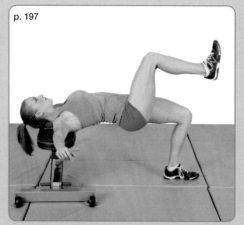

p. 197

A1: Bodyweight shoulder elevated single-leg hip thrust—3 sets of 8-20 reps (each side)

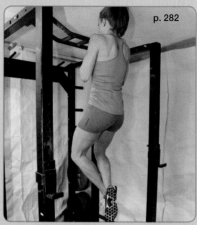

p. 282

A2: Bodyweight chin-up—3 sets of 3-10 reps

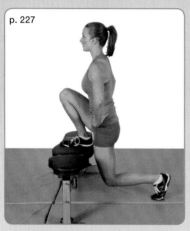

p. 227

B1: Bodyweight step up/reverse lunge combo—3 sets of 10-15 reps (each side)

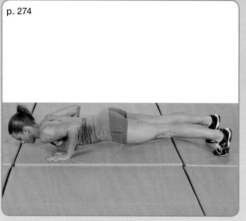

p. 274

B2: Push-up—3 sets of 5-10 reps

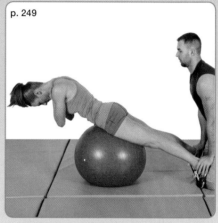

p. 249

Bodyweight Swiss ball back extension—3 sets of 8-20 reps (each side)

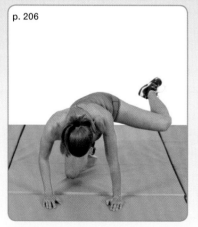

p. 206

Double-quadruped hip abduction—1 set of 6 reps (each side—slow and controlled)

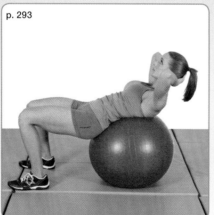

p. 293

Swiss ball crunch—1 set of 10-30 reps

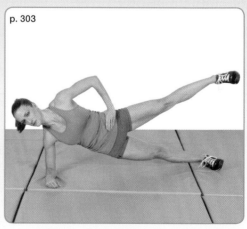

p. 303

Side plank with abduction—1 set of 20-60 seconds (each side)

Date:_____ Weight:_____

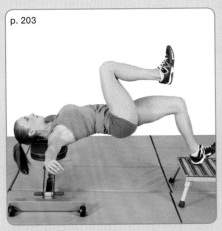

p. 203

A1: Bodyweight shoulder and foot elevated single-leg hip thrust
—3 sets of 6-20 reps (each side)

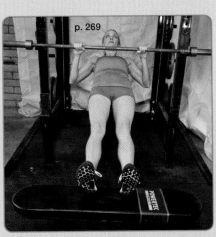

p. 269

A2: Bodyweight feet elevated inverted row
—3 sets of 6-12 reps

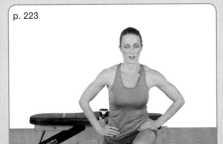

p. 223

B1: Bodyweight Bulgarian split squat
—3 sets of 5-30 reps (each side)

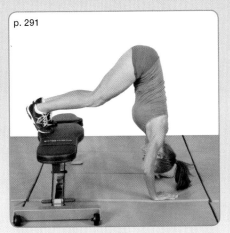

p. 291

B2: Bodyweight feet elevated pike push-up
—3 sets of 6-20 reps

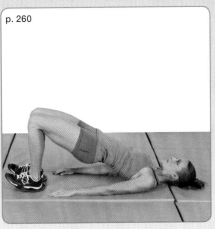

p. 260

Bodyweight sliding leg curl
—2 sets of 10-20 reps

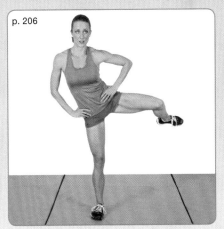

p. 206

Double-standing hip abduction—1 set of 6 reps (each side—slow and controlled)

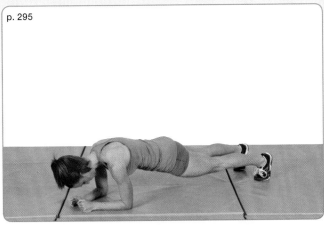

p. 295

RKC plank
—1 set of 30-60 sec

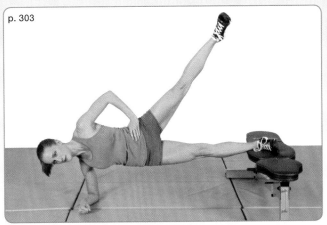

p. 303

Feet elevated side plank with abduction
—1 set of 20-60 seconds

Date:_____ Weight:_____

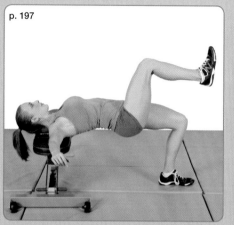
p. 197

A1: Bodyweight shoulder elevated single-leg hip thrust (pause reps)—3 sets of 5-15 reps (each side with 3 second pause at top)

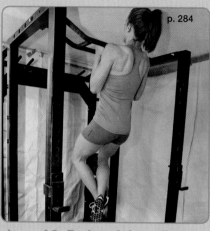
p. 284

A2: Bodyweight pull-up—3 sets of 3-10 reps

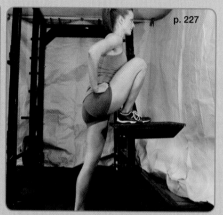
p. 227

B1: Bodyweight high step up—3 sets of 10-15 reps (each side)

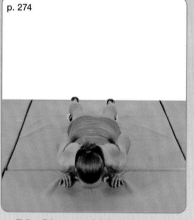
p. 274

B2: Close-width push-up—3 sets of 3-8 reps

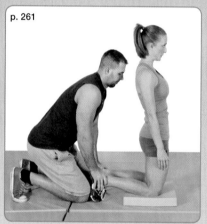
p. 261

Russian leg curls—3 sets of 3-5 reps

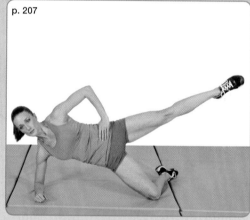
p. 207

Side lying hip raise—1 set of 10-20 reps (each side)

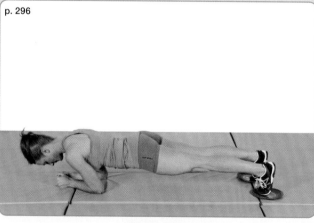
p. 296

Body saw—1 set of 10-15 reps

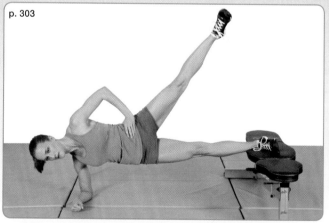
p. 303

Feet-elevated side plank with abduction—1 set of 20-60 seconds (each side)

Name: _____ Date: _____ Weight: _____

Exercise	Set 1	Set 2	Set 3
A1: Bodyweight glute bridge 3 sets, 10-20 reps	Weight Reps	Weight Reps	Weight Reps
A2: Bodyweight modified inverted row 3 sets, 8-12 reps	Weight Reps	Weight Reps	Weight Reps
B1: Bodyweight box squat 3 sets, 10-20 reps	Reps left Reps right	Reps left Reps right	Reps left Reps right
B2: Bodyweight torso-inclined push-up 3 sets, 8-12 reps	Weight Reps	Weight Reps	Weight Reps
Bodyweight hip hinge with dowel 3 sets, 10-20 reps	Weight Reps	Weight Reps	Weight Reps
Side lying abduction 1 set, 10-30 reps (each)	Reps left Reps right		
Front plank 1 set, 30-120 seconds	Seconds		
Side plank from knees 1 set, 20-60 sec (each)	Seconds left Seconds right		
Notes:			

Note: Perform one set of A1, and immediately follow it with one set of A2. Rest 30-90 seconds and repeat until all sets are completed. Do the same for B1 and B2.

Name:_____ Date:_____ Weight:_____

Exercise	Set 1	Set 2	Set 3
A1: Bodyweight foot elevated single-leg glute bridge 3 sets, 10-20 reps (each)	Weight Reps	Weight Reps	Weight Reps
A2: Bodyweight chin-up (negative) 3 sets, 1-3 reps	Weight Reps	Weight Reps	Weight Reps
B1: Bodyweight step up 3 sets, 10-20 reps (each)	Reps left Reps right	Reps left Reps right	Reps left Reps right
B2: Bodyweight knee push-up 3 sets, 5-15 reps	Weight Reps	Weight Reps	Weight Reps
Bodyweight Swiss ball 45-degree back extension 3 sets, 10-20 reps	Weight Reps	Weight Reps	Weight Reps
Side lying clam 1 set, 20-30 reps (each)	Reps left Reps right		
Crunch 1 set, 20-30 reps	Reps		
Side crunch 1 set, 20-30 reps (each)	Reps left Reps right		
Notes:			

Note: Perform one set of A1, and immediately follow it with one set of A2. Rest 30-90 seconds and repeat until all sets are completed. Do the same for B1 and B2.

Name:_____ Date:_____ Weight:_____

Exercise	Set 1	Set 2	Set 3
A1: Glute march (alternate legs in marching fashion) 3 sets, 30-60 sec	Weight Reps	Weight Reps	Weight Reps
A2: Bodyweight inverted row 3 sets, 8-12 reps	Weight Reps	Weight Reps	Weight Reps
B1: Bodyweight box squat 3 sets, 10-20 reps	Reps left Reps right	Reps left Reps right	Reps left Reps right
B2: Bodyweight negative push-up 3 sets, 3-5 reps	Weight Reps	Weight Reps	Weight Reps
Bodyweight hip hinge with dowel 3 sets, 10-20 reps	Weight Reps	Weight Reps	Weight Reps
Side lying abduction 1 set, 10-30 reps (each)	Reps left Reps right		
Straight-leg sit-up 1 set, 15-30 reps	Reps		
Swiss ball side crunch 1 set, 15-30 reps (each)	Reps left Reps right		
Notes:			

Note: Perform one set of A1, and immediately follow it with one set of A2. Rest 30-90 seconds and repeat until all sets are completed. Do the same for B1 and B2.

Name:_____ Date:_____ Weight:_____

Exercise	Set 1	Set 2	Set 3
A1: Bodyweight hip thrust 3 sets, 10-30 reps	Weight Reps	Weight Reps	Weight Reps
A2: Bodyweight inverted row (less torso angle) 3 sets, 8-12 reps	Weight Reps	Weight Reps	Weight Reps
B1: Bodyweight full squat 3 sets, 10-30 reps	Reps left Reps right	Reps left Reps right	Reps left Reps right
B2: Bodyweight push-up 3 sets, 1 rep (strict singles)	Weight Reps	Weight Reps	Weight Reps
Bodyweight single-leg RDL 3 sets, 10-20 reps (each)	Weight Reps	Weight Reps	Weight Reps
Side lying abduction 1 set, 20-30 reps (each)	Reps left Reps right		
RKC plank 1 set, 20-60 seconds	Seconds		
Side plank 1 set, 20-60 sec (each)	Seconds left Seconds right		
Notes:			

Note: Perform one set of A1, and immediately follow it with one set of A2. Rest 30-90 seconds and repeat until all sets are completed. Do the same for B1 and B2.

Name:_____ Date:_____ Weight:_____

Exercise	Set 1	Set 2	Set 3
A1: Bodyweight single-leg glute bridge 3 sets, 10-20 reps (each)	Weight Reps	Weight Reps	Weight Reps
A2: Bodyweight chin-up (single rep) 3 sets, 1 rep	Weight Reps	Weight Reps	Weight Reps
B1: Bodyweight walk lunge 3 sets, 10-20 reps (each)	Reps left Reps right	Reps left Reps right	Reps left Reps right
B2: Bodyweight knee push-up with elbows tucked 3 sets, 6-20 reps	Weight Reps	Weight Reps	Weight Reps
Bodyweight reverse hyper extension 3 sets, 10-30 reps	Weight Reps	Weight Reps	Weight Reps
Side lying clam 1 set, 10-30 reps (each)	Reps left Reps right		
Swiss ball crunch 1 set, 15-30 reps	Reps		
Swiss ball side crunch 1 set, 15-30 reps (each)	Reps left Reps right		
Notes:			

Note: Perform one set of A1, and immediately follow it with one set of A2. Rest 30-90 seconds and repeat until all sets are completed. Do the same for B1 and B2.

Name:_____ Date:_____ Weight:_____

Exercise	Set 1	Set 2	Set 3
A1: Bodyweight hip thrust 3 sets, 10-30 reps	Weight Reps	Weight Reps	Weight Reps
A2: Bodyweight inverted row (steep torso angle) 3 sets, 8-12 reps	Weight Reps	Weight Reps	Weight Reps
B1: Bodyweight high step up 3 sets, 10-20 reps (each)	Reps left Reps right	Reps left Reps right	Reps left Reps right
B2: Bodyweight torso elevated push-up 3 sets, 8-12 reps	Weight Reps	Weight Reps	Weight Reps
Bodyweight back extension 3 sets, 20-30 reps	Weight Reps	Weight Reps	Weight Reps
Side lying hip raise 1 set, 10-20 reps (each)	Reps left Reps right		
Feet elevated plank 1 set, 60-120 sec	Reps		
Swiss ball side crunch 1 set, 20 reps (each)	Reps left Reps right		
Notes:			

Note: Perform one set of A1, and immediately follow it with one set of A2. Rest 30-90 seconds and repeat until all sets are completed. Do the same for B1 and B2.

Name:_____ Date:_____ Weight:_____

Exercise	Set 1	Set 2	Set 3
A1: Bodyweight shoulder elevated single-leg hip thrust 3 sets, 8-20 reps (each)	Weight Reps	Weight Reps	Weight Reps
A2: Bodyweight chin-up 3 sets, 3-10 reps	Weight Reps	Weight Reps	Weight Reps
B1: Bodyweight step up/ reverse lunge combo 3 sets, 10-15 reps (each)	Reps left Reps right	Reps left Reps right	Reps left Reps right
B2: Bodyweight push-up 3 sets, 5-10 reps	Weight Reps	Weight Reps	Weight Reps
Bodyweight Swiss ball back extension 3 sets, 8-20 reps (each)	Weight Reps	Weight Reps	Weight Reps
Quadruped double transverse abduction 1 set, 6 reps (each side, slow and controlled)	Reps left Reps right		
Prisoner Swiss ball crunch 1 set, 10-30 reps	Reps		
Side plank with abduction 1 set, 20-60 sec (each)	Seconds left Seconds right		
Notes:			

Note: Perform one set of A1, and immediately follow it with one set of A2. Rest 30-90 seconds and repeat until all sets are completed. Do the same for B1 and B2.

Name:_____ Date:_____ Weight:_____

Exercise	Set 1	Set 2	Set 3
A1: Bodyweight shoulder and foot elevated single-leg hip thrust 3 sets, 6-20 reps (each)	Weight Reps	Weight Reps	Weight Reps
A2: Bodyweight feet elevated inverted row 3 sets, 6-12 reps	Weight Reps	Weight Reps	Weight Reps
B1: Bodyweight Bulgarian split squat 3 sets, 5-30 reps (each)	Reps left Reps right	Reps left Reps right	Reps left Reps right
B2: Bodyweight feet elevated pike push-up 3 sets, 6-20 reps	Weight Reps	Weight Reps	Weight Reps
Bodyweight sliding leg curls 2 sets, 10-20 reps	Weight Reps	Weight Reps	
Side double abduction 1 set, 1-6 reps (each, slow and controlled)	Reps left Reps right		
RKC plank 1 set, 30-60 sec	Reps		
Feet elevated side plank with abduction 1 set, 20-60 secs (each)	Seconds left Seconds right		
Notes:			

Note: Perform one set of A1, and immediately follow it with one set of A2. Rest 30-90 seconds and repeat until all sets are completed. Do the same for B1 and B2.

Name:_____ Date:_____ Weight:_____

Exercise	Set 1	Set 2	Set 3
A1: Bodyweight shoulder elevated single-leg hip thrust (pause reps) 3 sets of 5-15 reps (each side with 3 second pause at top)	Weight Reps	Weight Reps	Weight Reps
A2: Bodyweight pull-up 3 sets of 3-10 reps	Weight Reps	Weight Reps	Weight Reps
B1: Bodyweight high step up 3 sets of 10-15 reps	Reps left Reps right	Reps left Reps right	Reps left Reps right
B2: Bodyweight narrow base push-up 3 sets of 3-8 reps	Weight Reps	Weight Reps	Weight Reps
Russian leg curls 3 sets of 3-5 reps	Weight Reps	Weight Reps	Weight Reps
Side lying hip raise 1 set of 10-20 reps (each side)	Reps left Reps right		
Body saw 1 set of 10-15 rep	Reps		
Feet elevated side plank with abduction 1 set of 20-60 seconds (each side)	Seconds left Seconds right		
Notes:			

Note: Perform one set of A1, and immediately follow it with one set of A2. Rest 30-90 seconds and repeat until all sets are completed. Do the same for B1 and B2.

Chapter 13:

Twelve-Week Gorgeous Glutes Program (lower body only)

I've worked with plenty of clients who came to me for booty makeovers. They were perfectly happy with the rest of their bodies, but wanted me to work my magic for their glutes. If this sounds like you, the Gorgeous Glutes Program is the perfect match.

When you go through this program, its simplicity may throw you off. But once you learn to activate those glutes properly, you will find that the Gorgeous Glutes Program is very challenging. Each workout consists of four glute-taxing exercises with varying reps and intensity. Notice that unlike the other programs, there are no paired supersets. It's very important to rest between sets with this program to ensure your glutes work hard with each consecutive exercise.

This program uses the largest muscles in your body throughout the duration of your workout, so you will not only sculpt a great behind but will also turn your body into a fat incinerator. As your glutes grow and take on a nice round shape, you will experience notice-able fat reduction. Though I enjoy full body workouts, this is by far my favorite workout for women because you can achieve incredible results while spending little time in the gym. The caveat is that your diet needs to be spot-on for this program to work.

Movement matters in this program. Read through the information on glute activation and movement patterns so that you make the most of your time in the gym. The Exercise Index offers common mistakes and how to correct them. Go through each one, and determine the issues you might have with the movement patterns. The better you are at moving and activating, the greater results you will see with these workouts.

Twelve-Week Gorgeous Glutes Program

- Goal is to first master the movement patterns.
- Once coordinated and feeling the correct muscles doing the job, then increase in repetitions and learn to make the movement more challenging.

Equipment needed week 1-4:

- *Exercise mat*
- *Back extension or Swiss ball*
- *Dumbbells*
- *Barbell with weights*
- *Hampton thick bar pad*

Weeks 1-4: Workout A
(perform on day one of workout week)

Date:_____ Weight:_____

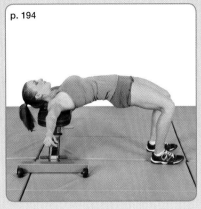

p. 194

Bodyweight hip thrust
—3 sets of 20 reps

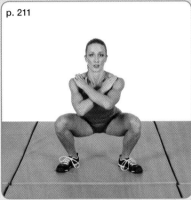

p. 211

Bodyweight full squat
—3 sets of 20 reps

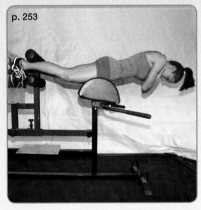

p. 253

Bodyweight back extension
—3 sets of 20 reps

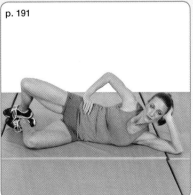

p. 191

Side lying clam
—1 set of 30 reps (each side)

Weeks 1-4: Workout B

(perform on day three of workout week)

Date:_____ Weight:_____

Bodyweight single-leg glute bridge
—3 sets of 20 (each side)

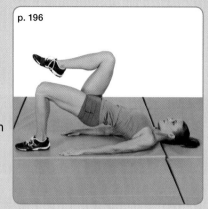

p. 196

Bodyweight walking lunge
—3 sets of 10-20 reps (each side)

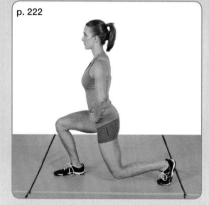

p. 222

Bodyweight reverse hyper
—3 sets of 20 reps

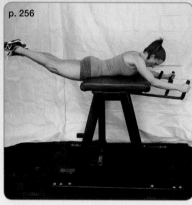

p. 256

Side lying abduction
—1 set of 30 reps (each side)

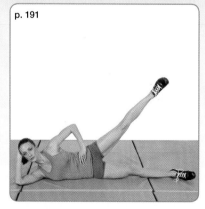

p. 191

Weeks 1-4: Workout C

(perform on day five of workout week)

Date:_____ Weight:_____

Barbell glute bridge
—3 sets of 10 reps

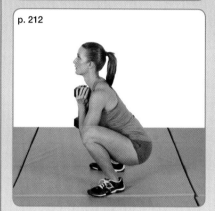

p. 198

Goblet full squat
—3 sets of 10reps

p. 212

Dumbbell Romanian deadlift
—3 sets of 10 reps

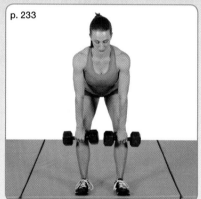

p. 233

Cable hip rotation
—1 set of 10 reps (each side)

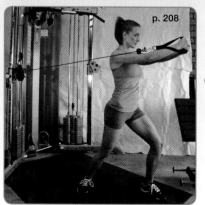

p. 208

Weeks 5-8: Workout A

(perform on day one of workout week)

Date:_____ Weight:_____

Equipment needed week 5-8:
- *Exercise mat*
- *Barbell with weights*
- *Dumbbells*
- *Cable with ankle cuff*
- *Band*

Barbell hip thrust
—3 sets of 8-12 reps

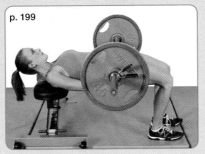

p. 199

Barbell front squat
—3 sets of 8-12 reps

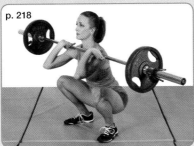

p. 218

Barbell Romanian deadlift
—3 sets of 8-12 reps

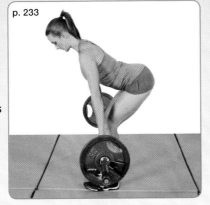

p. 233

Band seated abduction
—1 set of 30 reps

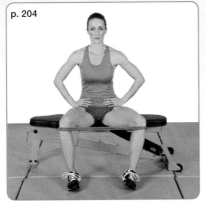

p. 204

Weeks 5-8: Workout B

(perform on day three of workout week)

Date:_____ Weight:_____

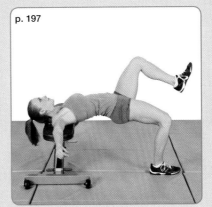

p. 197

Shoulders-elevated single leg hip thrust—3 sets of 8-12 reps (each side)

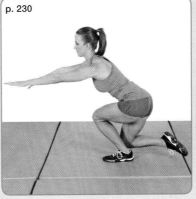

p. 230

Bodyweight skater squat
—3 sets of 8-12 reps (each side)

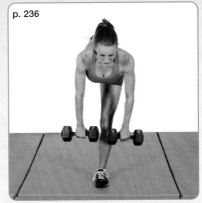

p. 236

Dumbbell single-leg Romanian deadlift
—3 sets of 8-12 reps (each side)

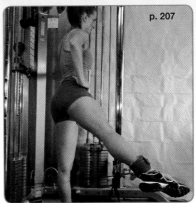

p. 207

Cable standing abduction
—1 set of 30 reps (each side)

Weeks 5-8: Workout C

(perform on day five of workout week)

Date:_____ Weight:_____

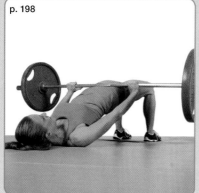

p. 198

Barbell glute bridge
—3 sets of 10 reps

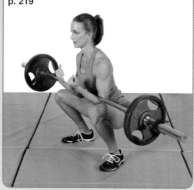

p. 219

Barbell Zercher squat
—3 sets of 10 reps

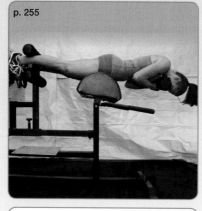

p. 255

Dumbbell back extension
—3 sets of 10 reps

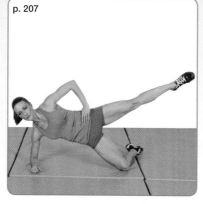

p. 207

Side lying hip raise
—1 set of 12 reps

Weeks 9-12: Workout A

(perform on day one of workout week)

Date:_____ Weight:_____

Equipment needed for week 9-12:

- Exercise mat
- Dumbbells
- Bench and plyometrics box, or short platform
- Barbell with weights
- Cable with Cook bar
- High plyometrics box
- Back extension
- Band
- Kettlebell

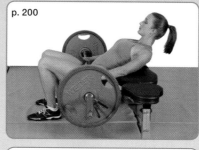

p. 200

Barbell American hip thrust (constant tension method)
—3 sets of 20 reps (nonstop)

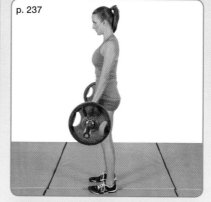

p. 224

Dumbbell deficit Bulgarian split squat
—3 sets of 12 reps (each side)

p. 237

Barbell American deadlift
—3 sets of 8 reps

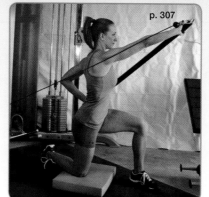

p. 307

Bar half-kneeling horizontal chop
—1 set of 15 reps (each side)

Weeks 9-12: Workout B
(perform on day three of workout week)

Date:_____ Weight:_____

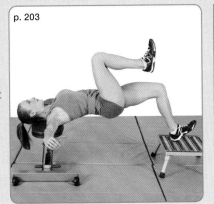
p. 203

Bodyweight shoulder and foot elevated single-leg hip thrust (pause rep method)
—3 sets of 6 reps (3 second pause at top, each side)

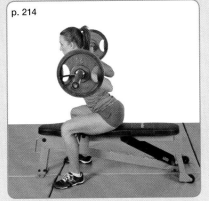
p. 214

Barbell high box squat
—3 sets of 6 reps

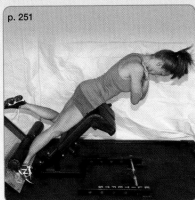
p. 251

Single-leg 45-degree hyperextension
—3 sets of 12 reps (each side)

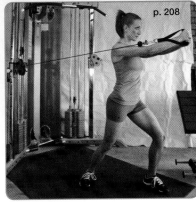
p. 208

Cable hip rotation
—1 set of 15 reps

Weeks 9-12: Workout C
(perform on day five of workout week)

Date:_____ Weight:_____

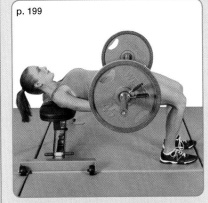
p. 199

Barbell hip thrust (rest pause method)
—3 sets of 10 reps (perform 6 reps, then 1, 1, 1, and 1)

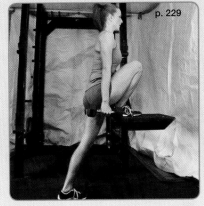
p. 229

Dumbbell high step up
—3 sets of 8 reps (each side)

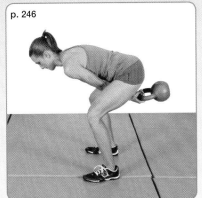
p. 246

Russian kettlebell swing
3 sets of 20 reps

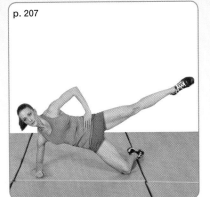
p. 207

Side lying hip raise
—1 set of 15 reps (each side)

Name:_____ Date:_____ Weight:_____

Exercise	Set 1	Set 2	Set 3
Bodyweight hip thrust 3 sets, 20 reps	Weight Reps	Weight Reps	Weight Reps
Bodyweight full squat 3 sets, 20 reps	Weight Reps	Weight Reps	Weight Reps
Bodyweight back extension 3 sets, 20 reps	Reps left Reps right	Reps left Reps right	Reps left Reps right
Side lying clam 1 set, 30 reps (each side)	Weight Reps		
Notes:			

Gorgeous Glutes (only) Workout B: Week 1-4 Training Log

Name:_____   Date:_____   Weight:_____

Exercise	Set 1	Set 2	Set 3
Bodyweight single-leg glute bridge 3 sets, 20 reps (each side)	Weight Reps	Weight Reps	Weight Reps
Bodyweight walking lunge 3 sets, 10-20 reps (each side)	Weight Reps	Weight Reps	Weight Reps
Bodyweight reverse hyper extension 3 sets, 20 reps	Reps left Reps right	Reps left Reps right	Reps left Reps right
Side lying abduction 1 set of 30 reps (each side)	Weight Reps		
Notes:			

Name:_____ Date:_____ Weight:_____

Exercise	Set 1	Set 2	Set 3
Barbell glute bridge 3 sets, 10 reps	Weight Reps	Weight Reps	Weight Reps
Goblet full squat 3 sets, 10 reps	Weight Reps	Weight Reps	Weight Reps
Dumbbell Romanian deadlift 3 sets, 10 reps	Reps left Reps right	Reps left Reps right	Reps left Reps right
Cable hip rotation 1 set, 10 reps (each side)	Weight Reps		
Notes:			

Name:_____ Date:_____ Weight:_____

Exercise	Set 1	Set 2	Set 3
Barbell hip thrust 3 sets, 8-12 reps	Weight Reps	Weight Reps	Weight Reps
Barbell front squat 3 sets, 8-12 reps	Weight Reps	Weight Reps	Weight Reps
Barbell Romanian deadlift 3 sets, 8-12 reps	Reps left Reps right	Reps left Reps right	Reps left Reps right
Band seated abduction 1 set of 30 reps	Weight Reps		
Notes:			

Gorgeous Glutes (only) Workout B: Week 5-8 Training Log

Name:_____ Date:_____ Weight:_____

Exercise	Set 1	Set 2	Set 3
Bodyweight single-leg hip thrust 3 sets, 8-12 reps (each side)	Weight Reps	Weight Reps	Weight Reps
Bodyweight skater squat 3 sets, 8-12 reps (each side)	Weight Reps	Weight Reps	Weight Reps
Dumbbell single-leg Romanian deadlift 3 sets, 8-12 reps (each side)	Reps left Reps right	Reps left Reps right	Reps left Reps right
Cable standing abduction 1 set, 30 reps (each side)	Weight Reps		
Notes:			

Name: _____ Date: _____ Weight: _____

Exercise	Set 1	Set 2	Set 3
Barbell glute bridge 3 sets, 10 reps	Weight Reps	Weight Reps	Weight Reps
Barbell Zercher squat 3 sets, 10 reps	Weight Reps	Weight Reps	Weight Reps
Dumbbell back extension 3 sets, 10 reps	Reps left Reps right	Reps left Reps right	Reps left Reps right
Side lying hip raise 1 set, 12 reps	Weight Reps		
Notes:			

Name:_____ Date:_____ Weight:_____

Exercise	Set 1	Set 2	Set 3
Barbell American hip thrust (constant tension method) 3 sets, 20 reps	Weight Reps	Weight Reps	Weight Reps
Dumbbell deficit Bulgarian split squat 3 sets, 12 reps (each side)	Weight Reps	Weight Reps	Weight Reps
Barbell American deadlift 3 sets, 8 reps	Reps left Reps right	Reps left Reps right	Reps left Reps right
Half-kneeling anti-rotation press 1 set, 15 reps (each side)	Weight Reps		
Notes:			

Name:_____ Date:_____ Weight:_____

Exercise	Set 1	Set 2	Set 3
Bodyweight shoulder and foot elevated single-leg hip thrust (pause rep method) 3 sets, 6 reps (3 second pause at top, each side)	Weight Reps	Weight Reps	Weight Reps
Barbell high box squat 3 sets, 6 reps	Weight Reps	Weight Reps	Weight Reps
Single-leg 45-degree hyper extension 3 sets, 12 reps (each side)	Reps left Reps right	Reps left Reps right	Reps left Reps right
Cable hip rotation 1 set, 15 reps (each side)	Weight Reps		
Notes:			

Name:_____ Date:_____ Weight:_____

Exercise	Set 1	Set 2	Set 3
Barbell hip thrust (rest pause method) 3 sets, 10 reps (6 reps, 1,1,1, and 1)	Weight Reps	Weight Reps	Weight Reps
Dumbbell high step up 3 sets, 8 reps (each side)	Weight Reps	Weight Reps	Weight Reps
Russian kettlebell swing 3 sets, 20 reps	Reps left Reps right	Reps left Reps right	Reps left Reps right
Side lying hip raise 1 set, 15 reps (each side)	Weight Reps		
Notes:			

Chapter 14:

Living the *Strong Curves* Life

Now that you are well on your way to developing *Strong Curves*, it's time to learn how to fit exercise into your lifestyle. One of the largest setbacks women face when implementing a new workout program is finding the time to do it. The great thing about *Strong Curves* is that it doesn't take up a ton of space on your busy calendar. In fact, you can see amazing results in as little as three hours per week. Considering that you have about seventy-two non-sleeping, non-working hours during your week, this is only a small fraction of that.

Okay, so it isn't reasonable to think that those seventy-two hours aren't busy. In fact, you probably feel like you barely have time to breathe during your week. At the end of a hectic day, all you want to do is sit down with a good book or your favorite TV program. Maybe you don't even have time for that because you spend the evening at swim or piano lessons, baseball practice, PTA, and many other family-related activities.

Regardless of how busy you are, it's important to set aside a few hours for exercise. If you don't give yourself that luxury, you will fall into the trap of being too tired to work out. This lack of energy is actually caused by lack of exercise. It's a perpetual cycle that many people fall into, but the only way to get out of it is to start moving.

You may feel that adding a few workouts to your schedule is selfish because you're leaving your kids at home or in the gym childcare center. Your laundry might go unfolded, or your dishes may stay dirty for an extra hour that evening. Maybe on workout nights, you serve leftovers rather than a meal from scratch. I promise this is not a big deal to anyone but you. Going to the gym is not selfish. Taking that extra time during your week to nurture your body improves your quality of life. There is a huge difference between exercise obsession and healthy exercise. Three hours per week is a far cry from obsession. To be healthy, you should exercise at least three hours per week. My female clients have come to me countless times with stories of improved energy, decreased cravings, greater moods, enhanced sex lives, better relationships with their loved ones, and amazing self-confidence. In fact, improved self-esteem, confidence, mood, and attitude rival the gains in physique enhancement, strength, and health.

As far as I can see, this is a winning situation for everyone who cares about you. Your partner will thank you for being more pleasant to be around and spending more time between the sheets. Your kids will thank you for having more energy to play and for enjoying life a little more. Your boss will thank you for being sharper and more focused at work. Your friends will thank you for being an inspiration. Everyone has so much to gain when you turn to a healthy lifestyle—especially you.

I stated earlier that you only need three hours per week to see great improvements. I usually like for my clients to invest between three and six hours a week in their workouts, depending on their goals. My athletes train more often, but my clients who are looking to just improve their physiques invest those three hours. If you think this is too little time to make changes, you've probably been talking to someone who slaves away at the gym because he or she thinks it's the only way to get results. Trust me, this is counterproductive. Spending too much time training will decrease your energy, destroy your hormonal balance, and actually work against you over time.

The *Strong Curves Program* is very flexible to fit your needs. If you can only train twice a week, do it. If you can only train for thirty minutes five times per week, work it into your schedule. *Strong Curves* has no defined rule that you must train on specific days for specific amounts of time. The most important aspect of this entire program is that you are strength training multiple times per week while hammering away at the best glute exercises. And when you work on this program, you do so with your best effort.

The only thing holding you back from your success on this program is your own limitations. I've noticed many women begin training once or twice a week just to get involved with exercise. Then within a few months, they up it to three or four times per week. Next thing I know, they are signing up for races, preparing for figure competitions, or taking an interest in powerlifting. They start craving bigger and better challenges because the bar rises each time they set a personal record. Strength training is nothing short of empowering. You will see your greatest potential when you start squatting, hip thrusting, and deadlifting better each week—all while maintaining those amazing curves.

Kellie's Quick Tips: *After competing in my second figure competition, I took the time for a self-evaluation. I started competing for what I thought were the right reasons, but I realized that I was achieving my goals the wrong way. I over-trained. I ate too little. I obsessed about food constantly. I didn't want my "ideal self" to get in the way of my real self and knew that I was going down a path that was taking me further from my goal—optimum health and wellness. Essentially, I needed to stop letting the perception of a fit lifestyle control me.*

So, I came up with a personal philosophy to which I adhere to this day:

- *My body is the reward for my hard work. I don't work hard to build the ultimate body.*
- *I love my body. I eat to nourish it, to build and repair tissue, to improve the function of my vital organs, to provide energy for my day, and to increase my longevity. I do not eat to deprive, to malnourish, to obsess, or to damage my body.*
- *Training is a habit. It is a part of who I am. I go to the gym as part of my daily routine and do not alter my life around my gym schedule.*

Once I shifted my focus from going for a certain look to achieving a certain level of health and well being, everything changed. My energy improved because I wanted to eat for my health. My strength increased because I was eating better. In turn, my physique transformed because my strength and diet were better.

You must develop a symbiotic relationship with everything involved in this program in order to achieve the best results. Of course, you want the perfect butt, a slimmer physique, and a nice tapered waist. But if that's all you focus on, you become obsessed. Focus on the right things—a strong immune system, balanced hormones, greater confidence, and fewer health issues, and everything else will fall into place.

Family and Your Fit Lifestyle

One of the most valuable things you can do for your family is to get them involved in a fit lifestyle. This doesn't mean that everyone needs to follow the *Strong Curves* plan (although that would be awesome!) Incorporating your daily fitness and nutrition practices into your family rituals will make a huge difference, however. Still, this is sometimes easier said than done. Humans are creatures of habit and convincing your family to change might be as easy as extracting a tooth. So, here are a few tips to help you get started:

Nutrition

Don't take away what they love, but encourage them to try new things: If your husband or partner loves beer and pizza during his football game, don't switch it to lemon water and baby mixed greens with chicken. Rather than turning him completely off before he even tries a healthy diet, teach him what you learn and how it will make a difference. He is far more likely to jump on board if it's his idea rather than yours. Oh, and when he does decide to opt for the salmon and broccoli rather than ribs and fries, don't ever say, "I told you so." Just let him think he took the initiative.

Get your kids involved in a way that is enjoyable: If your kids see a plate of green beans and grilled skirt steak on the dinner table, they might tape their mouths shut. If they get involved from the start they will enjoy and appreciate their food more. Take them along to the market with you, and let them pick out the items. Get them involved in making the menu. Once you get home, have them put the groceries away and help prepare dinner. Another great way to get your kids involved is to find cookbooks and chef's utensils especially for them. If your kids make the salad, stir the rice, and season the chicken, they are going to want to enjoy the fruits of their labor.

Order first, and your friends will follow: You will often find that when dining out with friends, if you take the lead, they will follow. Order your healthy meal before anyone else at your table has a chance to speak up. Once your friends hear that you are eating well, they may opt for the salmon salad rather than the cheeseburger.

Fitness

Find activities that you enjoy together: If your partner can't stand the thought of the gym, find something you both love. Mountain biking, jogging, kayaking, or other outdoor activities are a great way to bond over fitness. If your gym offers more than just weights and aerobics classes, see if he will join you. Many gyms have basketball courts, racquetball courts, pools, and tennis courts. It's very likely that once he sees your transformation, he will want to know what *Strong Curves* is all about. I've coached many women whose partners started showing up for their own training sessions after they watched their wives or girlfriends squat and deadlift their own body weight.

Get out and play with your kids: Don't be the mom who sits on the bench at the park. Get out there and play! Start a game of tag, hop on the swings, or glide across the monkey bars. Not only is it great exercise, but it's also good for the your inner child. Acting like a kid decreases your stress levels and helps you bond with your children more. If your children are teens, there's no reason not to drag them along with you to the gym. Both Kellie and I had gym memberships by age fifteen, and we've been going ever since.

Invite your friends along: Set up meetings with your friends at the gym. If they aren't interested in strength training, take a class with them. Even walks on the beach or strolls through the park are great ways to get your friends into fitness. Also, buying your friends a copy of *Strong Curves* will encourage them to start strength training. After seeing your success on the program, they will beg you for your secrets.

Build a community of fit females: It's amazing to see the recent movement in female fitness. Women from all over the globe are joining together to spread the message of strength and wellness. Why not join them? Online communities through social media and forums are a great way to find fit-minded friends.

When Ugly Habits Creep Back In

The *Strong Curves Program* forces you outside of your comfort zone. After being on the program for a few weeks, you will realize its positive effects on your life. You'll get rid of ugly habits and replace them with healthy ones, but bad habits can sometimes creep back in when you least expect them. Something stressful may happen that sets you back, causing you to revert to your old comforts. You might skip a workout and stay home. You might reach for the ice cream rather than the carrots when you feel stressed out. We all do it from time to time, but your ability to recognize when ugly habits reappear will help you stop them dead in their tracks.

The most important thing to remember is that tomorrow is always a new day. If you eat something off your diet plan, miss a workout, or train with less intensity one day, don't let it get you down. That's when habits form. We all deserve a break sometimes, and minor slip-ups are not going to ruin your progress. They may even help you. But if you let these minor incidents turn into daily occurrences, you have to sit back and reevaluate your purpose. You must ask yourself, "Self, do you want perky, strong glutes?" Of course, you do! "Self, do you want incredible energy and a great mood?" That would be a resounding yes. Whether your slip-up was for one day, an entire week, or even longer, don't let it ruin your progress. Just get up, dust off your blues, and get back in the saddle to start where you left off.

Keep yourself motivated by being your own greatest

advocate and pep coach. If things get too ugly, turn to a fitness friend or contact Kellie and me so that we can get you back on the right track. No one wants you to succeed on this plan more than we do.

Handling Criticism

Most people will be supportive of your fitness endeavors, but occasional stragglers will do anything to bring you down. From the office bully to the gym rat who hands you a pair of pink dumbbells, these downers come from all walks of life and creep up on you at the most inopportune times. There's nothing like a rude comment to ruin your good mood. If this happens, just ask yourself if that person's opinion is more important than your success. Also, try not to take things personally. Usually, someone's criticism has more to do with them than it has to do with you.

Just for a good laugh, here are some common comments my clients and female colleagues have heard over the years:

"Just one cookie won't hurt you."

"Why do you take things so seriously?"

"I can't believe you have to eat and train the way you do for competition."

"You are so lucky to be in such good shape."

"You are so disciplined; I don't know how you do it."

"Why can't you just live a little?"

"You look too skinny. Is everything okay?"

"If you keep working out that way, you're going to look like a man."

"I can't wait for your diet to end so that you're normal again."

"How can you eat that way? Don't you miss good tasting food?"

"It isn't healthy to eat that way all the time."

"Once you stop working out, your muscles just turn to fat anyway."

"Eating that much fat will clog your arteries."

"Your organs will shut down with all of those vitamins you take."

"You lost all of your boobs when you lost weight."

"I'm worried about you. You hardly eat."

"I just want to enjoy my life and not be so serious all the time."

"Why don't you just run like normal women do?"

"You're obsessed!"

"One day away from the gym isn't going to kill you."

How many of those statements are positive and supportive? None of them. But if these women were to let the words of others get under their skin, they wouldn't be the powerhouses they are today. I encourage you to use harsh criticism as fuel to push you harder and drive you closer to your goals. You aren't striving to meet the standards that everyone else sets for you. Create your own standards, and never allow others to discourage you from achieving what you set out to do.

And remember that you can "splurge" a bit now and then if you want. Let's say you have a catered party, ballgame, or movie coming up. You can have some dessert, a hot dog, or popcorn as long as you work it into your daily allotment of calories and macronutrients. Just don't eat as many calories, fats, and carbohydrates during the day. This will serve as one of your two to three "free" meals for the week. But only do this if you desire; don't feel the need to conform do others' expectations just to fit in.

Loving the New You

The *Strong Curves Program* will provide the most incredible transformation both inside and out. You will develop incredible strength that most people think is impossible for women. You will shed pounds of fat while adding pounds of lean muscle. Curves will form from head to toe, giving you the most enviable shape imaginable. Your energy will skyrocket, your mood will greatly improve, you will sleep better, have better sex, and improve your relationships with your loved ones. And that's just the froth on the latté.

What goes on inside when you add the *Strong Curves* strength training program to your weekly lifestyle is nothing short of amazing. You will notice your aches and pains going away. Your heart health, brain function, and metabolism will improve. You will look and feel years younger and have the ability to perform tasks that were once too difficult (like pick up something that weighs as much as you).

The *Strong Curves Program* will also improve your self-esteem and emotional well being. Often, you don't realize how much our appearance affects how we feel about ourselves. But the stronger you become, the more confident you will feel because as your strength increases, your body composition will change to what you have always desired. I can't tell you how many of my female clients say, "You'd be so proud of me, I can now carry all of my bags of groceries up the stairs" or "I can finally make it up the entire mountain without my back hurting," or, "Bret, the other day I was dead-lifting more than the guy next to me."

The benefits with *Strong Curves* are only limited to what you believe is possible. You may begin the program just to get in shape but soon realize that you want more than a smaller dress size. So, never stop striving toward bigger and better goals because the sky is the limit for you with regard to strength training and fitness. Many of the women you admire in fitness today started out in the same place as you. In fact, most of them struggled with weight issues, unhealthy food relationships, and lack of exercise before they embarked on their fitness endeavors. Just like the women on the covers of fitness magazines, you can change your life for the positive if you believe anything is possible.

One thing you need to promise yourself is to never stop improving upon your health. Initially, when you start your journey with *Strong Curves*, you will have superficial intentions (don't worry; we all do). You may just want to lose ten pounds, drop two dress sizes, or finally have a round butt. That's perfectly fine. There is nothing wrong with wanting a better body. Kellie and I both started out with this exact goal and still work toward aesthetic goals along with strength goals. Just make sure your goals are concrete and defined.

Just saying you want to lose weight isn't enough. How much weight? How long will you give yourself? Start small, and build from there. Once you reach that goal, keep going. I hope that when you achieve the body you want, you'll strive toward athletic feats. Most women I know started out wanting a better body, but now the body is just a reward for meeting other goals. My friend, Nia Shanks, a fitness professional and competitive powerlifter, is currently working toward deadlifting three times her own bodyweight (she will probably have this accomplished by the time *Strong Curves* is published). That is no small feat, and most men can't come close to doing this. If you talked with Nia about strength training, her looks would never come up in the conversation. She is a lean, mean powerhouse stacked with perfect muscles, but her body maintains this look because she is constantly striving toward bigger athletic goals. After strength training and eating a diet rich in whole foods for a while, the physique is just second nature.

Final Thoughts from Kellie: *We both feel honored that you invested in the* Strong Curves *Program. We truly believe you will succeed if you take to heart the material provided in these pages.*

Just as we did while writing Strong Curves, *you will face many trials and triumphs along the way to a sexier, more vibrant you. When you face each trial—whether it's giving up junk food, learning to love your body, or stepping into the gym for the first time—remember to celebrate that end goal when you reach it.*

As women, we spend so much time thinking about how far we have to go and neglect to appreciate how far we've come. Give yourself the gift of recognizing just how amazing you are, whether you lost two pounds or added five pounds to your squat. Understand how powerful that is, and use it as fuel to achieve even greater things. Neither Bret nor I would be who we are if we didn't celebrate our successes. We want that for you, too. Stay strong. Stay beautiful. Stay true to yourself.

GLOSSARY

Here are some terms and concepts that you should know. Understanding these definitions and methods will allow you to create better programs, use better form, and achieve better results.

Activation. Muscle activation can be determined by EMG (see below for a definition of EMG). Some muscles fire more readily than others, and the glutes are a stubborn muscle group that tends to shut down in sedentary individuals. For this reason, it is beneficial to include "activation exercises" or simple, low-load exercises to "reeducate" the glutes and get them firing properly during movement.

Active Insufficiency. When a bi-articular (two-joint) muscle is shortened on one end, the amount of tension it can create is diminished due to the sub-optimal muscle length. This applies to the hip thrust exercise. During the hip thrust, the hamstring muscle is shortened due to the bent-knee position throughout the movement. Since the hamstring can't produce optimum force during the hip thrust, the gluteus maximus must take over and produce increased force to make up for the weakened hamstrings.

Adaptive Shortening. If a muscle is placed in a shortened position for sufficient time, it will adapt by decreasing in length. Chronic sitting places the hip flexor muscles in a shortened position, which causes them to decrease in length over time. Tight hip flexors are not conducive to proper gluteus maximus function.

Anterior Pelvic Tilt. A majority of the population is in anterior-pelvic tilt (APT). This means that their pelvises are tilted forward. In other words, the top of the pelvis is shifted forward while the bottom of the pelvis is shifted rearward. This can interfere with proper gluteal functioning. Some portions of exercises, such as the bottom of a deadlift, should be performed with a slight anterior pelvic tilt. It isn't easy to modify posture, but proper strength training is a powerful stimulus for posture improvements if good form is consistently adhered to.

Auto-Regulation. Some days, you will feel great, have sufficient energy, and your body will feel very strong. Other days, you will feel drained and weak. It's important to "auto-regulate" or adjust your workout according to "biofeedback" by listening to what your body is telling you. You should always go to the gym with a plan in mind, but this plan is not set in stone since there will be days when you will ramp things up or scale things down depending on how you feel. Don't force a personal record to happen by using sloppy form. When you're not feeling up to the task, ease up, and you'll rebound quickly.

Biofeedback. Your body will give you signals that are indicative of how your body is functioning at the moment. Your psychological state, how much stress you're under, how much sleep you received, what foods you consumed, and how fatigued you are from previous workouts combine to determine your "readiness." Some days you'll be ready, some days you'll be really ready, and other days you won't be ready to achieve amazing training sessions.

Compensation. When strength, stability, or mobility is impaired during movement, the body will attempt to execute the pattern by compensating at other joints or with other muscles. From a survival standpoint, this is a good thing (for example, if you're trying to escape from being trapped under a heavy object), but from a safety standpoint, it's a bad thing. Let's say you lack hamstring flexibility (and, therefore, hip extension mobility) and you try to perform a heavy deadlift. Your body will inevitably round at the lumbar spine in order to "compensate" for the lack of hamstring flexibility, as this is the only way to get into position to hoist the barbell. This places your lower back at considerable risk, which is why optimal form via ideal levels of mobility, stability, and motor control is paramount.

Concentric Contraction. A concentric action requires that the muscle contracts with sufficient force to shorten the muscle. For example, when you're at the bottom of a squat and you rise to a standing position, you performed the concentric portion of the movement since the glutes and quadriceps went from stretched to normal lengths.

Constant Tension Method. The constant tension method is valuable for the barbell hip thrust exercise. Here's what you do: First, make sure you load the barbell with smaller plates—twenty-five pounders maximum. This way, there won't be a gap at the bottom of the movement where you're not under any tension. Now, start performing your set. Pump out your repetitions in piston-like fashion, moving up and down at a fast and steady pace while moving through a full range of motion. You'll use higher rep ranges for this method—for example, twenty reps. At fifteen reps, your muscles will burn very badly, but you'll make sure to squeeze out an extra five reps so that you reach twenty non-stop reps where the tension on the glutes never diminished throughout the set.

Density. When you pack a training session full of activity and don't rest very much, the session is "dense." In my experience, women are much better than men in terms of being able to tolerate dense training sessions. They can push themselves very hard on a set and move right into the next exercise or next set without resting much. While it's important to have dense workouts, remember that resistance training shouldn't mimic non-stop circuit training. You do need to rest in between sets in order to allow for recovery if you want to build maximum strength and curves.

Dynamic. Dynamic is another term for "moving." Dynamic exercises require motion in contrast to static exercises, which require motionless holds. For example, a sit-up is a dynamic core exercise, while a plank is a static core exercise. Some exercises require dynamic and static muscle actions. For example, a push-up or chin-up require dynamic shoulder and scapular motions combined with simultaneous static lumbar and pelvic actions.

Eccentric Contraction. An eccentric action requires that the muscle contracts while the muscle is elongated. For example, when you lower yourself from a standing position to the bottom of a squat, you perform the eccentric portion of the movement since the glutes and quadriceps contract while the muscles are forcibly lengthened.

Electromyography. Electromyography or EMG examines the level of neural activation received by the muscles. I have conducted many EMG experiments which have given me a good idea as to which exercises activate the specific portions of the glutes the best. In general, the greater the activation, the greater the active tension on the muscles.

Endurance. Performing high repetitions along with "dense" workouts will build muscular endurance and stamina.

Energy Leaks. When the body can't maintain proper position in an exercise, certain muscles will fail in their endeavors to stabilize joints and will be forced into "eccentric contractions" or active-lengthening actions due to insufficient strength. Think of the knees caving in a squat (upper glutes failing to stabilize and falling into eccentric contractions), or the lower back rounding in a deadlift (erector spinae failing to stabilize and falling into eccentric contractions).

Exercise Progressions. When a certain movement becomes too easy, you should increase the difficulty in order to continually challenge the muscles. You can do this by using more weight or performing more reps, but another way is by moving on to a more challenging exercise progression. For example, you can increase an exercise's range of motion by performing deadlifts or reverse lunges off of a step (creating a deficit), or you can increase an exercise's lever arm by placing the arms overhead in a back extension (prisoner position), for example, or performing an ab wheel rollout from the feet rather than from the knees.

Exercise Regressions. When an exercise is too challenging to allow for proper execution, it is necessary to regress the exercise in order to allow for the mastery and motor learning of sound movement patterns. You must master bodyweight in a squat before placing a bar on your back. You must be able to hip hinge before holding onto a bar in a deadlift. You must master bodyweight hip thrusts before loading up with a barbell. You can regress by using smaller ranges of motion, less loading, or shortening the lever arms.

Flexibility. Flexibility refers to the muscles, specifically how much they can lengthen. For example, in order to deadlift properly, the hamstrings need to possess sufficient flexibility.

Frequency. Training frequency can refer to how many days you train per week or how many times you hit a particular movement or muscle group per week. The glutes can handle far more frequency than most people assume. In my experience, training the glutes three to five times per week is ideal, and four days per week is probably optimal for most.

Gluteal amnesia. Due to technological advances, we're forced to sit most of the day. For these reasons, our glutes have shut down, and most individuals are left with a thin slab of glute muscle that doesn't activate well. This has been appropriately coined "gluteal amnesia." Modern times have made us forget how to use our glutes!

Hip Abduction. The gluteus maximus has many roles, and one of these is to abduct the hip or move the hip straight out to the side. Hip abduction is a unique movement that requires activation of the upper gluteus maximus muscle in order to carry out the motion (the gluteus medius is heavily involved as well). During hip abduction exercises, the mid and lower gluteus maximus don't receive much activation. An example of hip abduction is a side lying hip abduction or a standing cable hip abduction. Even a side plank requires an isometric upper gluteal contraction to maintain hip abduction (or better yet, to prevent eccentric hip adduction from occurring). The same mechanism is required during gait to prevent the opposite hip from sagging.

Hip Extension. The most popular role of the gluteus maximus is hip extension, which involves moving the thigh rearward in relation to the hip or moving the hip forward in relation to the leg. The most popular glute exercises are all hip extension movements such as squats, lunges, deadlifts, and hip thrusts, which all involve hip extension. So does sprinting and jumping. Individuals are stronger in hip extension at deeper ranges of hip flexion (for example, the bottom of a squat) because the adductors are heavily involved in this zone,

and the gluteus maximus contributes to the strength of this zone due to its activation (active contribution) and considerable stretch (passive contribution). But the gluteus maximus actually has much better leverage on the hip joint at end ranges of hip extension (for example, the top of a hip thrust), and this is also the zone that receives maximum neural activation. For these reasons, a variety of hip extension exercises are necessary for optimal gluteal performance.

Hip External Rotation. A highly underrated role of the gluteus maximus is hip external rotation, which involves rotating the hip outward (sometimes called lateral rotation). The gluteus maximus is highly activated during this motion, and exercises such as cable hip rotations—in addition to sporting motions such as throwing, swinging, and striking—require sound gluteal functioning to properly execute the movement pattern. The gluteus maximus has excellent leverage on the hip to carry out external rotation. Unfortunately, lifters rarely include hip rotation exercises in their programs. A side lying clam is a basic beginner hip external rotation movement.

Hip Hyperextension. When the hip extends past neutral position, hip hyperextension occurs. This is a natural motion that occurs during gait. Sadly, many modern humans lack sufficient hip hyperextension mobility because their hip flexors have shortened from so much sitting. This is why it's important to include hip flexor stretches and mobility drills during the warm-up to prevent losses in hip extension mobility over time. The gluteus maximus has excellent leverage for hip hyperextension and is highly activated in this zone, which is why it's important to squeeze the glutes extra hard to rise sufficiently during glute bridges, hip thrusts, and back extensions.

Hip Transverse Abduction. Hip transverse abduction is an interesting joint action. It takes place when the hips are flexed forward (think of a squat position), and it requires outward movement on the thighs in relation to the hips. The band seated hip abduction exercise trains this motion dynamically, but it is trained statically every time you perform the squat exercise. While the hips are extending, the gluteals and deep hip external rotators exert force to keep the knees out and prevent valgus collapse.

Hypertrophy. Muscle hypertrophy is synonymous with muscle growth. There is a strong science to hypertrophy, and I went into great detail when I discussed this topic earlier in the book. There are different types of hypertrophy. Sarcomeric or myofibrillar hypertrophy involves the growth of the contractile elements that are required for increased force production. Sarcoplasmic hypertrophy involves the growth of the non-contractile elements such as the sarcoplasm and organelles inside the cell that help feed the contractile elements during movement. Both types of hypertrophy are required for maximal shape and curves. In general, for maximal hypertrophy, you want to utilize the shotgun approach and make sure you induce ideal levels of muscle damage, pump up the muscles, and place a ton of tension on the muscles through a variety of exercises, rep ranges, and methods.

Intensity. There are two types of intensity—intensity of load and intensity of effort. Intensity of load refers to the amount of weight you use in reference to your maximal strength. If your one-rep max is one hundred thirty-five pounds and you're using one hundred twenty-five pounds for your set, your "intensity of load" is quite high. Intensity of effort refers to how hard you push a set or a session. If you push yourself to failure on a particular set, your "intensity of effort" is quite high.

Iso-Hold Method. The iso-hold method is also valuable for the barbell hip thrust exercise. Simply raise the barbell to full extension, and hold the top position for time (for example, thirty seconds). Make sure your low back and pelvis stay in neutral and that your glutes are pushing the hips upward and preventing the pelvis from tilting rearward throughout the set. Make sure also that your feet stay planted firmly on the ground.

Isometric Contraction. An isometric action requires that the muscle contracts with just enough force to keep the muscle at a constant length. Sometimes, isometrics are referred to as "static holds," since there is no movement occurring at the joints. An example of an isometric contraction was described directly above for the "iso-hold method."

Lumbar Flexion. When the low back rounds, lumbar flexion occurs. This is not to be confused with lumbar extension, which is the opposite motion. During most gluteal movements, you want to learn to lock up the spine and move mostly at the hips. The pelvis will move

a bit, but you definitely don't want the spine to move through a significant range of motion during resistance exercise, as this can be damaging to the spine. In the case of lumbar flexion, the intervertebral discs are exposed to considerable risk if too much range of motion under load is reached. For example, losing the low back arch during a heavy deadlift is very dangerous.

Lumbar Hyperextension. When the low back arches past its normal position, lumbar hyperextension occurs. Lumber extension is the opposite of lumbar flexion, but lumbar hyperextension occurs when you keep extending past neutral position. This is dangerous for the spine as well. During certain lower body movements, hip hyperextension is fine, but make sure this isn't accompanied by lumbar hyperextension since it places the posterior parts of the spine at risk. For example, repeatedly hyperextending the spine during back extensions could be problematic over time, which is why you should always rotate around the hips via hip extension, not around the low back via lumbar extension.

Lumbopelvic-Hip Complex. The lumbopelvic-hip complex or LPH complex involves the lumbar spine, pelvis, and hips. The LPH is an intriguing unit that works together to produce coordinated movement, and various exercises require strategies to increase the gluteal contribution as well as the safety of the movement. For example, during deadlifts, you want very slight lumbar extension and very slight anterior pelvic tilt at the bottom of the movement. At the top of the movement, however, you want very slight lumbar flexion and very slight posterior pelvic tilt. This is a controversial topic, but this practice places more of the loading on the strong gluteal muscles and spares the spine. In general, anterior pelvic tilt and lumbar extension are related to each other, and posterior pelvic tilt and lumbar flexion are related to each other as the lumbar spine and pelvis are intimately linked.

Mechanical Tension. The most important aspect of hypertrophy (and, therefore, booty-building) is mechanical tension. The more tension you place on the muscle, the better. There is active tension created through muscle contractions, and there is passive tension created through stretch. Dynamic exercises combine both of these types of tension to produce maximum hypertrophy. For optimal results, it's important to perform exercises that induce maximal tension on the muscle and also place the muscle under considerable "time under tension" (TUT). Some exercises are better suited for maximally activating muscles, and some exercises are better suited for maximally stretching muscles, which is why it's important to perform a variety of movements.

Metabolic Stress. When you train a muscle, it creates metabolic stress. In fact, there are a lot of different metabolic mechanisms occurring in the muscles while you lift weights. Chemicals such as calcium, lactate, IGF-1, and cytokines will increase in concentration in the muscles, the muscles will start to swell, and oxygen deprivation will occur. These mechanisms can all lead to hypertrophy, which is why it's important to perform bodybuilding-type methods rather than just power-lifting-type methods. For example, higher rep ranges, lower rest periods, and advanced methods such as the constant tension and rest-pause method can all increase metabolic stress.

Mind-Muscle Connection. Your results are highly dependent upon your ability to formulate an intense mind-muscle connection. If you want your glutes to improve in shape, you had better learn to activate them maximally on call and during all types of movements. You can perform all the right exercises, but if you're not activating your gluteus maximus, it will not change in shape. Each exercise requires strategies for achieving maximal gluteal activation and tension.

Mobility. In contrast to flexibility, which only involves the muscles, mobility is the range of motion achieved during dynamic movement. This requires muscular contractions and often involves the interplay of multiple joints. For example, you can lie down on your back and lift a straightened leg to determine passive hip flexion range of motion (a good indicator of hamstring flexibility), or you can perform a Romanian deadlift to determine your active hip flexion range of motion (a good indicator of hip flexion mobility). Developing proper levels of mobility requires whole body coordination and joint stability, which is why it's critical to control exercises through full ranges of motion and perform athletic training methods.

Motor Control. The way the human body moves is highly complex, and our movement patterns are dependent upon habits, flexibility, mobility, stability, coordination, and efficiency. For example, most individuals pick something off the ground by flexing their ankles,

knees, hips, and spine. This is a cost-effective approach to carrying out the movement. During weight-training, however, we're interested in the safest and most effective movement strategies. This is why we teach people to deadlift heavy weight by keeping the spine relatively neutral while moving mostly at the hips. This requires increased gluteal and hamstring strength in addition to increased lumbar spine and pelvic stability. Furthermore, it isn't as efficient in terms of energy demands since it requires more energy (rounding the back requires less muscle activation because the spinal ligaments provide passive force when they are stretched), but it's much safer and more effective for muscle-building. As you increase your flexibility, mobility, strength, and stability, you will need to coordinate these qualities into your motor programming, and this is why you must always focus on using excellent form.

Muscle Damage. Resistance training creates microscopic damages in the muscle fibers, and this damage forces the muscles to grow back stronger through multiple mechanisms. The goal is not to annihilate the muscles and induce maximum soreness. Just a touch of soreness is good, which indicates that you adequately worked, stretched the fibers, and displayed adequate variety in your programming. Too much soreness can compromise recovery, prevent you from achieving personal records, and prevent you from progressively overloading the muscles.

Neural Drive. Not all gains in performance are related to muscle hypertrophy. The neuromuscular system has two components—the nervous system and the muscular system. Muscles will grow stronger and improve in shape, but as you continue to train, your ability to activate the muscles will improve dramatically as well. Over time, you want to be able to clench your glutes to maximal voluntary contraction at will. Many individuals are good at activating their glutes from a certain position but lack the ability to achieve impressive glute activation from other positions or movements. Well-rounded gluteal functioning requires optimal muscle activation in all movement patterns that require gluteal muscle contribution. This is why it's important to perform activation drills and focus on sound technical form during every repetition.

Neutral Spine. The concept of a "neutral spine" is a bit nebulous because there are multiple segments in the spine, and people exhibit varying degrees of spinal posture depending on their anatomy, previous injuries, strength levels, and motor control. Many people live in lumbar extension or lumbar flexion, which is not optimal. Ideally, low back posture would be relatively neutral (not extended or flexed), but regardless, we always want to maintain safe postures when resistance training. When core muscles contract, they produce considerable compressive forces on the spine. If the spine is kept relatively neutral, it can easily tolerate these forces. If the spine is flexed forward or extended rearward, however, the compression can become deleterious, and the more flexed or extended the spinal posture, the more potential for damage. For this reason, it's important to move at the hips and not so much at the spine during various gluteal exercises.

Pause Method.
The pause method is yet another advanced method for barbell hip thrust performance. It can also be used during other exercises such as back extensions, full squats, or deficit reverse lunges. Simply pause for time at the most difficult portion of the repetition for a predetermined period of time (for example three or five seconds). In the hip thrust and back extension, this means you'll hold the top portion of the movement, but in the full squat and reverse lunge, you'll hold the bottom portion of the movement.

Posterior Pelvic Tilt.
A final role of the gluteus maximus that is often overlooked is posterior tilting of the pelvis. Sometimes, you want to actively posterior-tilt the pelvis during exercise—for example, during the RKC plank and the American deadlift. Other times, you want to engage the posterior tilting mechanism just to prevent the pelvis from "energy leaking" or moving into eccentric anterior pelvic tilt—for example, at the top of a hip thrust or back extension. There are still other times when you want to avoid posterior pelvic tilting as much as possible by engaging the anterior tilting muscles—for example, the erector spinae. An example of this is the bottom of a full squat; the pelvis will want to tilt posteriorly, which is accompanied by lumbar flexion. At the bottom of a squat or deadlift, this is a terrible idea. Some individuals live in posterior pelvic tilt (PPT) due to their flexed lumbar spinal posture (PPT and lumbar flexion are related). This is exhibited by a flat-backed appearance where the top of the pelvis is pulled rearward and the bottom of the pelvis is pulled forward. While it's difficult to improve posture, proper strength training can and does do so. This is why it's important to learn and practice proper form.

Power.
Power can be thought of as force multiplied by velocity or as work divided by time. This means that you can improve power by increasing force capabilities at the same velocity, by increasing velocity capabilities at the same levels of force, by increasing the amount of work conducted during the same period of time, or by decreasing the time it takes to perform a certain amount of work. Think of power as the ability to "explode." Resistance training can improve power by increasing the rate (speed) at which you develop force (called RFD or rate of force development) and by improving coordination and movement efficiency or by improving neural output (decreasing inhibiting neural mechanisms and increasing potentiating mechanisms). For this reason, training the glutes tends to dramatically improve your power.

Progressive Overload.
If you want to achieve results from strength training, you need to keep doing more over time. This is coined "progressive overload," and there are many ways to improve as time ensues. Some ways in which you can overload the muscles as time passes are lifting heavier weights over time (for the same number of repetitions), performing more repetitions over time (with the same weight), improving form, increasing the speed of execution, using less rest time in between sets (while performing the same amount of work), and increasing your range of motion during movements (while using the same weight for the same number of reps). The caveat is that you cannot achieve any of this "progress" through form degradation. Sound program design will allow for progressive overload over the long haul.

Reciprocal Inhibition.
When a muscle is short or tight, a neural phenomenon will cause it to inhibit the opposing (antagonist) muscle. Some muscle groups possess reciprocal relationships (for example, the gluteus maximus and hip flexors). Excessive sitting is bad for the glutes because it induces shortening of the hip flexors, which subsequently decreases gluteal muscle firing and prevents the hips from extending sufficiently. This is why it's important to perform stretches, mobility drills, and full range of motion strengthening exercises for the hips.

Rest Pause Method.
The rest-pause method is a final advanced method for barbell hip thrust performance and is valuable for the deadlift exercise as well. To perform the rest-pause method, simply select

a heavy weight. Perform as many repetitions as possible (six reps, for example), rest for a certain period of time (say, ten seconds), perform a couple more repetitions (say, two more reps), rest for a certain period of time (say, twenty seconds), and perform a couple more repetitions (say, two more reps). In this manner, you'll be able to extend the set and increase the set's effectiveness.

Stability. You can possess sound flexibility, but if you don't have appropriate joint stability, your mobility will be impaired. In other words, your body won't allow your muscles to sufficiently stretch due to the perceived dangers associated with joint instability. This is a natural protective mechanism because your nervous system doesn't want you to injure yourself. Therefore, mobility is not always limited by flexibility, but by joint stability. For example, you may have sound passive hamstring flexibility but not be able to perform full range deadlifts due to impairments in lumbopelvic stability. Your core stability won't allow you to achieve appropriate depth. Optimal movement requires sufficient muscle flexibility and joint stability. This is why it's important to perform core stability exercises and learn and practice proper strength training technique. Moreover, there are different types of stability such as whole body balance/proprioception and dynamic joint stability.

Static. Static is another term for "isometric" and involves holding a motionless position. A plank is an example of a static exercise because there is no joint motion during the exercise's performance. During certain movements, some muscles function statically while others function dynamically. For example, the upper and lower traps, in addition to the serratus anterior muscles, help stabilize the rotation of the scapulae during a push-up to allow for proper scapulohumeral rhythm. As you can see, the neuromusculoskeletal system and human movement are quite complex!

Strength. Strength is the ability to produce force. In general, force is equal to mass multiplied by acceleration. Therefore, if you can accelerate a heavy load via muscular activity, you possess strength, which is what builds shape. If you want to build an impressive backside, you must continue to strengthen the glutes over time by progressively overloading the muscles and setting personal records.

Synergistic Dominance. When a muscle lacks sufficient strength, muscles that help out that muscle in various motor patterns (called synergists) take over and contribute what's needed to execute the movement. If you have "gluteal amnesia" and try deadlifting or sprinting, your hamstrings will work double duty during hip extension since your gluteals won't be able to produce much force. This explains why weak glutes lead to muscle pulls and tears in the synergists (such as the hamstrings and groin muscles) during hip extension. Often, lifters must focus on activating their glutes during bridging motions as their hamstrings dominate the motion (which often leads to cramping). Strong glutes prevents synergistic dominance of the hamstrings, groin, hip external rotators, and many other muscles.

Use/Disuse Theory. You've probably heard the term, "use it or lose it." This applies to human movement, and many individuals go through life rarely activating their glutes to sufficient degrees. Many individuals get out of bed, walk around a bit, sit for most of the day, walk a little bit, and go back to bed. At no point does glute activation reach more than thirty percent of maximal capacity. The glutes then begin to shut down and atrophy (shrink). If it took you ten years to lose your glutes, you won't build them back in a week. Building *Strong Curves* requires persistence, so be patient.

Valgus Collapse. Knee valgus or valgus collapse is very common in today's world. When people jump, squat, land, and even walk, their knees tend to cave inward. Some coaches characterize a typical newcomer's squat form as "the melting candle" effect because the joints appear like a melting candle as they cave inward. Valgus collapse is usually caused by weak glutes. It's very important while exercising to make sure the knees track over the mid-toes, as valgus collapse leads to patellofemoral (knee) pain if left unchecked.

Volume. Volume is typically determined by the number of sets and reps you perform. A high-volume routine employs a variety of exercises with a high number of sets and repetitions. You can train long or hard, but not both. For this reason, it's important to maintain a proper balance of volume and intensity during your training sessions.

Joint Articulations:

Abduction. Lateral movement away from the midline of the body. Example: Moving the thigh outward with the hip straight.

Adduction. Medial movement toward the midline of the body. Example: Moving the thigh inward with the hip straight.

Extension. Straightening the joint resulting in an increased angle. Example: Moving the thigh backward when it's flexed forward.

Flexion. Bending the joint resulting in a decreased angle. Example: Moving the lower leg toward the back of the thigh.

Internal Rotation (aka Medial Rotation). Rotary movement around the longitudinal axis of the bone toward the center of the body. Example: Turning the upper arm inward.

External Rotation (aka Lateral Rotation). Rotary movement around the longitudinal axis of the bone away from the center of the body. Example: Turning the upper arm outward.

Transverse Abduction (aka Transverse Extension). Lateral movement away from the midline of the body. Example: Moving the thigh outward with the hip flexed.

Transverse Adduction (aka Transverse Flexion). Medial movement toward the midline of the body in a horizontal plane. Example: Moving the upper arm toward and across the chest with the elbows facing out to the sides.

STRONG CURVES

CURVES

A WOMAN'S GUIDE TO BUILDING A BETTER BUTT AND BODY

Self-Myofascial Release

Purpose: Foam rollers resemble something we used to joust with our siblings when we were kids, but self-myofascial release (soft tissue work) has quickly become a staple in exercise programs. This type of work on your muscles isn't limited to the use of a foam roller. Tennis balls, golf balls, sticks, lacrosse balls—and for the brave, even PVC pipe—are a few other tools you can use to improve muscle tissue quality.

You can think of foam rolling or soft tissue work with these tools as a poor man's (or woman's) massage. Your daily lifestyle takes a pretty good toll on your muscles, even when you sit all day and while you're sleeping. Your muscles might feel tight and swollen after a good workout or tense and achy when you work at your desk all day. Sometimes, you may even wake up barely able to rotate your neck back and forth.

Self-myofascial release, which I'll call SMR, alleviates all of these issues in just a few short minutes a day. Unless you're lucky enough to have an on-site massage therapist eager to work on those muscles, it's a good idea to keep at least one, if not all of these SMR tools, in your house.

The first question you probably have is, "Why am I doing this, again?" One theory is that adhesions and scar tissue buildup in the muscles as a result of strength training, and SMR helps to remove the adhesions and fibrotic tissue. Perhaps you've noticed that some areas feel knotted up and tender from strength training. Indeed, "trigger points," which are really just hyperac-tive and tight spots in the muscle that elicit miniature spasms, can wreak havoc on surrounding areas in the body. For example, trigger points in the upper glutes can refer pain or lead to alterations in movement, and that is never a good thing. SMR can alleviate trigger points and help restore natural muscle function.

A final theory is that the tension placed on the muscles when performing SMR causes the mechanical receptors found between muscles and tendons to send out inhibitory signals, which facilitates relaxation and allows them to stretch further.

Even though these theories lack scientific support, we can't ignore the countless number of lifters who swear that SMR helps them. Foam rolling is an excellent way to improve the quality and tone of your muscles. As resistance training builds the muscles, SMR will help to keep them pliable and smooth. A relaxed muscle should feel like water, not like a bag of marbles. So, you can think of foam rolling and the other SMR techniques offered in this book as cheaper, less talkative, and more convenient alternatives to daily massage therapy.

Medicine Ball Chest and Front Shoulder

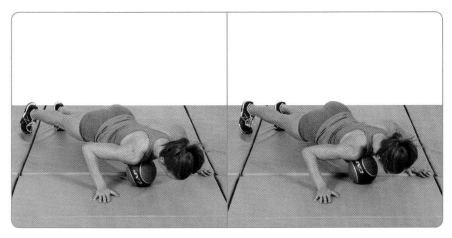

1. Lie on the floor face down, or stand facing a wall. Place a medicine ball, tennis ball, or lacrosse ball at the top of your chest.
2. Push your chest into the ball while supporting most of your weight with your arms and lower body.
3. Roll in a circular motion, going from the middle of your upper chest over the front of your shoulder.
4. If you find a tender spot, hold the ball in place for a few seconds to get extra release.

Medicine Ball Upper Glutes

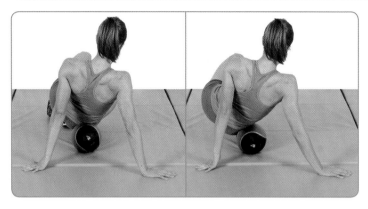

1. In a seated position on the ground, place the medicine ball, tennis ball, or lacrosse ball under one hip.
2. Support most of your weight with your hand behind you and your feet planted on the floor.
3. Roll back and forth over the top part of your butt, hitting the upper and upper-outer glutes from multiple angles.
4. This tends to be very tender with lots of trigger points for women. If you find a sore spot, hold the ball in place for a few extra seconds.

Golf ball Foot (Plantar Fascia)

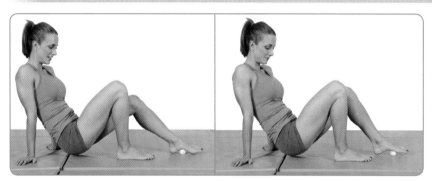

1. In a seated or standing position, place a golf ball, tennis ball, or lacrosse ball on the ground next to your bare foot.
2. Supporting your weight, place the sole of one foot on the ball.
3. Roll the ball back and forth along the entire bottom of your foot, pressing into the ball for increased pressure.

Stick SMR Work (Tibialis Anterior, Calves, Quadriceps, TFL)

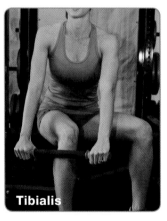 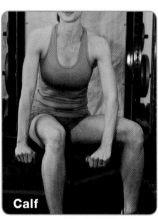 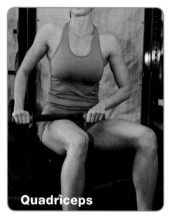 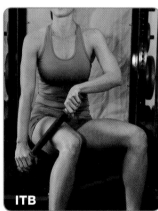

Tibialis **Calf** **Quadriceps** **ITB**

Before you rush out into your backyard and break a tree branch, go out and get The Stick Muscle Massager or a Tiger Tail Rolling Muscle Massager. You will go through far fewer Band-Aids. I like to group this all together because you're using the same motion with each drill, while working on different muscles.

1. Sit on a bench, and place the stick on the front outer part of your lower leg with your palms facing inward.
2. Roll the stick up and down your lower leg along the muscle just outside the shin bone.
3. Do this for the back of your calf muscle, the top front of your thigh, the outer part of your thigh, and the inner part of your thigh.
4. Roll the stick over the entire length of the muscle. For instance, if you're working the outer part of your thigh, start at the hip, and work down to your knee joint.

A foam roller is a fun gadget to keep in your home. It can easily travel with you to the gym or office. I recommend keeping some SMR tools at your work desk or in your gym bag. Balls and sticks are probably best for these environments since they store in small spaces, though smaller foam rollers are available.

Foam rollers come in various densities based on your level of experience and tolerance. Softer foam rollers are great for beginners or those with sensitive muscles. The denser foam rollers work well for those who have been practicing SMR for a while and need to up the intensity.

Always remember that you don't need to be in excruciating pain while doing these exercises. Some pain is fine, but don't overdo it. Foam rollers alone are pretty good workouts because you're using your entire body to manipulate over them. Go at your own pace, and slowly increase the amount of pressure and intensity you spend working with them each week. You don't need to spend all day long rolling around. Just five to ten passes over a muscle is sufficient.

Foam Roller SMR Work — Calves

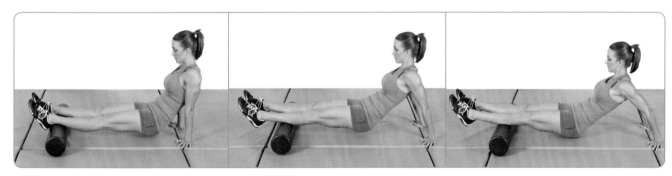

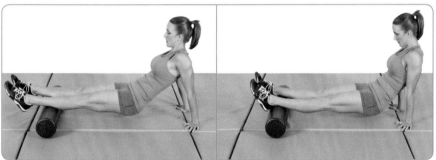

1. Sit on the ground with your legs straight and with the bottom of your calves draped over the foam roller.
2. Supporting yourself with your arms, lift your hips off the floor.
3. Lock your knees, and roll back and forth from your ankles all the way up to your knee joint.
4. Put pressure on the middle, inside, and outside portions of your calves as you move by turning your feet in and out to cover the entire calf area.
5. To increase pressure, cross one leg over the other, and roll only the bottom leg. Then, repeat with the other leg.

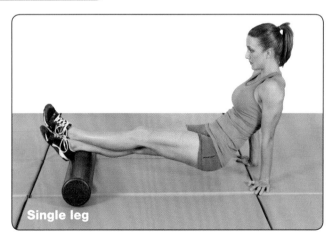

Single leg

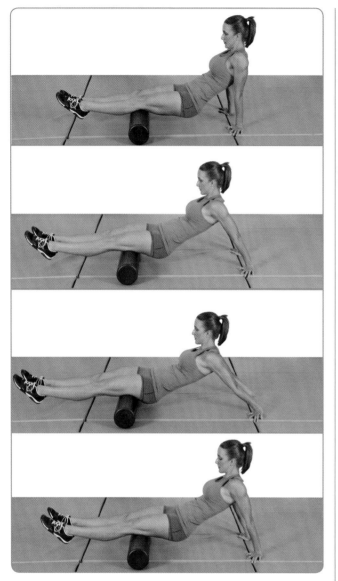

1. Sit on top of the foam roller with your hands on the floor behind you and your feet in front of you.
2. Roll back, keeping your hips off of the floor, until you come to the top of your knee joint.
3. To increase pressure, cross one leg over the other, and roll only the bottom leg. Then, repeat with the other leg.

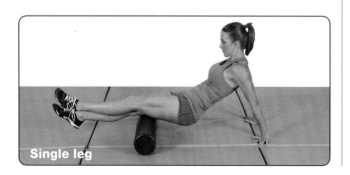

Single leg

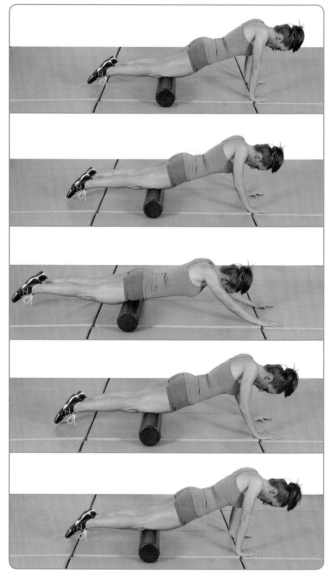

1. Lie facing down with the foam roller beneath your hips.
2. Support your body with your hands on the floor, and keep your feet elevated off the ground.
3. Roll forward, moving the foam roller from the tops of your thighs to the tops of your knees.
4. To increase pressure, cross one leg behind the other, and roll only the bottom leg. Repeat with the other leg.

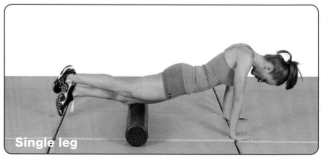

Single leg

Foam Roller SMR Work
Outer Thigh (IT Band)

Foam Roller SMR Work
Inner Thigh (Adductors)

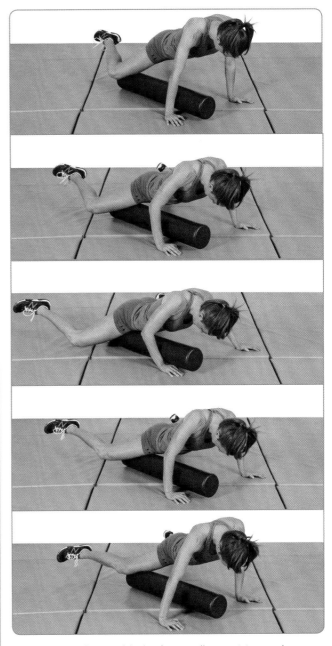

1. Lie on your side, placing the foam roller underneath the outer part of your thigh.
2. Rest on your bottom elbow, using your top hand and foot for support.
3. Press up and roll back over the outer part of your thigh.
4. You may need to reposition from top to middle and then the middle to lower portion.
5. The tissue surrounding the IT band is often knotted up and painful to roll. Take it slowly, and ease into the exercise over time.

1. Lie facing down with the foam roller next to you in a parallel position.
2. Place one leg over the roller so that you are lying over it with the roller positioned at the top inner part of your thigh.
3. Support your upper body with your hands planted on the floor.
4. Press up and roll back and forth over the inside portion of your thigh.

Foam Roller SMR Work
Back (Erector Spinae)

Foam Roller SMR Work
Sides of Back (Latissimus Dorsi)

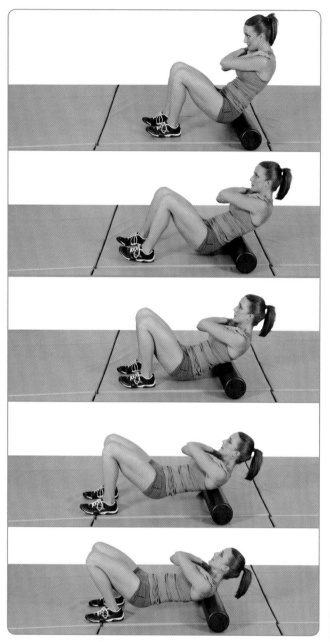

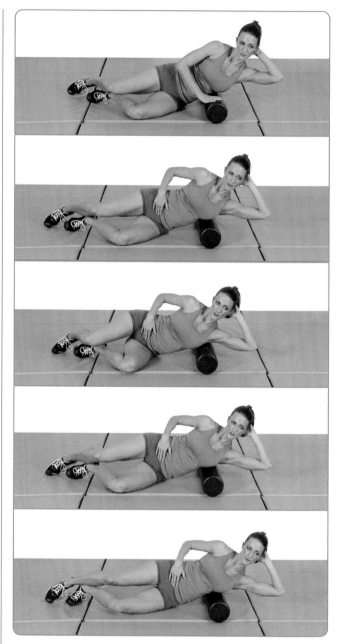

1. Sit on top of the foam roller with your feet planted on the floor and your hands behind your head or arms across your chest.

2. Roll forward, walking out with your feet.

3. The foam roller should move over your low back and up your middle back toward your shoulder blades toward the upper back.

4. Lean to one side to increase the pressure as you roll up and down.

1. Lie on your side with the foam roller under your armpit and your bottom arm straight at an angle above your head.

2. Use your top hand to support your weight while keeping your feet and butt on the floor.

3. Move the roller up and down the outer portion of your upper back.

4. Rotate your arm up to stretch the outer back muscles.

Static Stretches

If SMR improves the tone and texture of your muscle tissue, static stretches improve the *tolerance* of your muscles to stretch. We all learned static stretches as kids when we counted at the tops of our lungs during gym class, so you are probably familiar with the ones used in the *Strong Curves* warm-up programs.

Single-Leg Hamstring Stretch

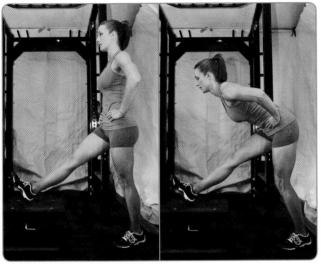

1. Place your foot on top of a chair or bench, keeping the elevated leg straight.
2. Maintaining a neutral spine with your hands on your hips, lean into the elevated leg until you feel tension in the hamstrings.

Double-Leg Hamstring Stretch

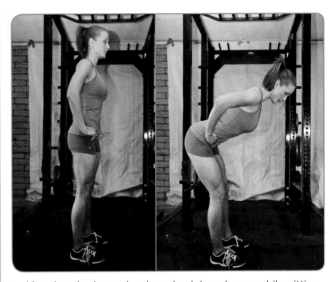

1. Keeping the lower back arched, bend over while sitting back.
2. Descend until your hamstring flexibility "runs out" and hold for time.

Thigh Stretch (Quadriceps)

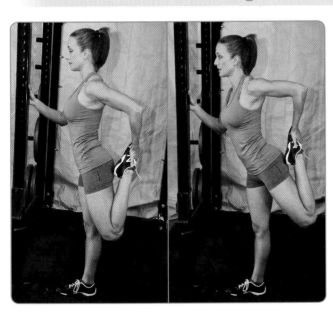

1. Stand next to a support with your weight on one leg and one hand holding the support.
2. Bend the non-weight-bearing leg back, holding your foot in your free hand.
3. Pull your foot toward your butt while squeezing the rear glute and maintaining an upright position.
4. You should feel the stretch mostly in the rectus femoris (middle upper thigh).

Single-Arm Chest Stretch
(pectoral muscles)

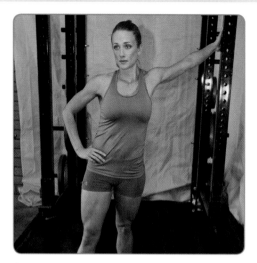

1. Stand at an angle facing away from a support.
2. Reach one arm back, grasping the support at head level.
3. Pull just enough to feel tension in your chest muscles.

Single-Arm Back Stretch
(Latissimus dorsi)

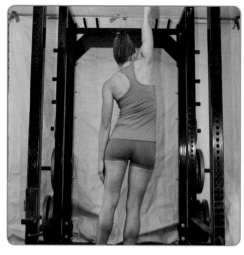

1. Reach overhead, grabbing a bar support with one arm.
2. With your feet planted on the floor, lean in the direction of the stretched arm, and sink down into the stretch.
3. You should feel the stretch in your lats.

Double-Arm Back Stretch

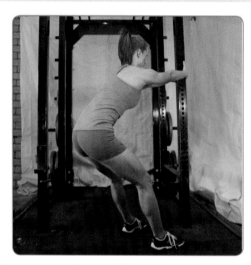

1. Grab a support in front of you.
2. Lean back, and spread your shoulder blades apart to stretch the upper back muscles, namely the mid-traps and rhomboids.

Single-Leg Calf Stretch

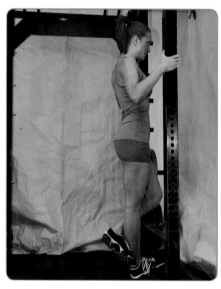

1. Stand on an elevated support with one foot, placing the other foot over your standing ankle.
2. Holding the support, lower your body down while keeping your leg straight to get a good stretch in the calf muscles.

Standing Inner-Thigh Stretch (adductors)

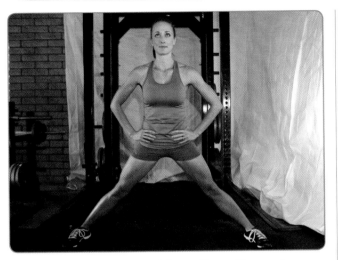

1. Place your legs in a straddle position with your toes facing forward.
2. Slowly slide down, and spread the legs apart further and further while maintaining upright posture with your hands on your hips until you feel tension in the adductors.

Flexed Inner-Thigh Stretch (adductors)

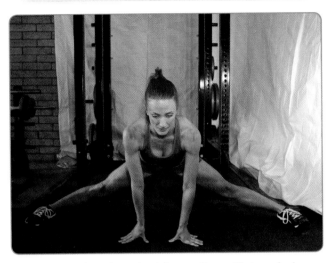

1. Place your legs in a straddle position with toes facing forward.
2. Lean over so that your torso is parallel to the floor, supporting your upper body with your arms.
3. Slide down, and spread the legs apart further and further until you feel tension in the adductors.

Child's Pose

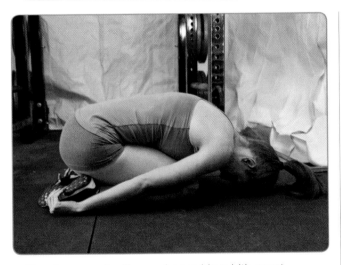

1. Kneel on a mat with your knees hip-width apart.
2. Lean forward, draping your body over your thighs until your forehead rests on the floor.
3. Reach your arms behind you along your sides, feeling a stretch in the lower back muscles.

Cobra

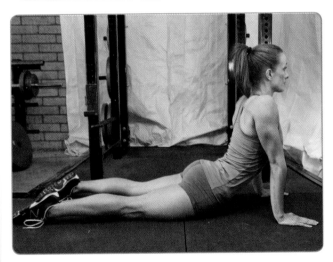

1. Lie face down with your hands and shoulders in the bottom of a push-up position.
2. With the hips staying in contact with the ground, point your feet downward, and very slowly push your torso up as far as you feel comfortable.
3. You should feel the stretch in the abdominals.

Mobility

You probably took mobility for granted while growing up. Everything came with ease. You could squat down to pick up a toy or slide under a fence. You squeezed into tiny spaces for hide and seek without grunting. Now, you may find yourself picking up toys with your toes and taking the easy route with regard to playing with your kids.

Mobility is joint-related movement, and the mobility drills in this book work to improve movement within the ankles, hips, and thoracic spine. The topic of mobility was discussed in depth in Chapter Four. Feel free to refer back to that section for more detail on the importance of mobility.

Rocking Rectus Femoris

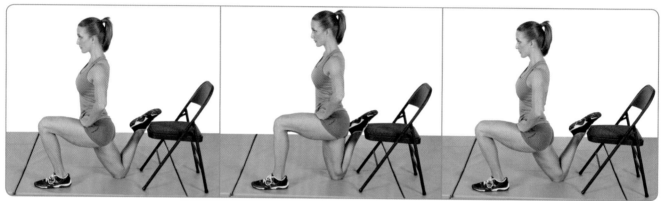

1. From a half-kneeling position, place your back foot on a chair or bench.

2. Lean back so that your butt touches your heel, while remaining upright and squeezing the rear glute.

3. Lean forward, bringing your knee over your front ankle and your butt away from your back heel.

Rotational Squat

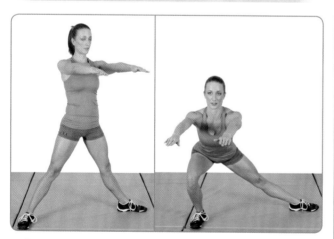

1. Stand in a straddle position with toes pointed out and arms straight out in front of you.

2. Rotate right into a side lunge position, but rather than shifting the body to the side, sink the hip into the stretch by rotating inward on the leaning side.

3. Return to the starting position and repeat on the left side.

Scap Wall Slide

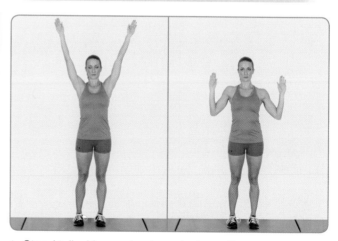

1. Stand tall with your back against a wall.

2. Raise your arms overhead in a Y position with palms facing out.

3. Keeping contact with the wall without bending your wrists, slide your arms straight down into a W formation as deep as you can without coming off of the wall.

This drill increases shoulder mobility.

Deep Lunge with Rotation

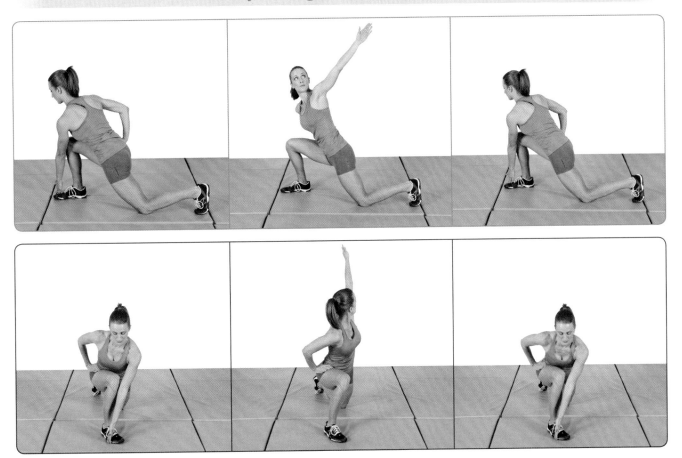

1. Drop down into a deep half-kneeling position, aligning your right knee over your ankle.
2. Rotate forward and inward, bringing your left hand to your right toe with palms facing in.
3. Rotate upward and outward, reaching up while opening your chest.

Squat to Stand

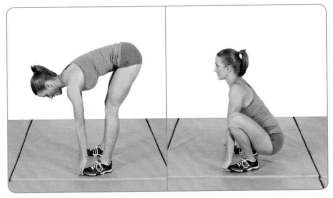 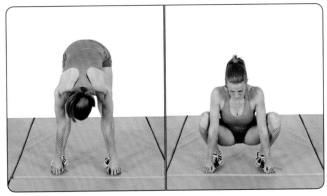

1. Stand with your feet hip-width apart. Lean down, and grab your toes while keeping your back as flat as possible.
2. Squat straight down as deep as you can go, forcing the knees out while holding your chest up.
3. Stand straight up, holding the front of your toes if possible until you feel a big stretch in the hamstrings.

Walking Knee Hug

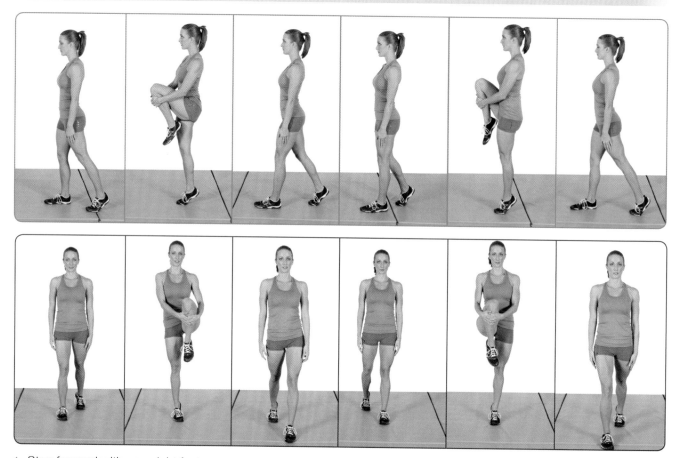

1. Step forward with your right foot.
2. Bring your left knee up toward your chest while rising up on the ball of your right toe.
3. Stand tall, grab your left knee with your hands, and pull it into your chest. Squeeze the rear glute at the same time.
4. Continue walking forward, alternating knees.

This will increase your hip flexor flexibility and hip flexion mobility.

Rocking Psoas

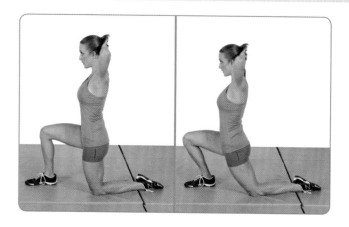

1. Drop to a half-kneeling position with your hands behind your head.
2. Lean forward, moving your knee past your ankle until you feel a good stretch in the front of your back hip.
3. Squeeze the rear glute, and keep a tall chest throughout the set.

This drill increases your hip flexor flexibility and hip flexion mobility.

Hip Hinge with Dowel

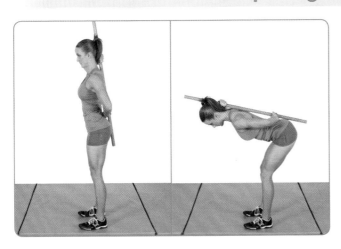

1. Stand with feet shoulder-width apart.
2. Run a dowel along your spine; and grasp the top behind your neck and the bottom near your low back.
3. Bend forward at the hips with a slight knee bend.
4. Sit back, moving at the hips, not the spine.
5. Keep the dowel in contact with your head, middle back, and top glutes throughout the duration of the movement.
6. Alternate hand positions between sets.

This drill teaches you how to sit back and move at the hips while keeping your spine stable.

YTWL

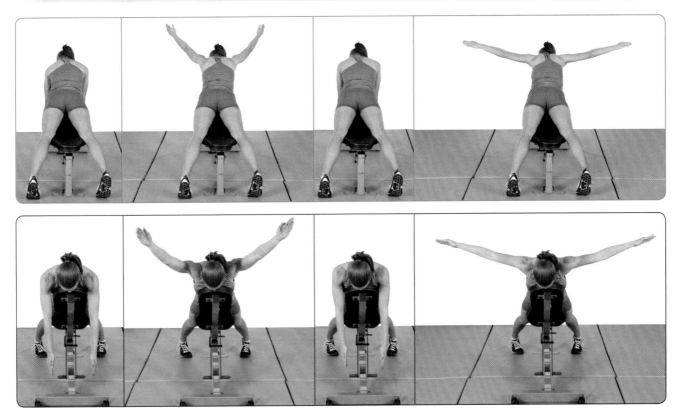

1. Lie face down on a bench with your legs fully extended to support your weight.
2. Extend your arms straight down in front of you with palms facing in.
3. Move your arms up overhead into a Y position, keeping your palms facing in and thumbs pointed upward. Lower back down and repeat ten times.
4. Return to the starting position. Raise your arms straight out to the side in a T position with palms facing the floor. Repeat ten times.

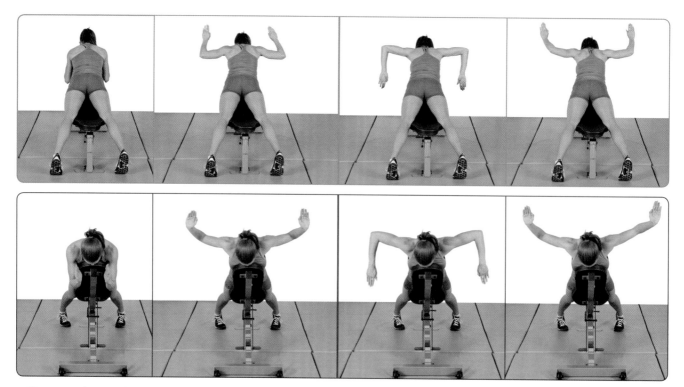

5. From starting position, flex your elbows, bringing your hands near the top of the bench. Keeping your arms in this position, raise them to the sides by squeezing the shoulder blades together. Repeat ten times.

6. From the top of the previous position with the elbows out, rotate your shoulders upward so that your upper arms are in line with your torso. Repeat ten times.

This drill will activate the mid and lower traps, the rear delts, and the shoulder external rotators.

Quadruped Thoracic Extension Rotation

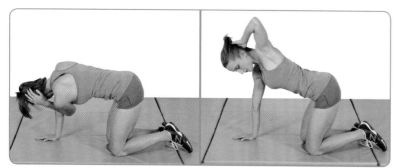

1. Get on all fours with your arms straight under your shoulders, your knees hip-width apart, and your back flat.

2. Place your right hand on the back of your neck, and rotate your elbow inward.

3. Extend and rotate your upper back by moving your elbow outward.

4. Repeat for 6 reps, and repeat on the opposite side.

Dowel Ankle Mobility Drill

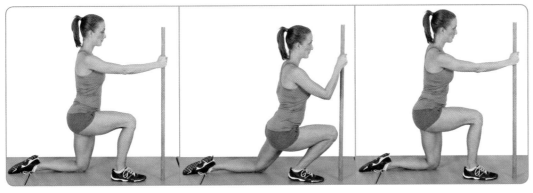

1. In a half-kneeling position with your right knee up, hold a dowel vertically out in front of your toe.
2. Lean into the dowel pushing your knee toward the dowel.
3. Repeat on both sides.

Wall RDL

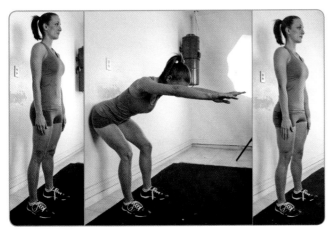

1. Stand with your feet hip-width apart about two feet out from the wall.
2. Place your hands on your hips, sit back, and bend at the hips by trying to stretch the hamstring.
3. Return to the starting position, and repeat for 6-8 reps.

Wall RDL with Rack

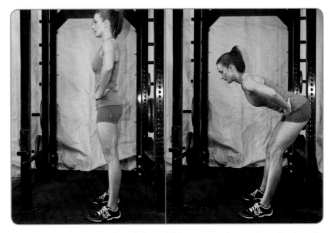

1. Stand with your feet hip-width apart about two feet out from the rack.
2. Place your hands on your hips, sit back, and bend forward until your butt touches the rack behind you.
3. Relax your knees by slightly bending them, but most of the movement should come from your hips.
4. Return to the starting position, and repeat for 6-8 reps.

Hip Internal Rotation

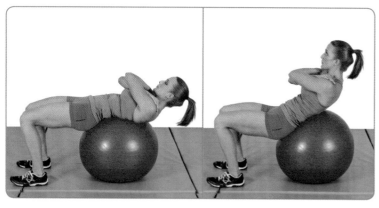
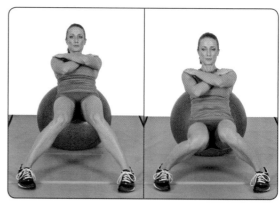

1. Lie on a Swiss ball with your feet planted on the floor and arms crossed over your chest.
2. Walk your feet out to the side while keeping your knees facing forward.
3. Your knees will cave inward, which is the opposite of what you want for a squat.

4. Roll forward, and sink down into the hips.
5. Roll back to starting position, and repeat for 6-8 reps.

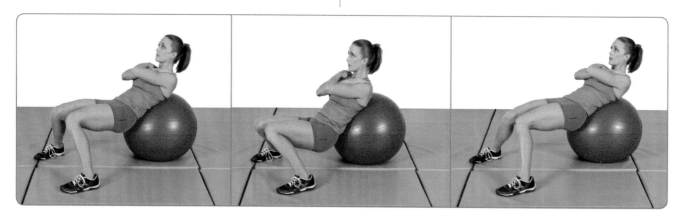

Reaching Single-Leg RDL

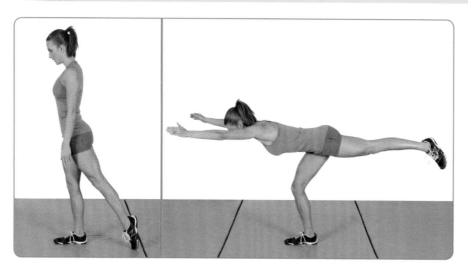

1. Stand on your right foot with your knee slightly bent.
2. Sit back, and bend over at the hips.
3. As you bend forward, move your arms directly out in front of you, and raise your back leg to create a straight line from your fingertips to your left toes.
4. Repeat for 6-8 reps, and repeat on the opposite leg.

Activation

Muscle activation drills help prime your muscles for the workload they are about to take on. Imagine baking a cake without preheating the oven. It would take far longer, and your cake wouldn't turn out quite right. Activation drills prep your body in the same way that preheating the oven preps for baking.

Activation drills target muscles that are prone to inhibition, which means that they shut down by receiving distorted or no neurological input. The body contains many muscles, and some muscles tend to fire incredibly well throughout life, while others tend to shut down and weaken if not consistently activated. Everyday life requires us to activate our quads and calf muscles, but muscles like the gluteus maximus aren't highly activated throughout the course of your day. Performing these activation drills regularly will prevent their tendency to shut down and help them fire optimally throughout your daily activities.

When performing activation drills, focus on quality, not quantity. A strong woman might be able to perform one hundred non-stop bodyweight glute bridges, but when performing activation drills, she will only perform about ten repetitions with the goal of highly activating the glutes and minimizing the activity of the erector spinae and hamstrings during the movement.

Bird Dog

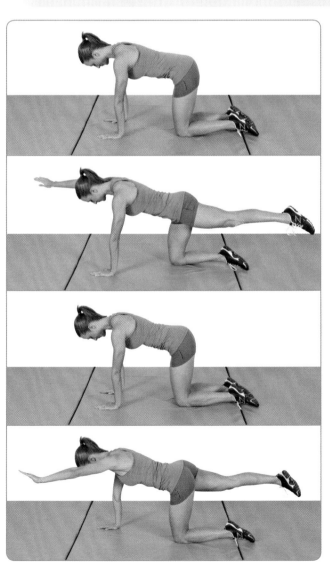

1. Get on all fours with your arms straight under your shoulders, your knees hip-width apart, and your back flat.
2. Raise your right arm and left leg up.
3. Avoid shifting from side to side or twisting laterally.
4. Stabilize your core while moving at the hips and shoulders only.
5. Lower back down, and alternate to the left arm and right leg.
6. Perform 6-8 reps on each side.

This drill **activates the gluteus maximus muscle.**

Fire Hydrant

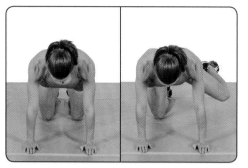

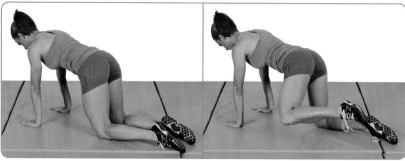

1. Get on all fours with your arms straight under your shoulders, your knees hip-width apart, and your back flat.
2. Keeping your knee bent, raise your right leg out to the side to a height that allows you to keep your shoulders and pelvis parallel to the floor.
3. Return to the starting position, and repeat for 6-8 reps before switching sides.

This drill activates the hip external rotators and upper glutes.

Quadruped Hip Extension

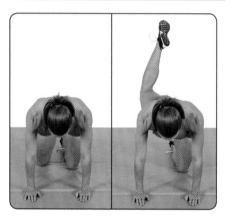

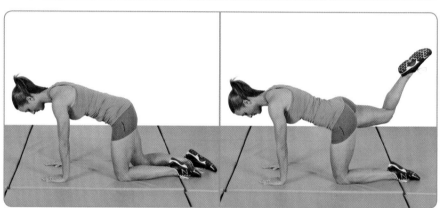

1. Get on all fours with your arms straight under your shoulders, your knees hip-width apart, and your back flat.
2. Keeping your knee bent, raise your right leg up rearward toward the ceiling.
3. Bring your leg to a height that allows you to maintain spinal alignment without over-extending your lower back.
4. Return to the starting position, and repeat for 6-8 reps before switching sides.

This drill activates the gluteus maximus muscle.

Push-Up Plus

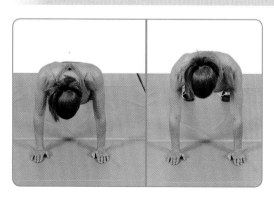

1. Get in push-up position with your hands shoulder-width apart.
2. Form a straight line with your body from your head to your ankles by engaging your core and glutes.
3. Keeping your arms straight, drop your chest down while squeezing your shoulder blades together.
4. From this position, push your back toward the ceiling, spreading your shoulder blades apart.
5. Return to the starting position, and repeat for 6-8 reps.

This drill activates the serratus anterior muscle.

Side Lying Hip Abduction

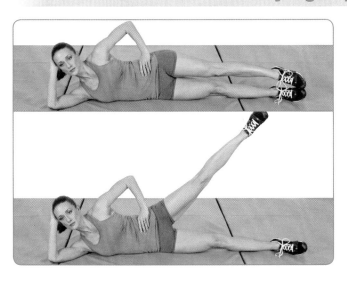

1. Lie on your side with your legs straight and feet stacked in neutral position.
2. Rest your head on your bottom arm, and rest your top arm along your side.
3. Raise the upper leg until you get a nice squeeze on the side of your butt, keeping your knees straight and your hips neutral. Do not allow your hips to roll forward or backward.
4. Return to the starting position, and repeat for the desired number of reps before switching to the other side.

This drill activates the upper glutes.

Side Lying Clam

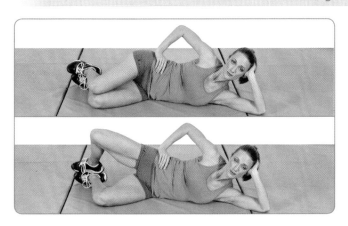

1. Lie on your side with both knees bent at 90-degrees and hips flexed to a 135-degree angle.
2. Rest your head on your bottom arm with your top arm out in front of you.
3. Keeping your heels together, and open your knees by rotating at the hips.
4. Avoid shifting or twisting the lower back.
5. Return to the starting position, and perform 6-8 reps before switching sides.

This drill activates the hip external rotators and upper glutes.

Superman

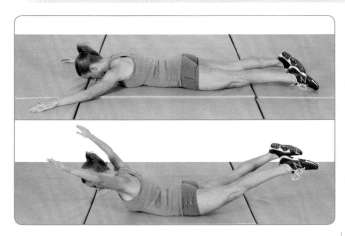
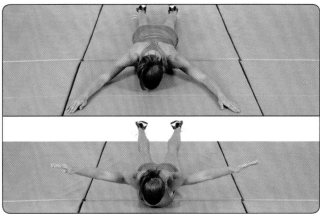

1. Lie on the floor facedown with your body straight.
2. Fully extend your arms in front of you with palms facing down.
3. Simultaneously raise your arms, legs, and chest off the floor, holding the contraction for a moment up top.
4. Squeeze your glutes hard to raise your legs off the ground.
5. Perform 6-8 reps.

This drill activates the gluteus maximus and spinal erectors.

Supine Posterior Pelvic Tilt

1. Using a bench or box, get into a table position by placing your shoulders on the bench with your feet flat on the floor, your hips level, and your knees at a 90-degree angle.

2. Keeping your shoulders on the bench, lower your butt toward the floor while arching your back and tilting your pelvis backward.

3. Bring your hips and pelvis back to starting position by squeezing your glutes and tilting your pelvis forward, making sure to focus on rhythmic pelvic motion.

4. Perform 8-12 reps.

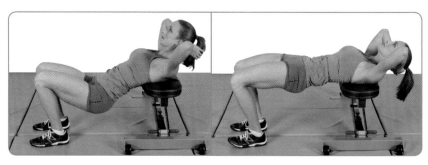

This drill activates the gluteus maximus, although its critical role is as a posterior pelvic-tilter, which is unfamiliar and underdeveloped in most people.

Bodyweight Glute Bridge

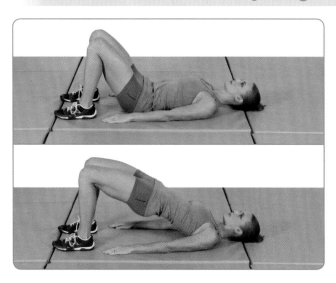

1. Lie on your back with your feet flat on the floor and arms at your side.

2. At the bottom of the movement, your knees will form a 90-degree angle or so, and your hips will form a 135-degree angle or so.

3. Push through your heels, and raise your hips as high as possible without arching your lower back, feeling the movement mostly in the glutes.

4. At the top of the movement, your hips will form a straight line from the knees to the shoulders.

5. Perform 8-12 reps.

This drill activates the gluteus maximus muscle.

Glute Dominant

Glute dominant exercises are critical if you want to possess a bodacious booty. If you bend your knees and slacken the hamstrings, thereby limiting the amount of force they can produce during hip extension, guess which muscle now has to pick up the slack? The gluteus maximus! See the term "active insufficiency" in the glossary section for more information on this topic.

Glute dominant exercises involve bent-knee hip extension. Unlike quad dominant exercises, which mainly strengthen the glutes down low when the hips are flexed, these exercises strengthen the glutes through a full range of motion—especially when the hips are locked out into full extension. In other words, they give you "full spectrum glute strength."

Due to the fact that they place maximum tension on the glutes at lockout (end-range hip extension), these exercises maximize glute activation since this is the zone that elicits the highest neural drive to the glutes. This is also the region where the glutes have the best leverage for moving the thigh rearward (extending the hip). For this reason, women tend to love this category of exercise because they like feeling a muscle working through its full range. This also explains why exercises like hip thrusts can produce a pump—known as "cell swelling" to scientists—and assist in making muscles grow larger.

Another benefit to glute dominant exercises is that the bilateral (double-leg) variations are incredibly stable, which allows you to lift heavy loads to create greater muscle tension. A benefit to unilateral (single-leg) variations is that they can be performed anywhere and can also be quite challenging when performed correctly. Bodyweight resistance alone can provide an amazing glute workout for this category of movements.

Glute dominant exercises lend themselves well to a myriad of different advanced techniques. See the glossary section for information regarding the constant tension method, rest-pause method, pause method, and isohold method.

I'm often asked if the barbell glute bridge or barbell hip thrust is a better exercise for glute-building. The hip thrust still reigns supreme in this category due to an increased range of motion at the hips, but the barbell glute bridge can maximize glute activation because your body can take a heavier load. That's why I advocate having both in your program. Do the hip thrust more often, but every once in a while, go from the floor and bridge as heavy as possible for maximum gluteus maximus activation. A good program incorporates both exercises to help build a beautiful, strong backside.

Just remember the *Strong Curves* motto: The stronger the booty, the better the booty. The stronger your hip thrust and barbell glute bridge get, the better your butt will look. The same can't always be said of the squat and deadlift because depending on your specific goals, there may come a point when squats can build up the quads too much and deadlifts can build up the back too much. This is not meant to scare you away from squats or deadlifts. It's quite rare for women to become overly muscular, especially if body weight is kept in check. But it can and does happen from time to time. Over the course of a year of hard training, I've had everyday women build their strength levels up to one hundred eight-five pounds on the full squat and two hundred seventy-five pounds on the deadlift, and their physiques looked incredible. But these women didn't allow their bodies to accumulate fat or extra weight. An excellent goal over the long haul is to be able to hip thrust two hundred twenty-five pounds for ten repetitions.

Glute dominant movements can work wonders for those suffering from back pain. The exercises teach your body to rely on the glutes during hip extension and not the low back or hamstrings. Moving at the hips while keeping the spine stiff is critical for preventing back stress.

In addition, glute dominant exercises are very important for sports. A well-developed muscle has more potential for force development, as muscle size is indeed related to force. Since power is force multiplied by velocity, strong glutes can improve power by way of increased force production (assuming velocity stays constant). Glute dominant movements also strengthen end-range hip extension, which is the zone involved in ground contact while sprinting—the most important zone for producing force and propelling the body forward. Speed and acceleration are absolutely critical in most sports, so glute dominant exercises are a mainstay due to their ability to target the glutes and strengthen a critical zone involved in sporting action.

Feet-Elevated Hip Thrust

The feet-elevated hip thrust targets the glutes in addition to the hamstrings musculature. This variation increases the range of motion, but due to the angle of the body at the top of the motion, a lower percentage of body weight is utilized. This is a very effective method for learning glute activation for those who have quad dominance. If you feel your quads take over during hip thrusts, try performing two sets of thirty reps twice a week.

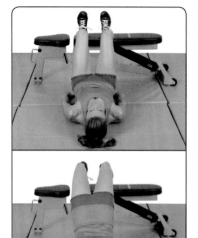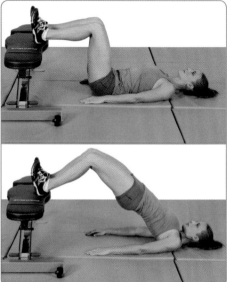

What You Feel: Glutes, hamstrings

Tips

- *Drive through your heels on the bench, keeping your toes pointed toward the ceiling.*
- *Push your weight up with your glutes, not your lower back.*
- *Lie back from the bench so that your knee is at slightly greater than a 90-degree angle.*
- *Keep a strong back by not allowing overarching or curving inward of the lumbar spine.*
- *At the top of the motion, your torso is parallel to the ground.*

What to Do

1. Lie on your back in front of a bench with your feet on the floor.
2. Place both heels on a bench with your toes pointed toward the ceiling.
3. Shift back so that your knees are at slightly greater than a 90-degree angle.
4. Push your hips up toward the ceiling, driving through your heels until a straight line runs from your middle back through your right knee.
5. Lower back down to starting position.

Bodyweight Hip Thrust

This hip thrust elevates the shoulders rather than the feet. Compared to the standard floor version, this increases how much range of motion your hips move from start to finish, promoting more glute strengthening and quadriceps activation for stabilization.

What You Feel: Glutes, quadriceps

Tips

- *Drive through your heels, keeping your toes on the floor and your knees in line with your toes.*
- *Push your body up with your glutes, not your lower back or hamstrings. You will feel these muscles working to an extent, but they should not overcompensate for your glute muscles.*
- *Use a fluid motion all the way up and down.*
- *Keep a strong back by not allowing overarching or curving inward of the lumbar spine.*
- *At the top of the motion, your torso is parallel to the ground..*

What to Do

1. Sit with your back up against a bench and your feet planted on the floor.
2. Push through your heels, and lift your shoulders onto the bench, raising your hips upward with the glutes until your hips are in line with your shoulders and your knees are at a 90-degree angle.
3. Return to the starting position.

Feet and Shoulder-Elevated Hip Thrust

This variation elevates the shoulders and feet, increasing the intensity and range of motion. It promotes increased glute strengthening, and hamstring activation increases as you force them to extend the hip and stabilize the knee.

What You Feel: hamstrings

Tips

- *Drive through your heels, keeping your toes on the floor and your knees in line with your toes.*
- *Push your body up with your glutes, not your lower back or hamstrings. You will feel these muscles working to an extent, but they should not overcompensate for your glute muscles.*
- *Use a fluid motion all the way up and down.*
- *Keep a strong back by not allowing overarching or curving inward of the lumbar spine.*
- *At the top of the motion, your torso is parallel to the ground.*

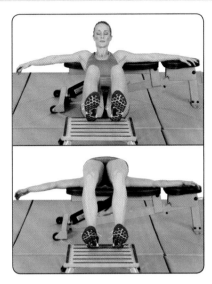
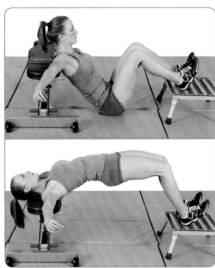

What to Do

1. Sit with your back against a bench and your feet planted on the floor.
2. Place both heels onto a bench that is about 16 inches from your hips.
3. Push through your heels, and lift your shoulders onto the bench, raising your hips upward until your hips are aligned with your shoulders and your knees are at a 90-degree angle.
4. Return to the starting position.

Foot-Elevated Single-Leg Hip Thrust

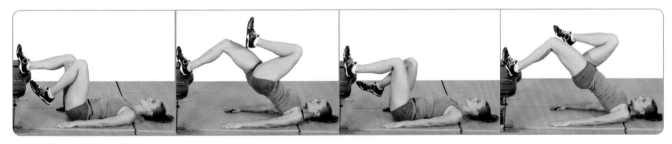

The foot-elevated single-leg hip thrust is the easiest single-leg bridging variation, but it's definitely worth performing since it works the hips through a large range of motion and brings the hamstrings more into play.

What You Feel: Glutes, hamstrings

Tips

- *Drive through your heel on the bench, keeping your toes pointed toward the ceiling.*
- *Push the weight up with your glutes, not your lower back.*
- *Lie back from the bench so that your knee is at slightly greater than a 90-degree angle.*
- *Keep a strong back by not allowing overarching or curving inward of the lumbar spine.*
- *At the top of the motion, your torso is parallel to the ground.*

What to Do

1. Lie on your back in front of a bench with your feet on the floor.
2. Place your right heel on the bench with your toe pointed toward the ceiling, keeping your left foot on the floor.
3. Shift back so that your elevated knee is at slightly greater than a 90-degree angle.
4. Lift your planted left foot off the floor slightly so that your leg is pulled in toward your chest.
5. Push your hips up toward the ceiling with your right heel until you create a straight line that runs from your middle back through your right knee.
6. Lower back down to starting position, and repeat for the desired number of reps. Then, switch sides.

Single-Leg Glute Bridge

This is a great exercise to work the glutes to impressive levels of activation without the use of any equipment. Many people mistakenly underestimate its difficulty. When performed correctly, it's surprisingly challenging. Yet, it can be performed anywhere. I still bust out a couple sets of twenty reps from time to time to give my glutes a simple but effective workout.

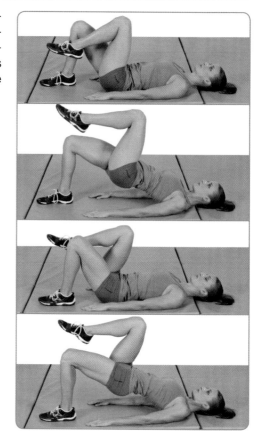

What You Feel: Glutes

Tips

- *Push through your heel, keeping no weight on your toes.*
- *Do not arch your back so that you feel the exercise in your back muscles.*
- *Feel the exercise in your glutes, not your hamstrings. This may take a few sessions to figure out, so keep trying.*
- *Keep your hips and shoulders aligned to avoid shifting from one side to the other.*
- *Pause for a brief moment when at the top of the movement.*

What to Do

1. Lie on your back with your feet flat on the floor and your arms down at your sides.
2. Keep your knee bent, and elevate your left leg by raising the knee toward your chest.
3. Push-upward with your hips, driving your right heel into the floor to rise into a bridge position.
4. Return to the starting position, repeat for the desired number of reps, and switch sides.

Shoulder-Elevated Glute March

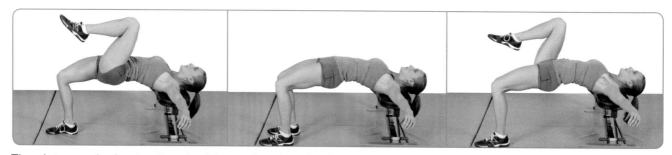

The glute march elevates the shoulders rather than the feet and is intensified through working one leg at a time by alternating legs in a marching fashion. This builds considerable end-range hip strength and stability.

What You Feel: Glutes, quadriceps

Tips

- *Push through your heels, and keep your knees in line with your toes.*
- *Push your body up with your glutes, not your lower back or hamstrings. You will feel these muscles working to an extent, but they should not overcompensate for your glute muscles.*
- *Keep a strong back by not allowing overarching or curving inward of the lumbar spine.*
- *At the top of the motion, your torso is parallel to the ground.*

What to Do

1. Sit with your back up against a bench and your feet planted on the floor.
2. Push through your heels, and lift your shoulders onto the bench, raising your hips upward until your hips align with your shoulders and your knees are at a 90-degree angle.
3. Remaining in top position, lift your left leg off the floor, bringing your knee toward your chest, and hold the position for two seconds.
4. Return to the starting position, and raise the right leg, holding the position for two seconds.
5. Repeat for the desired number of reps.

Shoulder-Elevated Single-Leg Hip Thrust

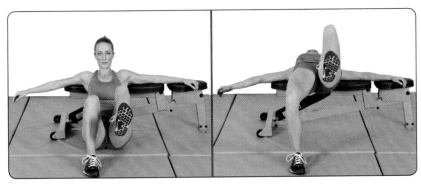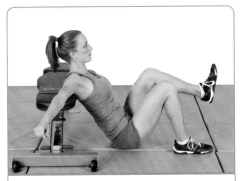

The shoulder-elevated single-leg hip thrust elevates the shoulders rather than the feet and is intensified by working one leg at a time. This increases the range of motion your hips move from start to finish, promoting more glute strengthening, and quadriceps activation is increased for stabilization purposes.

What You Feel: Glutes, hamstrings

Tips

- *Drive through your heel on the bench, keeping your toes pointed toward the ceiling.*
- *Push the weight up with your glutes, not your lower back.*
- *Lie back from the bench so that your knee is at slightly greater than a 90-degree angle.*
- *Keep a strong back by not allowing overarching or curving inward of the lumbar spine.*
- *At the top of the motion, your torso is parallel to the ground.*

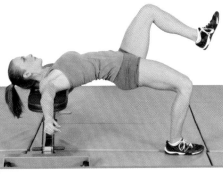

What to Do

1. Sit with your back up against a bench and your feet planted on the floor.
2. Lift your left knee so that your leg is pulled in toward your chest.
3. Push through your right heel, and lift your shoulders onto the bench, raising your hips upward with the glutes until your hips are in line with your shoulders and your knee is at a 90-degree angle.
4. Return to the starting position.
5. Repeat for the desired number of reps before switching legs.

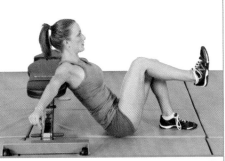

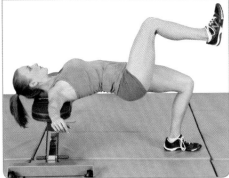

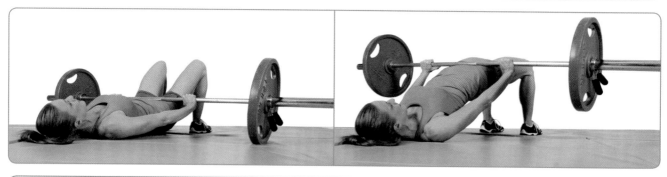

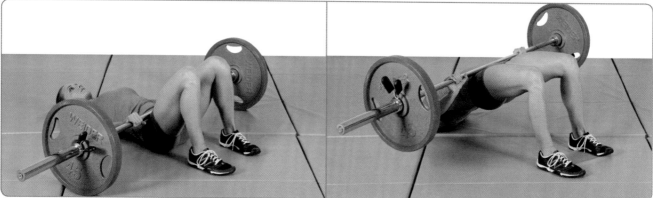

The barbell glute bridge is a progression from a bodyweight glute bridge (found in the activation section). Adding weight to this exercise helps to develop stronger glutes using a shorter range of motion. This exercise allows you to use extremely heavy weight from a stable position. Many individuals benefit from mastering this movement prior to performing the barbell hip thrust because it's simpler with less range of motion and easier in terms of activating the glutes.

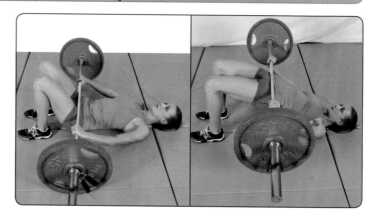

What You Feel: Glutes

Tips

- *Drive through your heels. You may find it easier to push your heels into the ground by lifting your toes up.*
- *Push the weight up with your glutes, not your lower back or hamstrings. You will feel these muscles working to an extent, but they should not overcompensate for your glute muscles.*
- *Keep a stable core by not allowing overarching or curving inward of the lumbar spine.*
- *Pause for a brief moment when at the top of the movement.*

What to Do

1. Sit straight-legged on an exercise mat with the loaded barbell straight out in front of you.
2. Roll the bar over your legs up to your pelvis.
3. Lie back, and bring your feet to the floor, bending your knees close to your butt.
4. Grasp the bar so that it stays on your hips as you move up.
5. Push through your heels, raising your hips off the floor so that a straight line runs from your upper back through your knees.
6. Return to the starting position.

Barbell Hip Thrust

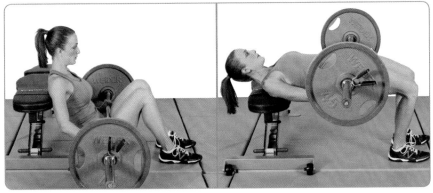

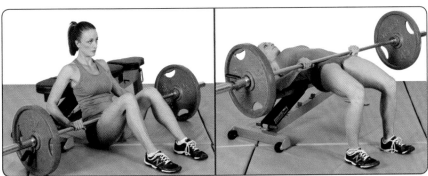

Tips

- *Drive through your heels, keeping your toes on the floor and your knees in line with your toes.*
- *Push your weight up with your glutes, not your lower back or hamstrings. You will feel these muscles working to an extent, but they should not overcompensate for your glute muscles.*
- *Use a fluid motion all the way up and down.*
- *Keep a strong core by not allowing overarching or curving inward of the lumbar spine.*
- *At the top of the motion, your torso is parallel to the ground.*
- *Pause for a brief moment when at the top of the movement.*

The hip thrust is the premier glute-building movement. The knees stay bent so that the hamstrings are inhibited, forcing the glutes to work harder. Tension doesn't let off the glutes throughout the movement like it does in other popular glute exercises. This constant tension causes a deep burn in the glutes, letting you know how much your booty is working. Muscle activation reaches a high point due to the end-range glute muscle force requirements which is the range of maximal neural activation for the gluteus maximus.

The hips move through a good range of motion, and the glutes produce incredible force due to the inherent stability involved in the exercise. Since the core (back strength) isn't a limiting factor like it is in other movements, the hip thrust allows the gluteus maximus to "do its thing" and maximize its output.

Increasing glute strength and glute muscle will not only improve aesthetics, but it will improve the leverage and power that the glutes produce during exercise and positively impact the way your body moves and transfers force throughout.

What to Do

1. From a seated position on the floor, position your upper back across a bench (should be lined up at around the bottom of the shoulder blades). Make sure the bench is secure and doesn't slide.

2. Place a barbell across the hips (should be lined up just above the pubic bone), and grasp the bar to keep it in place throughout the movement. A Hampton bar pad or Airex Balance pad can be used to reduce the bar pressure on the abdomen.

3. If sufficient weight is used (example: 135 pounds), the larger plates will allow for the bar to simply roll over the legs and onto the hips.

4. Bend the hips and knees so that the feet are positioned toward the buttocks and are flat on the ground.

5. Make sure your back "hinges" around the bench; don't allow it to slide back and forth during the movement, and don't allow the barbell to slide forward or backward during the movement.

6. Take a deep breath, and raise your hips, making sure to push through the heels and keep the knees tracking over the middle toes.

7. As the hips rise, your lumbar spine will want to hyperextend (overarch), and your pelvis will want to tilt anteriorly (forward), but you cannot let this happen.

8. Make sure that the glutes push the hips upward so that the movement occurs at the hips and not the spine, and make sure that the glutes prevent the pelvis from tilting forward.

9. Raise your hips as high as possible while keeping the spine in a neutral position.

10. If observing the lockout of the movement from the side view, the hips should be at full extension (or slightly hyperextended), the knees should be at right angles or 90 degrees, and your feet should be flat on the ground.

11. Lower the weight under control, and return to the starting position.

American Hip Thrust

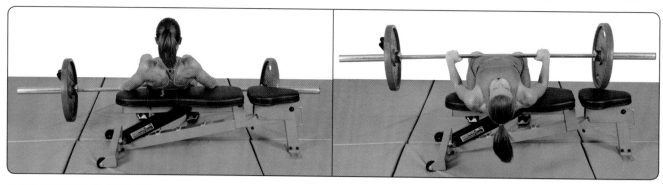

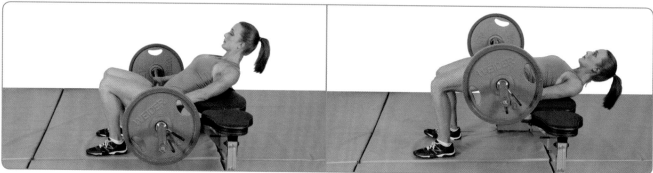

This is a variation of the barbell hip thrust that shifts the fulcrum so that heavier loads can be used, and less pressure is placed on the back with possibly even more loading on the glutes. It naturally leads to posterior pelvic tilting in addition to hip extension, which adds more glute activation since the glutes are serving multiple roles. The American hip thrust is probably the best exercise for glute activation, but I prefer the standard version most of the time because it's easier to standardize. This is because the upper back is placed on the bench in the same position each time. You should definitely perform the American hip thrust regularly, however, as it's an excellent variation.

What You Feel: Glutes, quadriceps

Tips

- *Drive through your heels, keeping your toes on the floor and your knees in line with the toes.*
- *Push the weight up with your glutes, not your lower back or hamstrings. You will feel these muscles working to an extent, but they should not overcompensate for your glute muscles.*
- *Use a fluid motion all the way up and down.*
- *Keep a strong back by not allowing overarching or curving inward of the lumbar spine. In fact, at the top of the movement you should tilt the pelvis slightly posteriorly to work the glutes more.*
- *At the top of the motion, your torso is parallel to the ground.*

What to Do

1. Sit up right against a bench with your legs straight out in front of you and the bar over your shins.
2. Roll the bar up to your hips, and bring your feet to the floor with your knees bent at a comfortable angle.
3. Grasp the bar so that it stays on your hips as you move up.
4. Slide upward so that the middle of your back is positioned across the bench, and your elbows are resting on the top of the bench while still gripping the barbell.
5. Push through your heels, and raise the hips by squeezing the glutes.
6. At the top of the movement, your hips are aligned with your shoulders, and your knees are at a 90-degree angle.
7. Sink your hips down without allowing the bar to touch the ground, and repeat for the desired number of reps.

Hip Thrust Mistakes and How to Fix Them

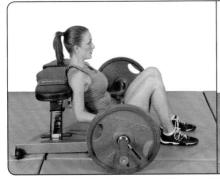
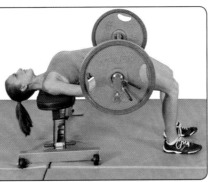

Overarching Low Back—Notice in the picture that Kellie is overarching (also known as hyperextending her lumbar spine). This is accompanied by an anterior pelvic tilt, where the front of the pelvis drops downward and the back of the pelvis rises upward. You can spot this because her chest isn't in neutral; it's too arched, as is the arch in her lumbar spine. This happens if you have weak glutes and try to substitute lumbopelvic motion for hip motion. The solution is to reduce the load and learn to keep your spine stable in the neutral position, while moving entirely at the hip joint and using the glutes to push the hips upward and prevent the pelvis from tilting.

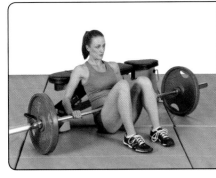
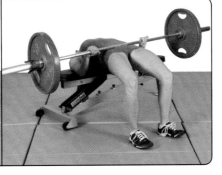

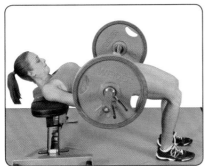
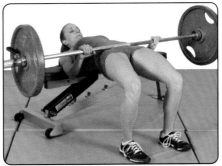

Improper Neck Alignment—As you can see in the picture, Kellie is failing to maintain proper neck alignment and is flexing her cervical spine. The neck should stay in line with the spine throughout the hip thrust motion.

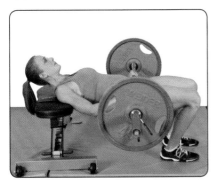
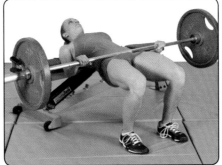

Insufficient Hip Extension—In this picture, Kellie isn't reaching full hip extension. This happens when you use too much weight and are unable to complete the full range of motion. It's very important that you achieve full hip extension on each repetition, as this is the range of motion that activates the glutes the best. The solution is to drop down in weight and feel the glutes pushing the hips forward to end-range.

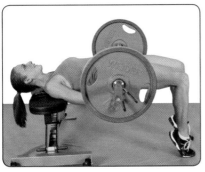
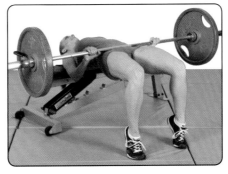

Rising Onto Toes—Notice in the picture that Kellie has risen up onto her toes. This typically occurs in individuals who display "quad-dominant" movement strategies. Keep your toes on the ground, and push through the heels. Eventually, this will feel natural.

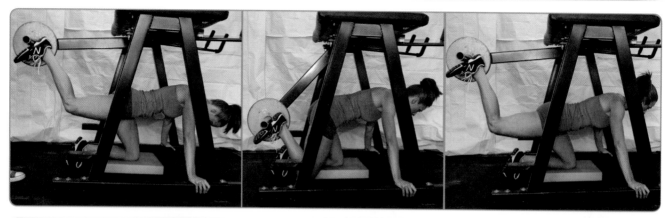

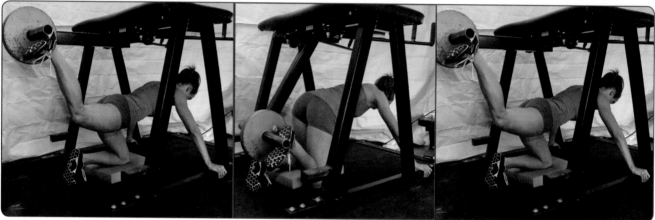

This exercise maintains constant tension on the glutes and requires considerable core stability to prevent your core from shifting or twisting. I prescribed the pendulum quadruped movement frequently when I owned my studio, and it was a favorite of many of my female clients. It's very rare for a gym to contain a reverse hyper machine, but if you have access to one, you should definitely perform this exercise because it's highly effective for the glutes.

What You Feel: Glutes, hamstrings, core

Tips

- *Maintain alignment without shifting your torso left or right or twisting.*
- *Push through the middle of the foot.*
- *Hold the side rails for support.*
- *Control your core by keeping it tight.*

What to Do

1. Get on your hands and knees beneath a reverse hyper machine. Note where the hands grip the siderails.
2. Center your right foot onto the pendulum.
3. Push your weight upward until your leg is aligned with your torso, keeping your knee bent the entire time.
4. Squeeze the glute at the top of the lift.
5. Return to start position, and repeat. Then, switch legs.

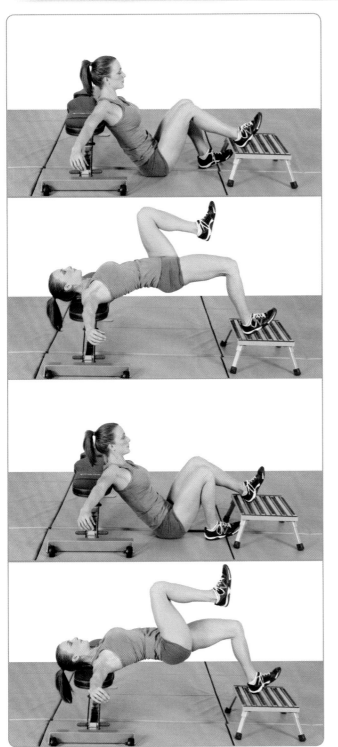

This exercise elevates the shoulders and one foot, increasing the intensity and range of motion while working one leg at a time. This builds rotary stability in the hips and effectively works the glutes. The hamstrings are heavily worked as you force them to do two things in this movement—extend the hip and stabilize the knee. This is the most challenging hip thrust variation, and advanced exercisers can always perform this variation when they don't have access to a gym by using a couch and a chair. Just make sure they don't slide apart in the middle of the set.

What You Feel: Glutes, hamstrings

Tips

- Drive through your heel, keeping your toes on the floor and your knee in line with your toes.
- Push your body up with your glutes, not your lower back or hamstrings. You will feel these muscles working to an extent, but they should not overcompensate for your glute muscles.
- Use a fluid motion all the way up and down.
- Keep a strong back by not allowing overarching or curving inward of the lumbar spine.
- At the top of the motion, your torso is parallel to the ground.

What to Do

1. Sit with your back up against a bench and your feet planted on the floor.
2. Place your right heel onto a bench that it is about 16 inches from your hips.
3. Lift your left knee slightly so that your leg is pulled in toward your chest.
4. Push through your right heel, and lift your shoulders onto the bench, raising your hips upward with the glutes until your hips are in line with your shoulders and your knee is at a 90-degree angle.
5. Return to the starting position.
6. Repeat all reps before switching legs.

Glute Accessory

The glute accessory category is an important but often overlooked group of exercises for glute development. Many programs focus solely on hip extension exercises such as those found in the quad dominant, hip dominant, or glute dominant categories. While it's certainly wise to focus on hip extension exercises, especially those that let you load up the glutes, it's unwise to leave glute accessory exercises out of your program altogether.

Glute accessory exercises involve hip abduction, hip transverse abduction, and hip external rotation movements (see glossary for terms). While hip abduction movements focus more on the upper glutes, hip external rotation movements activate the entire glute. In fact, the gluteus maximus is highly activated by hip external rotation movements—something missing from many programs. The gluteus maximus has excellent leverage for rotating the hip outward, and it's important to learn how to feel the glute twisting the hips during exercises like band hip rotations.

Each of the exercises in this category also strengthens other important hip muscles such as the hip external rotators, the gluteus medius, and the gluteus minimus. These muscles are critical for proper lumbopelvic-hip motion during functional movement.

Every time you run, your hip works as an abductor (or better yet, an anti-adductor) during the stance phase. Since you're on one leg, your body would naturally want to cave inward, but the gluteus medius and upper gluteus maximus ensure that that doesn't happen. Furthermore, every time you pivot, cut from side to side, swing something, or throw something, you rely on these lateral and rotational movements at the hips. Finally, the abductor and external rotator muscles of the hip fire in proper amounts to prevent the knee from caving in during gait, squatting, stair climbing, jumping, and landing. For these reasons, the glute accessory category is a small but important group of exercises to include in your programming.

Band Seated Abduction

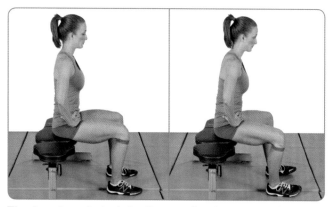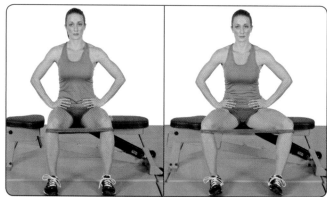

The band seated abduction works the upper glutes from a seated, hips-flexed position. This builds hip strength needed to force the knees out during squatting tasks. This exercise is very easy to perform, and when performed correctly, it produces a nice burn in the glutes.

What You Feel: Upper glutes

Tips

- *Start with the feet wider than the knees in a knock-kneed position, and move the knees in line with your feet.*
- *Alternatively, you can start with your feet aligned with your knees, pushing your knees out past your feet.*
- *Hold the contraction for a brief moment before returning to starting position.*

What to Do

1. Seated on a bench or chair, wrap a band around your legs so that it rests right below your knees. If you have a longer band, wrap it twice around your legs.
2. Position your feet wide with your knees caved inward.
3. Sit up straight, and push your knees out against the band to contract the upper glutes.
4. Return to the starting position, and repeat.

X-Band Walk

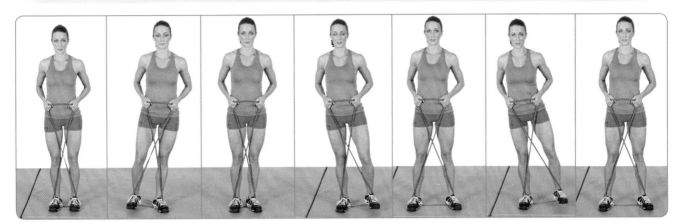

The x-band walk strengthens the upper glutes from a standing, athletic position that is common in sports. This exercise is a favorite glute-activator of many of my clients.

What You Feel: Upper glutes

Tips

- *You will feel both hips working at the same time.*
- *Stand tall.*
- *Keep your steps short and low to the ground.*
- *Focus on pushing through the grounded leg rather than reaching with the non-grounded leg.*

What to Do

1. Place the lower portion of the band on the floor, and step each foot on the band so that it is positioned in the middle of the foot.
2. Cross the band over in front of your knees to create an X.
3. Pull each side of the band up to your hips, locking your elbows into place.
4. Stand with good posture.
5. Keeping your leg straight, take short steps to the right for reps.
6. Repeat on the left side.

Standing Cable Abduction

The standing cable abduction targets the upper glutes and strengthens both hip abductors simultaneously. The grounded leg works isometrically, while the free leg works dynamically through a full range of motion. This is a challenging exercise, and its effectiveness shouldn't be underestimated.

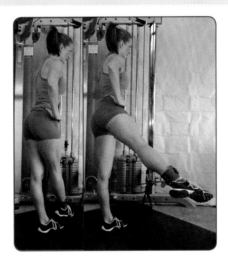

What You Feel: Upper glutes

Tips

- *Do not bend at your side as you lift your leg up.*
- *Maintain good posture, and only lift your leg high enough to feel a squeeze in your glutes.*
- *Your standing leg will definitely feel this exercise and may tire easily. Bend at the knee slightly to ease some of the stress.*

What to Do

1. Stand with your left side against a cable machine. Place an ankle cuff cable attachment around your right ankle. Adjust to appropriate weight.
2. Grasp a nearby handle or the cable bar for support, and move your right leg behind your left leg.
3. Keeping your torso aligned, lift up and slightly back with your right leg until you feel a contraction in your upper glute.
4. Return to the starting position, and repeat for reps on both sides.

Double-Quadruped Hip Abduction

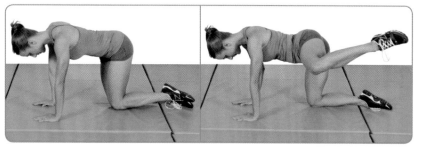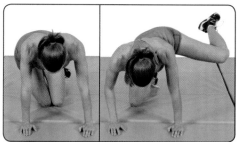

The double-quadruped hip abduction is a unique hip exercise that strengthens the upper glutes in a hips-flexed position, which is important for activities such as squatting. It takes some practice to get it right, but you'll definitely like this movement more than the standard fire-hydrant exercise that doesn't involve as much range of motion.

What You Feel: Glutes, hamstrings, core

Tips

- *Focus on spreading your hips outward as much as possible.*
- *Do the entire sequence in one fluid motion.*

What to Do

1. Get in position on your hands and knees, with your knees positioned under your hips and your arms positioned under your shoulders.
2. Shift your weight to sink into your left side without twisting your upper body. As you sink, your right leg hovers off the floor.
3. Push both hips outward, lifting your right leg up to the side and feeling your upper glute contract while also shifting toward the right side with your left leg.
4. Sink back down into your left hip.
5. Repeat for reps on both sides.

Double-Standing Hip Abduction

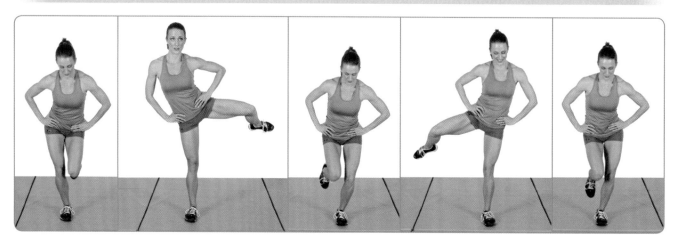

The double-standing hip abduction is another unique hip movement that strengthens the upper glutes and promotes balance and coordination. This movement is not as easy as it looks. You may benefit from initially holding onto something for balance until you get the hang of it. Then, you can try the hands-free version.

What You Feel: Glutes, hamstrings, core

Tips

- *Pause at the top, and squeeze for a brief moment.*
- *Do the entire sequence in one fluid motion.*
- *If you lose balance, reposition yourself from the starting position, and begin your repetition over.*

What to Do

1. Bend slightly at the hips while standing on your right leg.
2. Keep your right knee slightly bent, bringing your left leg off the floor with the knee bent.
3. From a quarter-squat position, sink your weight into your right hip, allowing the hip to collapse inward a bit.
4. Reverse the motion, and raise your left leg up to your side to hip height, shifting your weight to your left side.
5. Bring your leg back down, and repeat for reps on both sides.

Side Lying Hip Raise

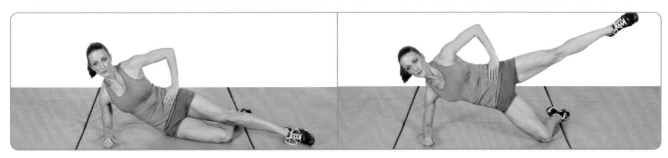

The side lying hip raise works the upper glutes from a lying position. You should master the side lying hip abduction and side plank before attempting the side lying hip raise because it's surprisingly challenging.

What You Feel: Upper glutes

Tips

- *Keep your spine aligned without leaning forward or backward.*
- *Use a fluid motion throughout the duration of the exercise.*
- *Both hips are worked simultaneously during this exercise.*

What to Do

1. Lie on your right side, supporting your weight on your elbow with your arm positioned under your shoulder.
2. Bend your knees, placing your feet behind you with your left leg on top of your right leg.
3. Align your spine so that you aren't arching back or leaning forward.
4. Lift your top leg, and move it up toward the ceiling slightly. You can leave your left leg bent or straighten it.
5. Press up with your right hip while keeping your left leg up the entire time.
6. Lower back to the floor, and repeat reps before switching sides.

Band Standing Abduction

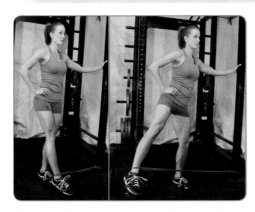 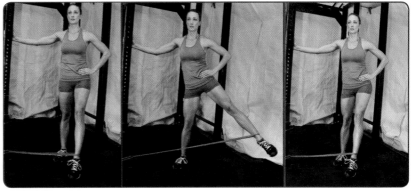

The band standing abduction targets the upper glutes and strengthens both hip abductors simultaneously. The grounded leg works isometrically, while the free leg works dynamically through a full range of motion. Make sure you practice the cable variation before attempting this exercise, as the band variation will most likely require some tinkering to get right. So, having some experience with cables will help.

What You Feel: Upper glutes

Tips

- *You may wrap a towel around the band to cushion your ankle so that the band doesn't slide.*
- *Do not bend at your side as you lift up your leg.*
- *Maintain good posture, and only lift your leg high enough to feel a squeeze in your glutes.*
- *Your standing leg will definitely feel this exercise and may tire easily. Bend at the knee slightly to ease some of the stress.*

What to Do

1. Stand with your left side against a rack or pole.
2. Loop a band around a support, weaving it through so that it is harnessed.
3. Place your right ankle inside of the band.
4. Grasp a nearby handle or the cable bar for support.
5. Move your right leg behind your left leg, and step out from the rack so that you create tension on the band.
6. Keeping your torso aligned, lift up and slightly back with your right leg until you feel a contraction in your upper glute.
7. Return to the starting position, and repeat for reps on both sides.

The cable hip rotation helps you build and strengthen the muscles in your hips that produce a twisting motion, especially the gluteus maximus because it has the best leverage for this pattern. This exercise is incredibly challenging, and many struggle to perform it properly. Once you get it right, it will activate your glutes to amazing levels, and you'll feel strong and powerful at rotational movements.

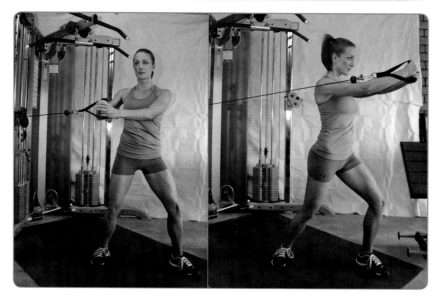

What You Feel: Glutes, obliques

Tips

- *As you rotate, your front hip will turn inward while your back hip will turn outward.*
- *Keep your arms out in front of your body to maintain a good lever length throughout the motion; don't let the cable get too close to the body or tension will diminish.*
- *Rotate at the hips, keeping your core in neutral.*
- *Push through the glute as you turn, getting a nice squeeze at the end of the movement before returning to starting position.*

What to Do

1. In an athletic stance, grasp the cable handle with both hands and arms extended out.
2. Turn diagonal to the cable, and create tension on the cable by stepping out away from the machine.
3. Keeping your arms straight, swivel at the hips, and twist your body so that the cable is furthest away from your body at the termination of the movement.
4. Return to the starting position, and finish the desired number of reps before repeating on the opposite side.

Quad Dominant

Quad dominant exercises all resemble squatting motions, either on one or two legs. The knee joint moves through a significant range of motion, and the hips usually flex considerably as well, stretching the glutes. When the knee is bent, the hamstrings slacken, which allows the hips to sink deeper into greater range of motion. For this reason, quad dominant exercises are best for stretching the glutes under heavy load, which is why they tend to induce the greatest amount of soreness among the glute exercises. If you have ever taken a break from full squatting or loaded walking lunges, you know how sore you can become when you resume performing them. Walking lunges are probably responsible for more sore glutes than any other exercise. In particular, the eccentric (lowering) portion of the exercise creates the most soreness, so it's important to load up the glutes and sink down into the hips when performing quad dominant exercises.

Many people who are new to this particular type of strength training avoid using their hips when performing quad dominant movements. They shift their weight forward and bend mostly at the knees when squatting, rather than sitting back and absorbing the load with their hips. They rise up on their toes and avoid going deep when lunging. The list of compensations goes on and on, but you're going to work very hard to avoid these pitfalls. Learn to push through the heels, and feel the hips producing power during these movements.

Quad dominant exercises also work the quads the best in terms of both activation and range of motion, and they hit the adductors hard as well. Nice thighs often sit high on the vanity priority list, and these exercises help you achieve that desired look.

Strength levels in quad dominant exercises are highly influenced by anthropometry, which means that you can naturally perform squats and lunges well, or it's something you have to work very hard to do. Don't feel bad if your squat is never impressive; some people simply aren't built to squat. But you should still work hard on them even if they don't come easy to you.

Don't make the mistake of thinking soreness is the end-all-be-all for muscle growth, though. Remember that some relative soreness is good, but too much inter-feres with strength gains. The goal is not to annihilate your muscles to the point that you move like a snail for a week. If you hit the glutes and other muscles frequently with a variety of movements, you will promote the best growth possible.

Quad dominant movements are also critical for preventing knee pain. When done correctly, they strengthen the quads, teach the hips to contribute to compound movement, and dramatically reduce knee stress by getting your knees tracking properly over your feet.

Just like glute dominant exercises, quad dominant movements are highly beneficial for sports. The quads are incredibly important for many sports actions, including running, jumping, and cutting from side to side. Quad dominant moves provide glute strength in deep positions, which is important for absorbing impact during jump landings. The squat is definitely at the top of the list for lower body exercises. It requires good core stability in the back muscles, excellent quad strength, good hip strength down low, and good lower body joint mobility. But the squat, along with other quad dominant exercises such as lunges, fail to activate the glutes to the same level of other exercises like the deadlift or hip thrust. This is why it's important to perform multiple glute movements for maximal results.

Bodyweight High Box Squat

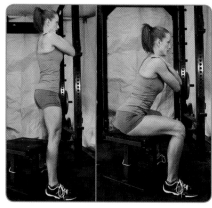

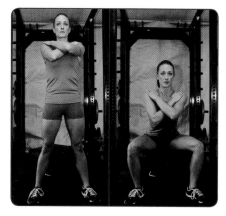

The box squat is an excellent variation that teaches people how to sit back and rely more on the hips during a squat. It's also a great option for people who have knee issues and find traditional squatting to be problematic. The higher the box, the easier it is to perform. Therefore, the higher box variation should be mastered prior to attempting lower box positions.

What You Feel: Quadriceps, glutes

Tips

- *Keep the chest up, and maintain a good low back arch.*
- *Push your knees out so that they track over your toes.*
- *Keep your weight on your heels.*
- *Sit way back in this variation, and keep your tibias upright so that your knees don't move forward.*
- *Squeeze the glutes to lockout.*

What to Do

1. Stand over a bench or a box that sits at knee level with a wide stance. Most people prefer to turn their toes out to about a 30 to 45-degree angle, but this depends on the person.
2. Place your arms in a "mummy" position crossed in front of your body.
3. Take a deep breath, and sit back in an exaggerated squat with your glutes extended back, keeping your tibias nearly vertical so that your knees don't move forward. This will require a considerable forward trunk lean.
4. Squat to the bench while forcing your knees out. Then, pause for a brief moment on the box without losing the neutral spinal position.
5. Rise upward, making sure to squeeze the glutes to lockout, and return to the starting position.

Bodyweight Box Squat

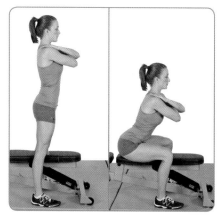

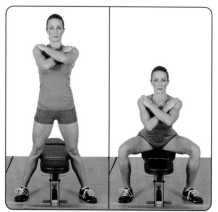

The box squat is an excellent variation that helps people learn how to sit back and rely more on the hips during a squat. It's also a great option for people who have knee issues and find traditional squatting to be problematic.

What You Feel: Quadriceps, glutes

Tips

- *Keep your chest up, and maintain a good lower back arch.*
- *Push your knees out so that they track over your toes.*
- *Keep your weight on your heels.*
- *Sit way back in this variation, and keep your tibias upright so that your knees don't move forward.*
- *Squeeze the glutes to lockout.*

What to Do

1. Stand over a bench or a box that sits at knee level and keep your legs at a wide stance. Most people prefer to turn their toes out to about a 30 to 45-degree angle, but this depends on the person.
2. Place your arms in a "mummy" position, crossed in front of your body.
3. Take a deep breath, and sit back in an exaggerated squat with your glutes extended back, keeping your tibias nearly vertical so that your knees don't move forward. This will require a considerable forward trunk lean.
4. Squat to the bench while forcing the knees out. Then, pause for a brief moment on the box without losing the neutral spinal position.
5. Rise upward, making sure to squeeze the glutes to lockout.
6. Return to the starting position.

Bodyweight Low Box Squat

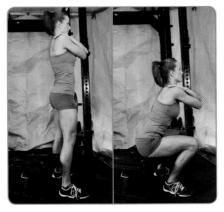
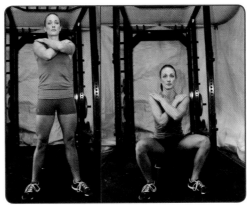

The low box squat is an excellent way to ensure that lifters reach proper depth while squatting. It also builds strength and improves form from the bottom position. In the high box squat, you sit back and don't allow for forward knee travel, while you sit back and down in the low box squat, allowing your knees to travel forward a bit and share the load equally between the hips and knees. You'll also use a shoulder-width stance in this variation, while you use a wide stance in the high box squat.

What You Feel: Quadriceps, glutes

Tips

- *Keep your chest up, and maintain a good lower back arch.*
- *Push your knees out so that they track over your toes.*
- *Keep your weight on your heels.*
- *Keep your trunk upright.*
- *Squeeze the glutes to lockout.*

What to Do

1. Stand over a bench or a box that sits below knee level and keep your legs at a shoulder-width stance. Most people prefer to turn their toes out to about a 30 to 45-degree angle, but this depends on the person.
2. Place your arms in the "mummy" position, crossed in front of your body.
3. Take a deep breath, and sit down, keeping your trunk mostly upright.
4. Squat to the bench while forcing your knees out. Then, pause for a brief moment on the box without losing the neutral spinal position.
5. Rise upward, making sure to squeeze the glutes to lockout.
6. Return to the starting position.

Bodyweight Squat

The bodyweight squat is a fundamental pattern in human movement, and it must be mastered before you start adding load. It is imperative that you learn to share the load between your hips and knees in order ensure optimal performance and joint health in the long-run.

What You Feel: Quads, glutes

Tips

- *Keep your chest up and your chin tucked so that your neck aligns with the rest of your spine.*
- *Sink your hips straight down between your knees, and keep the knees forced out so that they're aligned over your feet. The knees will travel over the toes, but do not allow your knees to cave inward.*
- *Keep your trunk mostly upright; it will lean forward, but don't allow for too much of a lean. Also, don't round your spine.*
- *As you move down, keep your lower back arched. Avoid curling your butt under.*
- *Push through your heels; don't rise up onto your toes.*

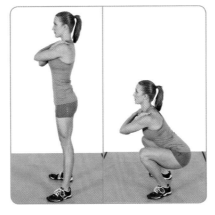
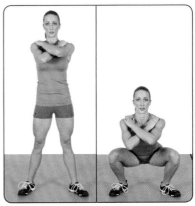

What to Do

1. Stand with your feet shoulder-width apart. Toe position depends on how you feel most comfortable. You can either point your toes forward or turn them slightly out to the sides. A 30-degree foot flare is typical.
2. Stand tall, and cross your arms over your chest.
3. Sit back by hinging at your hips.
4. Your hips begin the movement, followed by your knees.
5. Squat down as low as you can go without allowing your lower back to round; this depth will differ between individuals, but you want to at least squat until your hip joints reach below your knees.
6. Continue pushing your knees out throughout the duration of the movement, and continue to prevent too much forward trunk lean.
7. Return to the starting position.

Dumbbell Goblet Squat

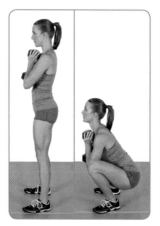
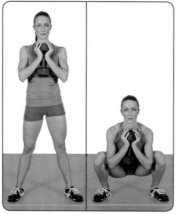

The goblet squat is a vital tool for beginners and intermediates. Placing the load at your chest in the goblet position is the best way to initially add weight when progressing from a bodyweight squat.

What You Feel: Quadriceps, glutes

Tips

- *Keep your chest up and your chin tucked so that your neck aligns with the rest of your spine.*
- *Keep your arms close to your body as you move down.*
- *Drop straight down while forcing your knees out over your toes.*
- *As you move down, keep the arch in your lower back, and avoid curling your butt under.*
- *When coming up, use the glutes.*

What to Do

1. Stand with your feet shoulder-width apart. Toe position depends on how you feel most comfortable. You can either point your toes forward or turn them slightly out to the sides.
2. Stand tall, and hold a dumbbell with both hands on one end.
3. Drop straight down while keeping your trunk mostly upright and not allowing for too much forward lean. Keep the chest tall.
4. Squat down until your hip joints come below your knees, pushing your knees out throughout the duration of the movement.
5. Push back up through your heels, continually pushing your knees out so that they don't cave inward.
6. Return to the starting position.

Kettlebell Goblet Squat

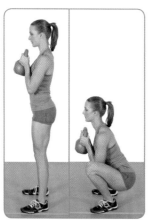
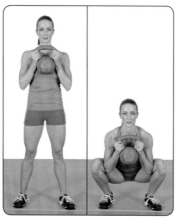

The goblet squat is a vital tool for beginners and intermediates. Placing the load at your chest in the goblet position is the best way to initially add weight when progressing from a bodyweight squat.

What You Feel: Quadriceps, glutes

Tips

- *Keep your chest up and your chin tucked so that your neck aligns with the rest of your spine.*
- *Keep your arms close to your body as you move down.*
- *Drop straight down while forcing your knees out over your toes.*
- *As you move down, keep the arch in your lower back, and avoid curling your butt under.*
- *When coming up, use the glutes.*

What to Do

1. Stand with your feet shoulder-width apart. Toe position depends on how you feel most comfortable. You can either point your toes forward or turn them slightly out to the sides.
2. Stand tall, and hold a kettlebell with both hands on the horn placed directly under the chin.
3. Drop straight down, while keeping your trunk mostly upright and not allowing for too much forward lean. Keep your chest tall.
4. Squat down until your hip joints come below your knees, pushing your knees out throughout the duration of the movement.
5. Push back up through your heels, continually pushing your knees out so they do not cave inward.
6. Return to the starting position.

Dumbbell Between-Bench Squat

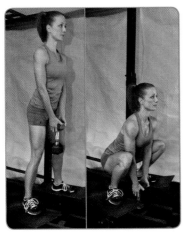 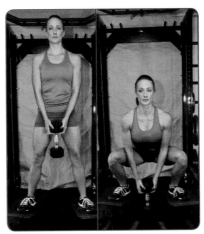

What You Feel: Quadriceps, glutes

Tips

- *Keep your chest up and your chin tucked so that your neck aligns with the rest of your spine.*
- *Keep your arms close to your body as you move down.*
- *Drop straight down while forcing your knees out over your toes.*
- *As you move down, keep the arch in your lower back, and avoid curling your butt under.*
- *When coming up, use the glutes.*

This exercise is a staple in my programs when I train women. It's an excellent squat variation that moves your hips through a wide range of motion and works the glutes well in the stretch position. It's also an excellent beginner and intermediate exercise for those just learning to squat with additional loading.

What to Do

1. Stand with your feet shoulder-width apart. Toe position depends on how you feel most comfortable. You can either point your toes forward or turn them slightly out to the sides.
2. Stand tall, and hold a dumbbell (or kettlebell) with your hands underneath the top bell.
3. Drop straight down, while keeping your trunk mostly upright and not allowing for too much forward lean. Keep your chest tall.
4. Squat down until your hip joints come below your knees, pushing your knees out throughout the duration of the movement.
5. Push back up through your heels, continually pushing your knees out so that they do not cave inward.
6. Return to the starting position.

Dumbbell Full Squat

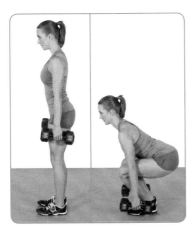 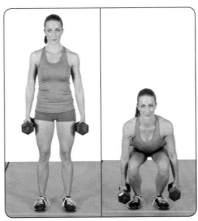

What You Feel: Quadriceps, glutes

Tips

- *Remember that this is a squat, not a deadlift. Your knees will bend, and you'll feel the movement in your quads.*
- *Keep your chest up with a narrow stance.*
- *Keep your arms straight as you descend with the dumbbells moving down to the floor out to the sides of your feet.*
- *Sit back while keeping your torso mostly upright.*
- *Do not let your knees cave in.*
- *Push through the heels.*

Many people struggle to perform this variation correctly, but when done properly, the dumbbell full squat is an effective way to squat.

What to Do

1. Stand with your feet shoulder-width apart. You can either point your toes forward or turn them slightly out to the sides.
2. In each hand, hold a dumbbell by your sides with palms facing in.
3. Sit back by hinging at your hips. Your hips begin the movement, followed by your knees.
4. Squat down until your hip joints come below your knees, pushing your knees out throughout the duration of the movement.
5. Push back up through your hips, continually pushing your knees out so that they do not cave inward.
6. Return to the starting position.

Barbell Half Squat

The barbell half squat is a good squat alternative for those who cannot squat to full depth due to injury or mobility issues. Furthermore, it allows for heavier loads, which can be useful from time to time. Many athletes and coaches prefer this squat variation, but I believe the full squat is superior if proper form can be achieved.

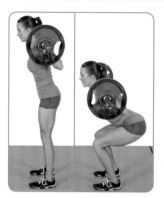

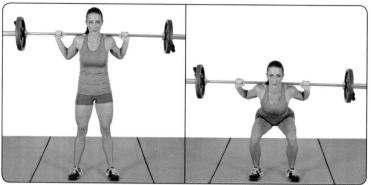

What You Feel:
Quadriceps, glutes

Tips

- *Sit back, and absorb the load with your hips. Feel the glutes contributing to the movement, not just the quads.*
- *Keep your weight on your heels.*

What to Do

1. Stand with your feet slightly wider than your shoulders.
2. Place a barbell across your upper back. You can place the bar above or below your shoulder blades. Just make sure it's comfortable and does not shift around.
3. Take a deep breath, and descend into the squat.
4. Descend by sitting back and down, and lower your body until your thighs reach about a 110-degree angle. (If your thighs reach parallel, you've dropped down too far).
5. Rise upward, making sure to squeeze the glutes to lockout.
6. Return to the starting position.

Barbell High Box Squat

The box squat is an excellent variation that helps people learn how to sit back and rely more on the hips during a squat. It's also a great option for people who have knee issues and find traditional squatting to be problematic.

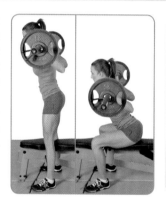

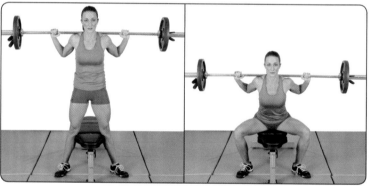

What You Feel: Quadriceps, glutes

Tips

- *Keep your chest up, and maintain a good lower back arch.*
- *Push your knees out so that they track over your toes.*
- *Keep your weight on your heels.*
- *Sit way back in this variation, and keep your tibias upright so that your knees don't move forward.*
- *Squeeze the glutes to lockout.*

What to Do

1. Stand over a bench or a box that sits at knee level, keeping your legs in a wide stance. Most people prefer to turn their toes out to about a 30 to 45-degree angle, but this depends on the person.
2. Place a barbell across your upper back. You can place the bar above or below your shoulder blades. Just make sure it's comfortable and does not shift around.
3. Take a deep breath, and sit back in an exaggerated squat with your glutes extended back, keeping your tibias nearly vertical so that your knees don't move forward. This will require a considerable forward trunk lean.
4. Squat to the bench while forcing your knees out. Then, pause for a brief moment on the box without losing the neutral spinal position.
5. Rise upward, making sure to squeeze the glutes to lockout.
6. Return to the starting position.

Barbell Parallel Squat

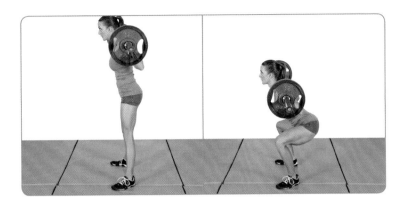

This variation uses slightly less ROM than the full squat and is ideal for those who lack sufficient ankle or hip mobility.

What You Feel: Quadriceps, glutes

Tips

- *Keep your chest up, and make sure your neck aligns with the rest of your spine.*
- *Sit back and absorb the load with your hips.*
- *Keep your trunk mostly upright; it will lean forward, but don't allow for too much of a lean. Also, don't round the spine.*
- *Push through your heels; don't rise up onto your toes.*

What to Do

1. Stand with your feet slightly wider than your shoulders. Most people prefer to turn their toes out to a 30-degree angle, but this is up to your personal preference.
2. Place a barbell across your upper back. You can place the bar above or below your shoulder blades. Just make sure it's comfortable and does not shift around.
3. Take a deep breath, and descend into the squat.
4. Squat down until your thighs are parallel with the ground, pushing your knees out over your toes.
5. Rise upward, making sure to squeeze the glutes to lockout.
6. Return to the starting position.

Barbell Wide Stance Squat

This "sumo" squat variation is often used in powerlifting and activates more glutes than narrower squatting. As you gain proficiency, this style allows you to use heavier loads as well. The barbell wide stance squat is similar in mechanics to the box squat except there's no box.

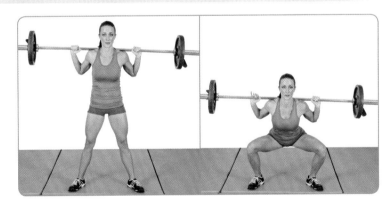

What You Feel: Quadriceps, glutes, adductors

Tips

- *Keep your chest up, and maintain a good lower back arch.*
- *Push your knees out so that they track over your toes.*
- *Keep your weight on your heels.*
- *Sit way back in this variation, and keep your tibias upright so that your knees don't move forward.*
- *Squeeze the glutes to lockout.*

What to Do

1. Standing with your feet in a wide position, turn your toes outward to a comfortable position (many prefer about a 45-degree angle).
2. Place a barbell across your upper back. You can place the bar above or below your shoulder blades. Just make sure it's comfortable and does not shift around.
3. Take a deep breath, and descend into the squat.
4. Squat to a depth where your hips are just below your knees.
5. Rise upward, making sure to squeeze the glutes to lockout.
6. Return to the starting position.

Barbell Low Box Squat

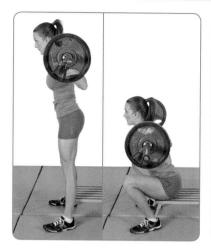
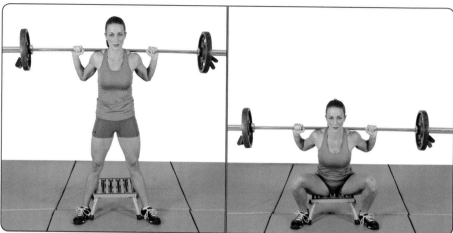

The low box squat is an excellent way to ensure that lifters reach proper depth while squatting. It also builds strength and improves form from the bottom position. In the high box squat, you sit back and don't allow for forward knee travel, while you sit straight down in the low box squat, allowing your knees to travel forward a bit while sharing the load equally between the hips and knees. You'll also be using a shoulder-width stance in this variation, while the high box squat uses a wide stance.

What You Feel: Quadriceps, glutes

Tips

- *Keep your chest up, and maintain a good lower back arch.*
- *Push your knees out so that they track over your toes.*
- *Keep your weight on your heels.*
- *Keep your trunk upright.*
- *Squeeze the glutes to lockout.*

What to Do

1. Stand over a bench or box that sits below knee level, keeping your legs at a shoulder-width stance. Most people prefer to turn their toes out to about a 30 to 45-degree angle, but this depends on the person.
2. Place a barbell across your upper back. You can place the bar above or below your shoulder blades. Just make sure it's comfortable and does not shift around.
3. Take a deep breath, and sit down, keeping your trunk mostly upright.
4. Squat to the bench while forcing your knees out. Then, pause for a brief moment on the box without losing the neutral spinal position.
5. Rise upward, making sure to squeeze the glutes to lockout.
6. Return to the starting position.

Barbell Full Squat

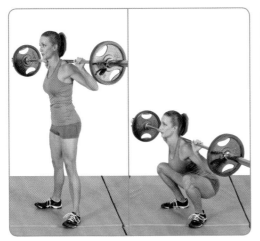

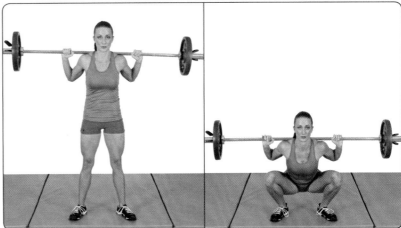

The full squat is a staple in any glute-training program, but squatting to a deep position isn't an easy task for many women. Poor ankle flexibility, limited hip movement, or upper back stiffness can cause issues with squatting. Poor core stability and strength within the back of your body (posterior chain) can also cause problems.

With the right coaching, many women can gain the ability to squat deeply over time, but some lifters may never be able to squat below a parallel position. For example, some lifters' hips are shaped in a way that prevents bending to a certain range at the hips. If this is an issue, this causes problems in the lower back and pelvis, and that nice outward arch starts to curve inward.

Improving mobility and stability while working on your squat pattern is a good idea no matter how great your squats. As you progress, your squat pattern will feel more natural, and you will be able to add more load. Not everyone is capable of safely and comfortably squatting deeply. If this is the case for you, it's perfectly fine to squat to a parallel position or slightly below parallel. Don't ever force yourself into a position that is potentially harmful.

The full squat works the glutes at the bottom of the movement when the hips are flexed and the glutes are stretched. It also works the quads and erectors, helping to build nice thighs and back muscles. For athletes, the squat can lead to increases in vertical jump and acceleration speed.

What You Feel: Quadriceps, glutes

Tips
- *Keep your chest up, and maintain a good lower back arch.*
- *Push your knees out so that they track over your toes.*
- *Keep your weight on your heels.*
- *Sink your hips straight down between your knees.*

What to Do
1. Stand with a stance just wider than shoulder-wide and your feet slightly flared to about a 30-degree angle.
2. Place a barbell across your upper back. The bar can be placed beneath the spine of the scapula (low bar position) or above the spine of the scapula (high bar position). Depending on your goals and comfort level, keep the bar tightly secured across the upper back (don't let it shift around).
3. Take a deep breath, and while keeping your chest up and a good lower back arch, descend into a full squat position.
4. Make sure to keep your knees out so that they track over the toes.
5. As you descend, the lower back will want to flex (round), and your pelvis will want to posteriorly tilt (tilt rearward). Do not let this happen.
6. Make sure your weight doesn't shift forward and that you push through the heels.
7. At the bottom position, your chest is up, your knees are out, your low back is arched, and your feet are flat on the ground.
8. Rise upward, making sure to squeeze the glutes to lockout.
9. Return to the starting position.

Barbell Front Squat

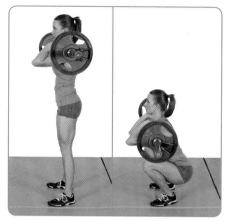

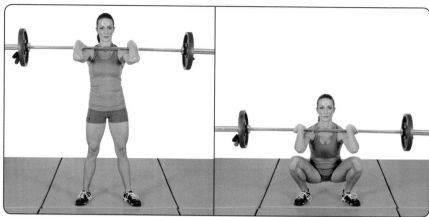

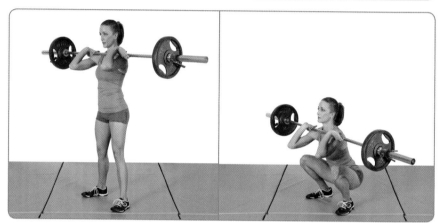

This squat variation keeps your trunk more upright, which spares the spine while still taxing the legs and core. Many coaches and athletes prefer this squat variation because they feel it's a safer alternative to the back squat. Some women initially complain that the barbell position on their shoulders is uncomfortable, but this diminishes over time.

What You Feel: Quadriceps, glutes

Tips

- *Keep your chest up, and maintain a good lower back arch.*
- *Rest the weight on your shoulders, not your wrists and hands.*
- *Keep your elbows high and tucked in.*
- *Push your knees out so that they track over your toes.*
- *Keep your weight on your heels.*
- *Sink your hips straight down between your knees.*

What to Do

1. Step up to the bar positioned at shoulder height. Create a shelf with your front shoulders. Place the bar on your shoulders close to your neck.
2. Keep your elbows up high, and step back from the rack. Stand slightly wider than shoulder width.
3. Sit down between your knees, and descend until your hip joints are below your knees, pushing your knees out over your toes.
4. When you reach a comfortable depth, push back up, making sure to keep your trunk upright.
5. Return to the starting position.

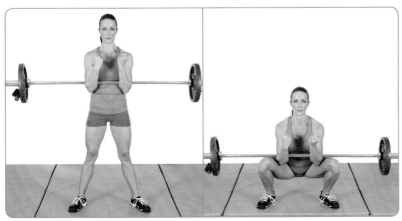
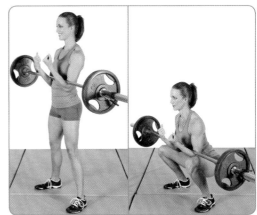

Out of all the standing squat variations, this type of squat maximizes gluteal and core muscle activation. Yet, it's probably the most uncomfortable variation because holding the load in the arms can be quite painful. Over time, this pain and discomfort subside, and you'll be able to up the intensity.

What You Feel: Quadriceps, glutes, core

Tips

- *Keep your chest up, and maintain a good lower back arch.*
- *Push your knees out so that they track over your toes.*
- *Keep your weight on your heels.*
- *Sit back, and use your hips.*

What to Do

1. Set the bar on the rack at waist height. Step up the bar, positioning it in the bend of your elbows.
2. Step back, and stand tall, keeping the bar tight against your body. Stand slightly wider than shoulder width.
3. Sit back and down, descending until your hip joints are below your knees, pushing your knees out over your toes.
4. Squat down until your elbows touch your thighs, keeping your core tight.
5. Return to the starting position.

Squat Mistakes and How to Fix Them

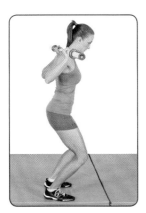
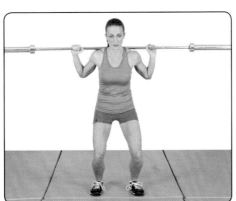

Knee Break/Forward Weight Shift—Notice in the picture how Kellie has an upright torso while initiating the bending at the knees and shifting her weight forward. You want to imagine that someone behind you has a rope around your hips and is pulling rearward, which allows you to initiate the movement by breaking at the hips. You also want to keep your weight on your heels, and sit back and down.

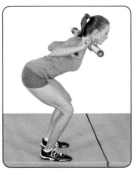
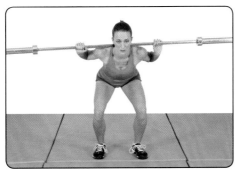

Too Much Torso Lean—Your torso will indeed lean forward in a squat, but you don't want to lean too far forward. Your anthropometry will play a large role in what your squat looks like, but you never want to fold in half during a squat.

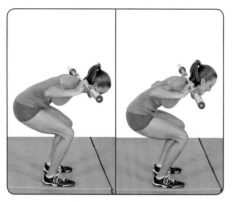
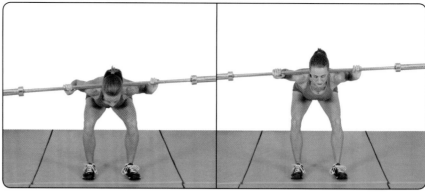

Low Back Rounding—Always keep your back arched in a squat; don't allow it to round. Often, individuals round at the bottom of a squat due to inadequate hip flexion mobility, which pulls the pelvis into posterior pelvic tilt. The spine then goes along for the ride and is pulled into flexion. So, only go as deep as you can while keeping the low back in neutral position.

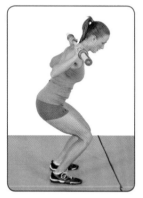
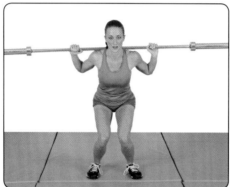

Knee Caving—Probably the most common error in a squat is valgus collapse or knee caving. This is due to weak glutes and external hip rotators. Force your knees out, especially at the bottom of the squat, so that they track properly over your feet.

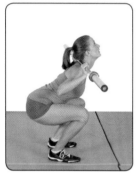
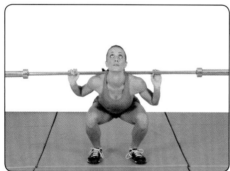

Improper Neck Alignment—Many individuals look up when they squat, and while this isn't the biggest deal in the world, it's probably safer and more efficient to maintain a neutral neck position. For this reason, avoid looking up, and keep your neck in line with your torso.

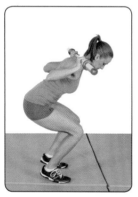
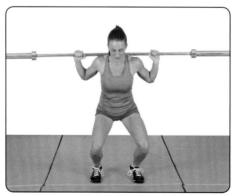

Rising Onto Toes—People often rise up onto their toes during a squat, particularly in the bottom position. This is usually a consequence of inadequate ankle dorsiflexion mobility or tight plantar flexors. Stay on your heels, and work on increasing ankle mobility to allow for proper squatting depth and performance.

Bodyweight Forward Lunge

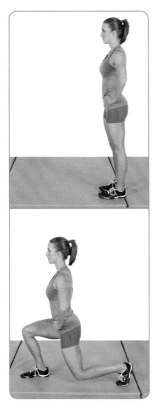
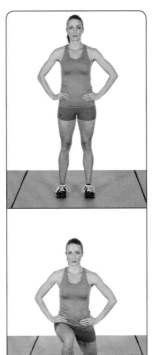

The bodyweight forward lunge targets the knee joint and works the quadriceps very well while still hitting the glutes. It's probably the best type of lunge for the quads, but the reverse lunge is better for the glutes.

What You Feel: Quadriceps, glutes

Tips

- *Step forward far enough so that your front knee aligns vertically with your ankle.*
- *Move straight down so that your front leg creates a 90-degree angle. Do not push your front knee forward.*

What to Do

1. Stand with your feet hip-width apart and your hand on your hips.
2. Step forward into a lunge with your right foot while staying upright.
3. Lower straight down until your left knee hovers just above the floor.
4. Spring back to starting position, and repeat for reps on both sides.

Bodyweight Reverse Lunge

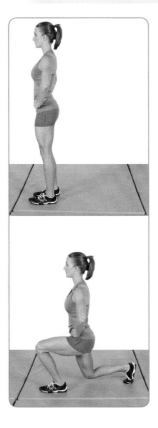
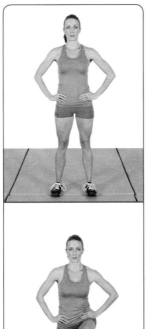

The bodyweight reverse lunge is the fundamental pattern that must be mastered before you start adding load. Stepping rearward targets the glutes and spares the knee joint, as does utilizing a slight forward trunk lean.

What You Feel: Quadriceps, glutes

Tips

- *Step back far enough so that your front knee aligns with your ankle.*
- *Move straight down so that your front leg creates a 90-degree angle. Do not push your front knee forward.*
- *Lean forward slightly while maintaining good spinal alignment.*
- *Sink into the hip of the front leg.*

What to Do

1. Stand with your feet hip-width apart and your hand on your hips.
2. Step backward into a lunge with your left foot while leaning forward slightly.
3. Lower straight down until your left knee hovers just above the floor.
4. Return to the starting position, and repeat for reps on both sides.

Dumbbell Walking Lunge

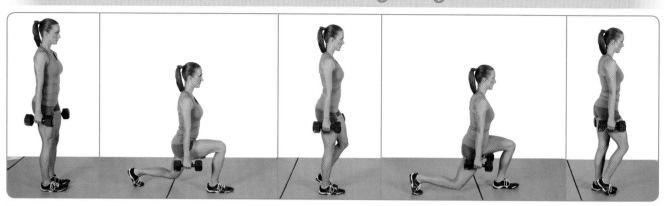

The dumbbell walking lunge is one of my favorite glute exercises. It's known to produce the most glute soreness due to the huge stretch load it induces on the lower glutes. So, don't overdo it with these. Remember that soreness isn't required for muscle growth and can do more harm than good. We all like to feel some residual soreness the next day just to remind us of our hard work and to envision adaptations taking place, but never forget that excessive muscle damage hampers performance and will diminish further gains by preventing new personal records. Don't shy away from the dumbbell walking lunge because it's an amazing movement, but there's no need to bust out five sets of parking lot lunges to failure so that you're out of commission for a week. Train smart!

What You Feel: Quadriceps, glutes

Tips

- *Step forward far enough so that your front knee aligns with your ankle.*
- *Move straight down so that your front leg creates a 90-degree angle. Do not push your front knee forward.*
- *Lean forward slightly while maintaining good spinal alignment.*
- *Contract your glutes during the stretch at the bottom, and spring up by keeping your torso in position. Don't let your hips rise before the shoulders; they should rise in unison.*

What to Do

1. Stand with your feet hip-width apart with a dumbbell in each hand down at your sides.
2. Step forward into a deep lunge with your right foot.
3. Lower straight down until your left knee hovers just above the floor.
4. Spring your body forward, alternating between right and left steps in a forward walking motion.

Dumbbell Deficit Reverse Lunge

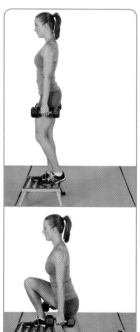

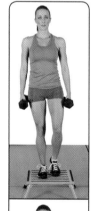

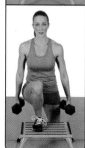

This is an incredibly effective hip and thigh exercise that works the quads well and also hits the glutes down low in a stretched position. The dumbbell loading placement is very stable, and the deficit allows for a greater range of motion.

What You Feel: Quadriceps, glutes

Tips

- *Step back far enough so that your front knee aligns with your ankle.*
- *Move straight down so that your front leg creates a 90-degree angle. Do not push your front knee forward.*
- *Lean forward slightly while maintaining good spinal alignment.*
- *Sink into the hip of your front leg.*

What to Do

1. Holding onto dumbbells, stand with your feet hip-width apart on top of a step.
2. Step backward into a lunge with your left foot while leaning forward slightly.
3. Lower straight down until your left knee hovers just above the floor.
4. Return to the starting position, and repeat for reps on both sides.

Barbell Reverse Lunge

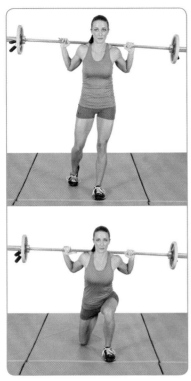
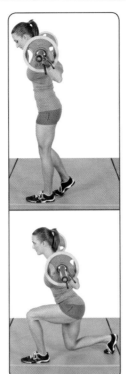

This is an incredibly effective hip and thigh exercise that works the quads and also works the glutes down low in a stretched position. Stepping rearward targets the glutes and spares the knee joint, as does utilizing a slight forward trunk lean.

What You Feel: Quadriceps, glutes

Tips

- *Step back far enough so that your front knee aligns with your ankle.*
- *Move straight down so that your front leg creates a 90-degree angle. Do not push your front knee forward.*
- *Lean forward slightly while maintaining good spinal alignment.*
- *Contract your glutes during the stretch at the bottom.*

What to Do

1. Stand with your feet hip-width apart. Place a barbell across your back, and step away from the rack.
2. Step backward into a lunge with your right foot.
3. Lower straight down until your left knee hovers just above the floor.
4. Spring back to starting position, and repeat for reps on both sides.

Bodyweight Bulgarian Split Squat

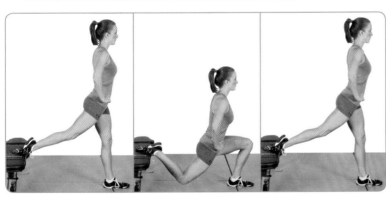
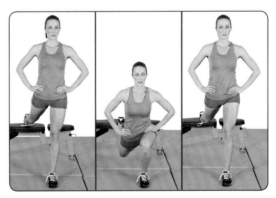

The bodyweight Bulgarian split squat is great for developing single-leg strength and hip stability and can be performed anywhere (with a chair, coffee table, or couch). I like to perform this movement for high reps when I'm training from home or on vacation, but beginners and intermediates can perform it for low to medium reps and still receive a significant challenge.

What You Feel: Quads, glutes

Tips

- *Maintain a slight forward lean, but don't let your hips shoot up faster than your shoulders.*
- *Keep most of your weight on the front foot, and try to use your back foot for balance instead of relying on it too much for support.*
- *Set up in a long stance so that when you drop straight down, the knee of your front leg doesn't travel too far forward.*
- *The knee of your back leg should come close to touching the ground.*
- *Make sure the knee of your front leg stays in line with the foot and doesn't cave inward or outward throughout the set.*

What to Do

1. Standing in front of a bench, place your hands on your hips.
2. Reach the right leg back, and hook the top of your foot over the top of the bench.
3. Sink straight down until your right knee almost touches the ground. Then, rise upward.
4. Repeat, and switch legs.

Bodyweight Deficit Bulgarian Split Squat

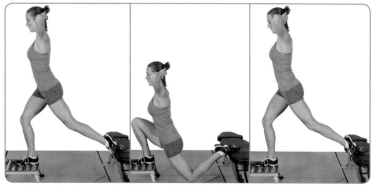 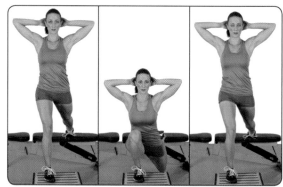

The Bulgarian split squat is great for developing single-leg strength and hip stability while also sparing your spine. The "deficit" allows for a greater range of motion, which places the glutes on stretch.

What You Feel: Quads, glutes

Tips

- *Maintain a slight forward lean, but don't let your hips shoot up faster than your shoulders.*
- *Keep most of your weight on your front foot, and try to use the back foot for balance instead of relying on it too much for support.*
- *Set up in a long stance so that when you drop straight down, the knee of your front leg doesn't travel too far forward.*
- *The knee of your back leg should come close to touching the ground.*
- *Make sure the knee of your front leg stays in line with your foot and doesn't cave inward or outward throughout the set.*

What to Do

1. Face away from the bench, and walk three to four steps out. Place your hands on your hips. Position your right foot in a rear lunge with your foot on the bench (shoelaces facing down).
2. Sink straight down until your right knee almost touches the ground. Then, rise upward.
3. Repeat, and switch legs.

Dumbbell Bulgarian Split Squat

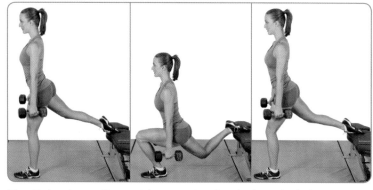 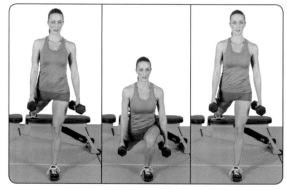

The Bulgarian split squat is great for developing single-leg strength and hip stability while also sparing your spine. The dumbbell placement is an extremely stable loading position, which allows for more tension to be placed on the muscles.

What You Feel: Quads, glutes

Tips

- *Maintain a slight forward lean, but don't let your hips shoot up faster than your shoulders.*
- *Keep most of your weight on the front foot, and try to use your back foot for balance instead of relying on it too much for support.*
- *Set up in a long stance so that when you drop straight down, the knee of your front leg doesn't travel too far forward.*
- *The knee of your back leg should come close to touching the ground.*
- *Make sure the knee of your front leg stays in line with your foot and doesn't cave inward or outward throughout the set.*

What to Do

1. Standing in front of a bench, grab hold of two dumbbells, and reach the right leg back, hooking the top of your foot over the top of the bench.
2. Sink straight down until your right knee almost touches the ground. Then, rise upward.
3. Repeat, and switch legs.

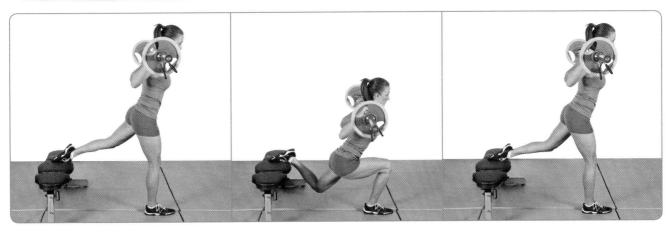

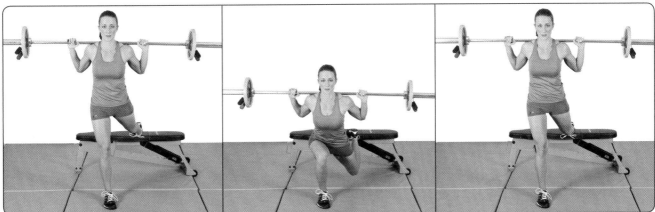

The Bulgarian split squat is great for developing single-leg strength and hip stability while also sparing the spine. The barbell placement is an advanced method for those who have mastered bodyweight and dumbbell variations. This exercise is a favorite of many athletes and coaches because it's a supreme method for developing leg strength.

What You Feel: Quads, glutes

Tips

- *Maintain a slight forward lean, but don't let your hips shoot up faster than your shoulders.*
- *Keep most of your weight on the front foot, and try to use your back foot for balance instead of relying on it too much for support.*
- *Set up in a long stance so that when you drop straight down, the knee of your front leg doesn't travel too far forward.*
- *The knee of your back leg should come close to touching the ground.*
- *Make sure the knee of your front leg stays in line with your foot and doesn't cave inward or outward throughout the set.*

What to Do

1. Standing in front of a bench, place a barbell across your upper back.
2. Reach your right leg back and hook the top of your foot over the top of the bench.
3. Sink straight down until your right knee almost touches the ground. Then, rise upward.
4. Repeat, and switch legs.

Bodyweight Step Up

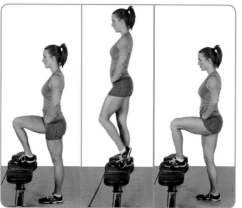
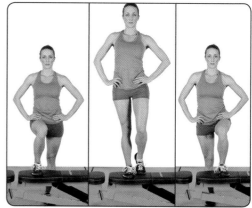

The bodyweight step up is an excellent variation, provided you perform the movement correctly. Pay close attention to your form so that your glutes and thighs achieve optimal loading. This is a fundamental movement that must be mastered by all beginners.

What You Feel: Quadriceps, glutes

Tips

- *Step up with your entire foot on the bench, not just your toes.*
- *Avoid leaning forward too far as you come up.*
- *Try to use mostly the working leg during the movement, and avoid providing too much assistance and "springiness" from the non-working leg.*
- *Return to the starting position in a slow and controlled manner so as to avoid crashing to the floor.*
- *Don't allow both feet to touch down on the box because this encourages cheating as the set progresses by catching your body in a quarter squat and using both legs to complete the movement. Rise to full lockout on one leg.*

What to Do

1. Place your hands on your hips. Stand about 3-6 inches in front of a bench.
2. Place your entire right foot onto the bench, keeping your left foot planted firmly on the ground.
3. Step up onto the bench, driving through the heel of your right foot.
4. Bring your left leg up so that your toe taps the bench, but do not rest tension on your left foot.
5. Return to the starting position, but keep your right foot on the bench.
6. Repeat for reps on both sides.

Dumbbell Step Up

The dumbbell step up is an excellent variation, but make sure you've mastered bodyweight prior to holding onto extra loading. This exercise is underutilized by athletes and coaches.

What You Feel: Quadriceps, glutes

Tips

- *Step up with your entire foot on the bench, not just your toes.*
- *Avoid leaning forward too far as you come up.*
- *Try to use mostly the working leg during the movement, and avoid providing too much assistance and "springiness" from the non-working leg.*
- *Return to the starting position in a slow and controlled manner so as to avoid crashing to the floor.*
- *Don't allow both feet to touch down on the box because this encourages cheating as the set progresses by catching your body in a quarter squat and using both legs to complete the movement. Rise to full lockout on one leg.*

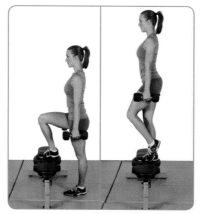
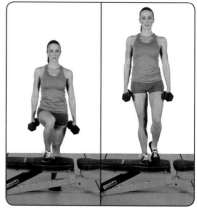

What to Do

1. Grab hold of two dumbbells. Stand about 3-6 inches in front of a bench.
2. Place your entire right foot onto the bench, keeping your left foot planted firmly on the ground.
3. Step up onto the bench, driving through the heel of the right foot.
4. Bring your left leg up so that your toe taps the bench, but do not rest tension on the left foot.
5. Return to the starting position, but keep your right foot on the bench.
6. Repeat for reps on both sides.

Step Up/Reverse Lunge Combo

This variation is a highly underrated glute and thigh exercise that can be performed at a gym or at home. All you need is a step, and the height of the step you use can vary from 12-24 inches in height. In fact, it's one of my favorite exercises to perform when I'm training from home or on vacation.

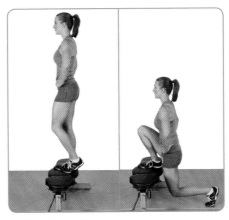
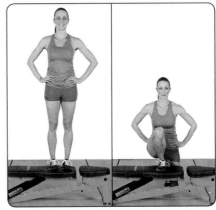

What You Feel: Quads, glutes

Tips

- *While this is a combination movement, perform the exercise in one fluid motion.*
- *Try to sink down into your hip to really work the glute.*
- *Step back far enough to allow you to lunge down.*
- *Stay balanced, and don't twist or shift from side to side.*

What to Do

1. Stand with both feet on a bench.
2. Plant on your right leg, and step back with your left leg, controlling the descent.
3. Land softly, and transition into a lunge movement. Lunge to where your left knee almost touches the ground.
4. Spring back up from the lunge while stepping back up onto the bench.
5. Repeat, and switch legs.

Bodyweight High Step Up

The high step up is an incredible glute-builder that you must work up to in order to perform the movement correctly. It is performed with the knee of your front leg higher than your hip, so you get a very large range of motion at the hip joint. The higher the elevation, the better. This is an exercise that can be performed by advanced lifters with just bodyweight loading. With proper height and tempo, you can achieve very high levels of glute activation.

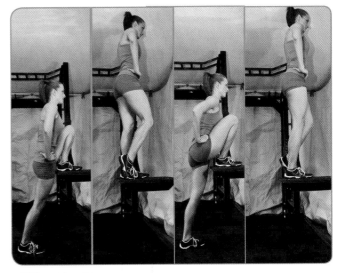

What You Feel: Quads, glutes

Tips

- *Step up with your entire foot on the bench, not just your toes.*
- *Avoid leaning forward too far as you rise.*
- *Do not elevate the step so high that it prevents you from maintaining a neutral lumbar spine when at the bottom of the movement with the leg elevated.*
- *Try to use mostly the working leg during the movement, and avoid providing too much assistance and "springiness" from the non-working leg.*
- *Return to the starting position in a slow and controlled manner so as to avoid crashing to the floor.*
- *Don't allow both feet to touch down on the box because this encourages cheating as the set progresses by catching your body in a quarter squat and using both legs to complete the movement. Rise to full lockout on one leg.*

What to Do

1. Place your hands at your hips. Stand about 3-6 inches in front of a bench.
2. Place your entire right foot onto the bench, keeping your left foot planted firmly on the ground.
3. Step up onto the bench, driving through the heel of your right foot.
4. Bring your left leg up so that your toe taps the bench, but do not rest tension on the left foot.
5. Return to the starting position, but keep your right foot on the bench.
6. Repeat for reps on both sides.

Zercher Step Up

The Zercher step up is a variation that often becomes a favorite over the traditional barbell step up. While holding the barbell in the elbows is at first uncomfortable, the discomfort diminishes over time. The Zercher position is very stable and makes the movement feel more coordinated and smooth.

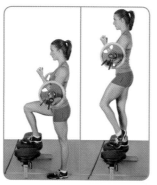 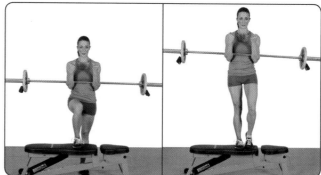

What You Feel: Quadriceps, glutes

Tips

- Step up with your entire foot on the bench, not just your toes.
- Avoid leaning forward too far as you come up.
- Try to use mostly the working leg during the movement, and avoid providing too much assistance and "springiness" from the non-working leg.
- Return to the starting position in a slow and controlled manner so as to avoid crashing to the floor.
- Don't allow both feet to touch down on the box because this encourages cheating as the set progresses by catching your body in a quarter squat and using both legs to complete the movement. Rise to full lockout on one leg.

What to Do

1. Set the bar on the rack at waist height. Step up the bar, positioning it in the bend of your elbows.
2. Step back, and stand tall, keeping the bar tight against your body.
3. Stand about 3-6 inches in front of a bench. Place your entire right foot onto the bench, keeping your left foot planted firmly on the ground.
4. Step up onto the bench, driving through the heel of your right foot.
5. Bring your left leg up so that your toe taps the bench, but do not rest tension on the left foot.
6. Return to the starting position, but keep your right foot on the bench.
7. Repeat for reps on both sides.

Barbell Step Up

The barbell step up is an excellent variation that works the legs incredibly well. Some athletes prefer heavy barbell step ups to squatting due to the decreased loading on the spine. I believe Bulgarian split squats are better in this regard, however. Nevertheless, the barbell step up is an effective exercise if performed correctly.

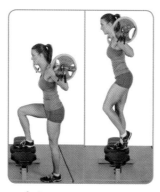

What You Feel: Quadriceps, glutes

Tips

- Step up with your entire foot on the bench, not just your toes.
- Avoid leaning forward too far as you come up.
- Try to use mostly the working leg during the movement, and avoid providing too much assistance and "springiness" from the non-working leg.
- Return to the starting position in a slow and controlled manner so as to avoid crashing down to the floor.
- Don't allow both feet to touch down on the box because this encourages cheating as the set progresses by catching your body in a quarter squat and using both legs to complete the movement. Rise to full lockout on one leg.

What to Do

1. Place a barbell across your upper back. You can place the bar above or below your shoulder blades. Just make sure it's comfortable and does not shift around.
2. Stand about 3-6 inches in front of a bench. Place your entire right foot onto the bench, keeping your left foot planted firmly on the ground.
3. Step up onto the bench, driving through the heel of your right foot.
4. Bring your left leg up so that your toe taps the bench, but do not rest tension on the left foot.
5. Return to the starting position, but keep your right foot on the bench.
6. Repeat for reps on both sides.

Dumbbell High Step Up

The high step up is an incredible glute-builder that you must work up to it in order to perform the movement correctly. It is performed with the knee of your front leg higher than your hip, so you get a very large range of motion at the hip joint. The higher the elevation, the better. Holding onto dumbbells makes the movement even more challenging, and holding onto just two five-pound dumbbells can make a world of difference. Just don't sacrifice form in order to use heavier loads.

What You Feel: Quads, glutes

Tips

- *Step up with your entire foot on the bench, not just your toes.*
- *Avoid leaning forward too far as you rise.*
- *Do not elevate the step so high that it prevents you from maintaining a neutral lumbar spine when at the bottom of the movement with the leg elevated.*
- *Try to use mostly the working leg during the movement, and avoid providing too much assistance and "springiness" from the non-working leg.*
- *Return to the starting position in a slow and controlled manner so as to avoid crashing to the floor.*
- *Don't allow both feet to touch down on the box because this encourages cheating as the set progresses by catching your body in a quarter squat and using both legs to complete the movement. Rise to full lockout on one leg.*

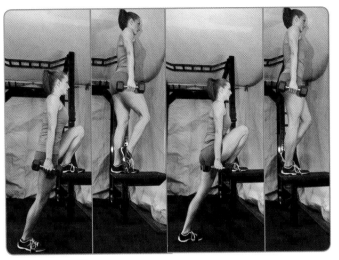

What to Do

1. Hold onto a pair of dumbbells.
2. Stand about 3-6 inches in front of a bench. Place your entire right foot onto the bench, keeping your left foot planted firmly on the ground.
3. Step up onto the bench, driving through the heel of your right foot.
4. Bring your left leg up so that your toe taps the bench, but do not rest tension on the left foot.
5. Return to the starting position, but keep your right foot on the bench.
6. Repeat for reps on both sides.

Single-Leg Box Squat

What You Feel: Quads, glutes

Tips

- *Avoid leaning to the right or left as you descend.*
- *Hold onto a light kettlebell, dumbbell, or plate in front of you for counterbalance.*
- *Keep your chest tall, and avoid rounding your lower back at the bottom of the movement.*
- *Don't plop onto the box; lower yourself under control.*

What to Do

1. Stand in front of a box with your feet shoulder-width apart. Balance on your right leg with your left leg straight out, hovering just above the floor.
2. Descend on your right leg by flexing the hip and knee.
3. As you move down, elevate your arms out in front of your torso, and keep your left leg locked out in front of you so that it remains off of the floor.
4. Sit back, and land softly onto the box.
5. Power back up through the glutes to return to the starting position.
6. Repeat for reps on both sides.

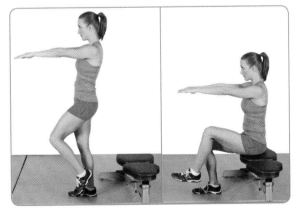

The single-leg box squat builds single-leg strength and stability. The box height can be adjusted and reduced over time to increase the challenge. This variation is ideal compared to the pistol squat because the pistol often leads to lower back rounding, which doesn't occur in a proper single-leg box squat. This is a true single-leg movement since it's performed one leg at a time.

Skater Squat

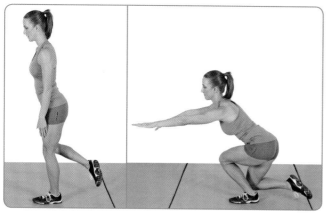
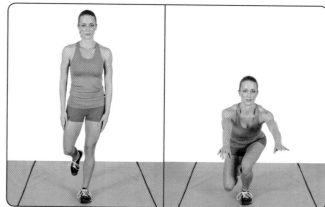

The skater squat builds single-leg strength and stability in addition to increasing balance and coordination. This is a very "knee-friendly" variation that should be incorporated into your workouts on a regular basis.

What You Feel: Quadriceps, glutes

Tips

- *Use a slow and controlled movement so that you don't crash onto the floor.*
- *You may want to place a pad under your back knee to signal when you've reached the appropriate depth.*

What to Do

1. Stand on your right leg with your left leg bent at a 90-degree angle. Rest your arms at your sides.
2. Squat straight down until your back knee hovers just above the floor, leaning forward with your torso.
3. As you descend, bring your arms straight out in front of you.
4. Power up through the hips, returning to the start position.
5. Repeat for reps on both sides.

Pistol Squat

This squat variation builds single-leg strength and stability in addition to increasing balance and coordination. It's probably the most challenging single-leg exercise in existence, and many folks do it with poor form. Make sure you look athletic and exhibit good posture when performing this movement.

What You Feel: Quadriceps, glutes

Tips

- *To ease into this exercise, start while standing on a box that has you descend until your thigh is parallel to the ground when the heel of the non-working foot reaches the ground. Gradually increase the height until full depth is reached and the box is no longer needed.*
- *Avoid leaning to the right or left as you descend.*
- *Hold onto a light kettlebell, dumbbell, or plate in front of you for counterbalance.*
- *Keep your chest tall, and avoid rounding your lower back at the bottom of the movement.*

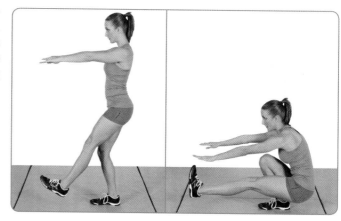

What to Do

1. Stand with your feet shoulder-width apart. Balance on your right leg with your left leg straight out hovering just above the floor.
2. Descend on your right leg by flexing the hip and knee.
3. As you move down, elevate your arms out in front of your torso, and keep your left leg locked out in front of you so that it remains off of the floor.
4. Power back up through the glutes to return to the starting position.
5. Repeat for reps on both sides.

Hip Dominant

The hip dominant category requires a certain level of experience to grasp, but you can transform from novice to master over time. When you squat or lunge, you feel the quads working very hard, and since your knees move through a large range of motion in those movements, they're categorized as quad dominant.

But what about deadlifts? The knees do bend, and the quads do contract very hard. But the knees don't bend as far, and the quads don't activate quite as high as they do in a squat. Since the knees are more straightened, however, the hamstrings are in a better position to produce force and are worked to greater degree during the deadlift compared to the squat. The hips move through a large range of motion, but the knees are only partially bent. So, the movement centers mostly on the hip joint. For these reasons, the deadlift, along with all of the exercises that resemble deadlifts, are considered to be hip dominant.

Hip dominant movements place the most stress on the hip extensors in a hips-flexed position, similar to squats. But one key difference between squatting movements and hip dominant movements is that the hamstrings are more highly activated and are at a better length to extend the hips and straighten out the body. The deadlift is easily the most popular hip dominant exercise. Since the barbell is held in your arms, muscle force must be produced to grip the barbell, hold the scapula and upper back in place, keep your core tight, and extend the hips, knees, and ankles. The deadlift is indeed a full body exercise and allows you to pull an incredible load, making it the more effective full body exercise.

When trained properly, most women can become incredible deadlifters, but they need to understand that the lift is not a squat. The hips stay higher, and the hamstrings are heavily involved in the lift. The glutes are also highly activated during the deadlift, as are the back extensors.

It's important to understand that there are many different ways to deadlift. The good morning has been called the Russian deadlift, as it closely resembles a deadlift but with the bar on the upper back instead of in the hands.

Hip dominant exercises do not produce as much glute soreness as quad dominant exercises because they're not stretched to the same degree. The glutes are activated to a higher degree during hip dominant exercises, however, compared to quad dominant exercises, though not quite as high as they are during glute dominant exercises. For this reason, hip dominant exercises are very well-rounded and lead to impressive levels of total body functional strength.

In fact, the hip-hinge pattern is paramount to lifting success, and it's very important to understand proper lumbopelvic-hip motion during this pattern. The deadlift is best at improving this motor skill down low in a hips-flexed position. Knowing how to move at the hips while keeping your core stable is critical for the prevention of low back pain, especially for long-term lifters.

Bent Knee Pull-through

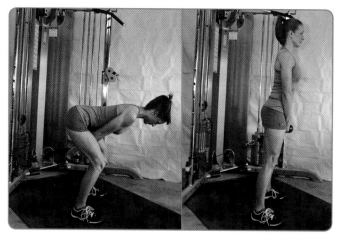

The pull-through is an underrated glute exercise that hits the glutes very well if performed properly. It's difficult to use heavy loads due to issues with balance and stability, but with practice, you'll gain coordination and improve upon your ability to use heavier loads.

What You Feel: Glutes, hamstrings

Tips

- *Keep your chest up, and bend at the hips while keeping your head and neck in a neutral position.*
- *Sit back, and push your hips forward with the glutes.*

What to Do

1. Grab hold of the cable implement (you can use a rope handle or v-bar handle) with the cable between your legs facing away from the cable column.
2. Step out a few steps to put the cable on tension, but don't step out too far to where the weight stack will "top out" and hit the top of the unit during the exercise.
3. Keeping the spine and neck in neutral, sit back, and bend at the hips.
4. Push your hips forward by squeezing the glutes, making sure to achieve full hip extension.
5. Repeat for the desired number of repetitions.

Hex Bar Deadlift

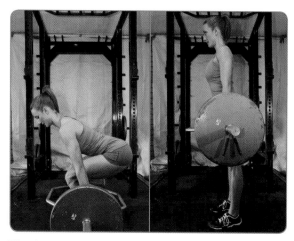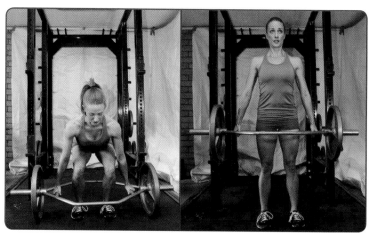

The hex bar deadlift is a favorite of many strength coaches around the world. It's really a mixture of a squat and a deadlift, and for this reason, it has been called the "squat lift." Since the knees won't be in the way of the traditional barbell, they're able to travel forward more, which increases the tension on the quads and slightly decreases tension on the hamstrings. People with poor hamstring flexibility are usually able to hex bar deadlift just fine, and this variation places slightly less loading on the spine. So, it's better tolerated by folks with back issues.

What You Feel: Back, quads, glutes, hamstrings

Tips

- *This lift is still a deadlift, not a squat, so keep your hips a bit higher than you would with a squat.*
- *Keep your spine in neutral, and hinge around the hips.*
- *Push through the heels, and squeeze the glutes to lockout.*
- *Make sure the eccentric (lowering) component mirrors the concentric (rising) component.*

What to Do

1. Stand in the center of a hex bar, making sure you're symmetrical with your arms in line with the handles.
2. Bend down, and grip the handles in the middle of the grips, keeping your spine and neck in a neutral position.
3. Raise the barbell, and squeeze the glutes to lockout.
4. Reverse the movement, and repeat for reps.

Dumbbell RDL

The dumbbell RDL is ideal for teaching the hip hinge pattern and can be used with beginners and more advanced lifters for variety.

What You Feel: Back, hamstrings, glutes

Tips

- *Sit back, and feel your hamstrings receiving the load, keeping the weight on your heels.*
- *Keep your spine in a neutral position, and don't allow your back to round.*
- *Don't be overly-concerned with loading on this exercise. If your form is strict, you can obtain an amazing workout without going too heavy on these.*

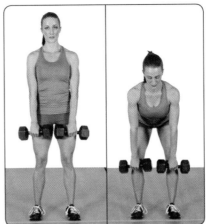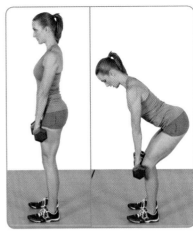

What to Do

1. Take the dumbbells out of the rack, and begin in a standing position.
2. Step back, and set your feet in a shoulder-width stance.
3. Sit back, and bend over at the hips. The knees will bend as you move your hips rearward. Try to feel the movement in your hamstrings as much as possible, and keep your core stable in a neutral position.
4. Reverse the movement, and squeeze the glutes to lockout.

Romanian Deadlift (RDL)

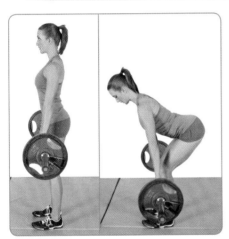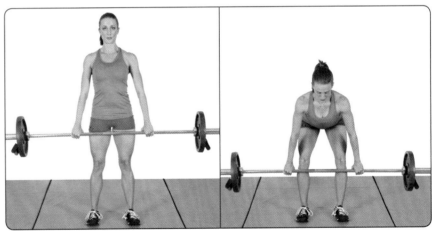

This variation is excellent for teaching individuals how to sit back and use the hips and hamstrings when lifting. The hip hinge pattern is essential for proper lifting performance, and the RDL is the premier exercise for teaching this pattern.

What You Feel: Back, hamstrings, glutes

Tips

- *Sit back, and feel your hamstrings receiving the load, keeping the weight on your heels.*
- *Keep your spine in a neutral position, and don't allow your back to round.*
- *Don't be overly-concerned with loading on this exercise. If your form is strict, you can obtain an amazing workout without going too heavy on these.*

What to Do

1. Take the bar out of the rack, making sure your grip is symmetrical. Begin in a standing position.
2. Step back, and set your feet in a shoulder-width stance.
3. Sit back, and bend over at the hips. The knees will bend as you move your hips rearward. Try to feel the movement in your hamstrings as much as possible, and keep your core stable in a neutral position.
4. Reverse the movement, and squeeze the glutes to lockout.

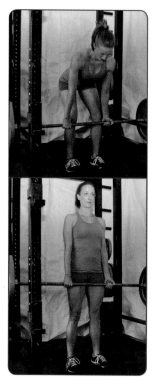
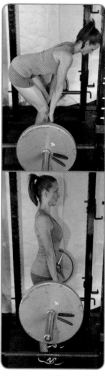
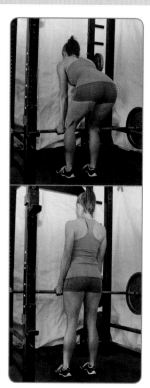

What You Feel: Back, hamstrings, glutes

Tips

* *Do not "squat" the weight up; it's a hip hinge movement. Sit back, and bend at the hips. The knees will bend, but your hamstrings will be put on stretch. Your knees won't move forward much.*
* *Keep your spine in a neutral position.*
* *Squeeze the glutes to lockout.*

What to Do

1. Stand inside the rack with a shoulder-width stance and your feet facing forward.
2. The barbell should be positioned somewhere below your kneecaps. Set up with the bar skimming your body.
3. Sit back, and bend over at the hips, while keeping your spine in a neutral position as you grab hold of the barbell. When the load gets heavy, you can switch from a double-overhand grip to a mixed grip.
4. Inhale, hold your breath, and raise the barbell.
5. Squeeze the glutes to lockout.
6. Reverse the movement by sitting back and having the barbell skim your legs.

The rack pull offers several key benefits. First, it's a great exercise for beginners due to the decreased hip ROM. Essentially, people with limited hamstring flexibility can still practice the hip hinge pattern while improving their core stability and hip mobility, allowing them to eventually move to full range deadlifts. Second, it allows for greater loads to be used, which is a good strategy to employ from time to time.

Dumbbell American Deadlift

The American deadlift (ADL) is one of my favorite glute exercises. It's like a Romanian deadlift (RDL), except that you posteriorly tilt the pelvis with a strong glute contraction at the top of the movement. You stress the hamstrings down low, and you stress the glutes up high. Most people have terrible motor control at the pelvis, and the ADL improves pelvic mechanics, which are important for core stability. Before using barbell loading, you may need to utilize dumbbells to master the pattern.

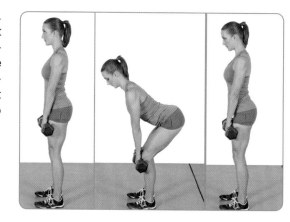

What You Feel: Back, hamstrings, glutes

Tips

* *Sit back, and get a strong arch and anterior pelvic tilt at the bottom of the movement to stress the hamstrings.*
* *As you rise upward, contract the glutes forcefully, and tilt the pelvis posteriorly to stress the glutes.*
* *Keep the dumbbells close to your body throughout the duration of the lift.*
* *Keep your neck in a neutral position.*

What to Do

1. Take the dumbbells out of the rack, and begin from a standing position with a shoulder-width stance.
2. Keeping your spine in a neutral position, sit back, and bend forward at the hips. Keep a good arch and anterior pelvic tilt so that you receive a good stretch in the hamstrings on the way down.
3. Reverse the movement, and raise the dumbbells. Start contracting the glutes forcefully to posteriorly tilt the pelvis.
4. Repeat for the desired number of reps.

Dumbbell Deadlift

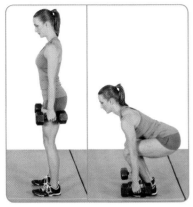 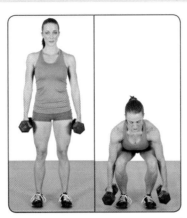

The dumbbell deadlift is a good variation, especially for beginners who may not be ready for barbell loading.

What You Feel: Back, hamstrings, glutes

Tips

- *The deadlift is not a squat; it's a hip hinge. The hips stay higher than they do in a squat.*
- *Don't let the dumbbells drift out in front of you. The bar skims the body.*
- *The eccentric component (lowering) should be a mirror image of the concentric component (rising). Don't neglect eccentric technique.*
- *Be concerned with neck position, and keep it in neutral throughout the deadlift ROM.*
- *Line up with your shoulders slightly in front of the dumbbells.*
- *Don't round your back down low or hyperextend your back up high. Keep your spine in a neutral position, and revolve around the hips.*

What to Do

1. Begin by standing with a narrow stance and your feet pointed straight ahead.
2. Sit back and down, bend over, and grasp hold of the dumbbells.
3. Make sure you keep your chest up, and hold a strong lower back arch. If a mirror were in front of you, you should be able to read your shirt in the mirror.
4. From a side view, your hips should be higher than your knees, and your shoulders should be higher than your hips. Your shoulders should be positioned slightly in front of the bar.
5. Before the lift begins, look down so that your neck is in a neutral position. (Obviously, you'll no longer be able to read your shirt in the mirror.)
6. Take a deep breath, and raise the dumbbells, making sure that the dumbbells skim the body throughout the entire repetition.
7. Your lower back will want to round (flex), and your pelvis will want to posteriorly tilt (roll rearward). Do not let this happen.
8. Rise to full extension, stand tall, and use the glutes to push your hips forward to lockout.
9. Begin the descent by sitting back as if performing an RDL. Keep a strong lower back arch, and keep the bar close to your body.
10. Once the dumbbells descend lower than your knees, bend the knees, and keep lowering until you return to the starting position.

Dumbbell Walking RDL

The dumbbell walking RDL is a variation that can be performed from time to time with success. Some people find it more natural than the single-leg RDL, and it's very easy on the knee-joint.

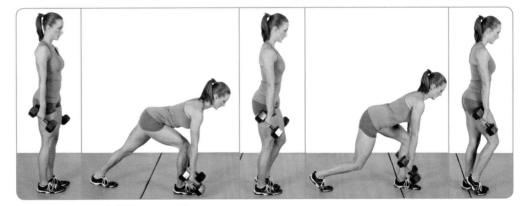

What You Feel: Hamstrings, glutes

Tips

- *Keep your chest tall; don't round your back.*
- *Find the sweet spot with stride distance. Don't take strides that are too short or too long.*

What to Do

1. Grab hold of the dumbbells, and begin in a standing position.
2. Step forward with your right leg, and bend over at the hips while keeping your spine in a neutral position.
3. Rise back to position, step forward with your left leg, and bend over at the hips while keeping your spine in a neutral position.
4. Continue alternating between legs until all repetitions are completed.

Dumbbell Single-Leg Abducted RDL

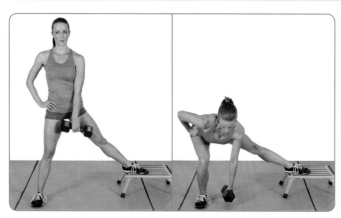

The single-leg abducted RDL is akin to the Bulgarian split squat. It isn't a "true" single-leg exercise since you're using the "non-working" leg for support. This variation provides increased balance and stability, which allows for heavier loads.

What You Feel: Hamstrings, glutes

Tips

- *Keep most of the load on your working leg, and use the other leg for balance/stability.*
- *Sink the dumbbell in between the hips.*

What to Do

1. Hold a dumbbell in your right hand. Plant on your left leg, and place your right leg on top of a small box with your leg straight out to the side.
2. Bend at the hips while keeping your spine in a neutral position.
3. Squeeze the glutes to lockout, and lower the load under control.
4. Perform all of the reps on your left leg.
5. Switch the dumbbell to the left hand, and repeat on the right leg.

Dumbbell Single-Leg RDL

The single-leg RDL is an excellent movement for teaching balance and proprioception. This movement requires a tremendous blend of balance, coordination, hamstring flexibility, and core stability. Initially, it will feel awkward, and you'll likely feel uncoordinated. But over time, it will feel more natural and comfortable.

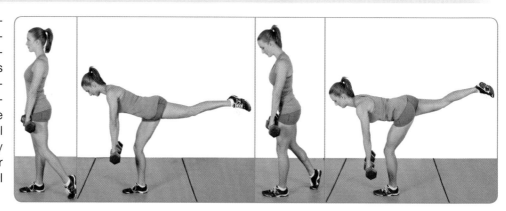

What You Feel: Hamstrings, glutes

Tips

- *Keep your back leg in line with your torso as you bend over.*
- *At the top of the movement, your back leg should be pointed straight back.*
- *Sit back just as you would with a bilateral RDL.*
- *Focus intensively on your balance. If you screw up on a repetition, just reset and continue.*
- *Keep your core stable while hinging at the hips; don't allow your back to round.*

What to Do

1. Grab hold of the dumbbells, and begin in a standing position with the weight shifted onto your right leg.
2. Squeeze the glute of your left leg, and lock it into position so that it stays in line with your torso as you bend over.
3. Sit back, and bend at the hips while keeping your spine and neck in a neutral position.
4. Receive a stretch in your hamstrings and then reverse back to starting position, firing the glute as you rise upward.
5. Repeat, and switch to the left leg.

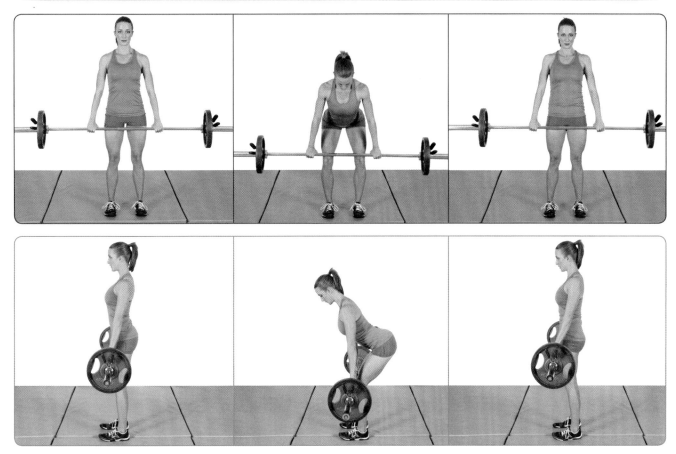

The American deadlift (ADL) is one of my favorite glute exercises. It's like a Romanian deadlift (RDL), except that you posteriorly tilt the pelvis with a strong glute contraction at the top of the movement. You stress the hamstrings down low, and you stress the glutes up high. Poor motor control at the pelvis is very common, and the ADL improves pelvic mechanics, which are important for core stability.

What You Feel: Back, hamstrings, glutes

Tips

- *Sit back, and get a strong arch and anterior pelvic tilt at the bottom of the movement to stress the hamstrings.*
- *As you rise upward, contract the glutes forcefully, and tilt your pelvis posteriorly to stress the glutes.*
- *Keep the bar close to your body throughout the duration of the lift.*
- *Keep your neck in a neutral position.*

What to Do

1. Take the bar out of the rack, and begin from a standing position with a shoulder-width stance.
2. Keeping your spine in a neutral position, sit back, and bend forward at the hips. Keep a good arch and anterior pelvic tilt so that you receive a good stretch in the hamstrings on the way down.
3. Reverse the movement, and raise the barbell.
4. Start contracting the glutes forcefully to posteriorly tilt the pelvis.
5. Repeat for the desired number of reps.

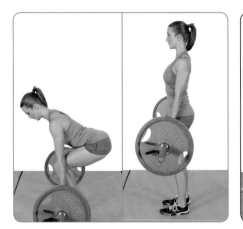
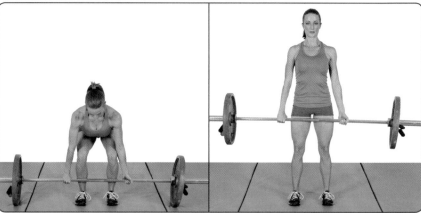

The deadlift is an incredible glute-builder when performed correctly. Most people are stronger when rounding the back, but this isn't the safest way to deadlift. Keeping the natural spinal arches in the deadlift will protect the spine and allow you to stay healthy over the long haul.

The glutes get worked thoroughly during the entire range of a deadlift, as they contribute to getting the bar off the ground as well as properly locking out the lift with good mechanics. The deadlift doesn't just work the glutes, however. It works the entire posterior chain, along with the grip muscles, including the calves, the hamstrings, the erector spinae, the lats, the rear delts, the rhomboids, and the traps.

For some, especially those with hamstring flexibility issues, maintaining good form at the bottom of the range of motion poses an issue. If this sounds like you, rack pulls or hex bar deadlifts are a better option until you improve your hip flexion and hamstring mobility.

Deadlifting will do wonders for functional, usable strength and will lead to considerable improvements in athleticism. Setting a personal record on a deadlift is a wonderful feeling that boosts confidence and improves self-esteem.

What You Feel: Back, hamstrings, glutes

Tips

- *The deadlift is not a squat; it's a hip hinge. The hips stay higher than they do in a squat.*
- *Don't let the bar drift out in front of you. The bar skims your body.*
- *The eccentric component (lowering) should be a mirror image of the concentric component (rising). Don't neglect eccentric technique.*
- *Be concerned with your neck position, and keep it neutral throughout the deadlift ROM.*
- *Line up with your shoulders slightly in front of the bar.*
- *Don't round your back down low or hyperextend your back up high. Keep your spine in a neutral position, and revolve around the hips.*

What to Do

1. Begin by standing with a narrow stance and your feet pointed straight ahead with your shins approximately 2-3 inches from the barbell.
2. Sit back and down, bend over, and grasp hold of the barbell, making sure to keep an even grip. (A double overhand grip can be used, or a mixed grip can be used if going heavy.)
3. Make sure you keep your chest up, and hold a strong lower back arch. If a mirror were in front of you, you should be able to read your shirt in the mirror.
4. From a side view, your hips should be higher than your knees, and your shoulders should be higher than your hips. Your shoulders should be positioned slightly in front of the bar.
5. Before the lift begins, look down so that your neck is in a neutral position. (Obviously, you'll no longer be able to read your shirt in the mirror.)
6. Take a deep breath, and raise the barbell, making sure that the bar skims your body throughout the entire repetition.
7. Your lower back will want to round (flex), and your pelvis will want to posteriorly tilt (roll rearward). Don't let this happen.
8. Rise to full extension, stand tall, and use the glutes to push your hips forward to lockout.
9. Begin the descent by sitting back as if performing an RDL. Keep a strong lower back arch, and keep the bar close to your body.
10. Once the bar descends lower than your knees, bend the knees, and keep lowering until you return to the starting position.

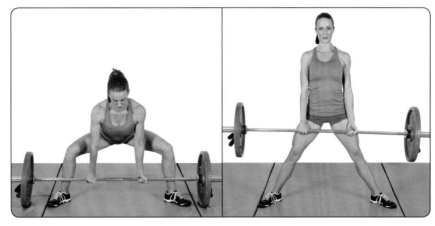

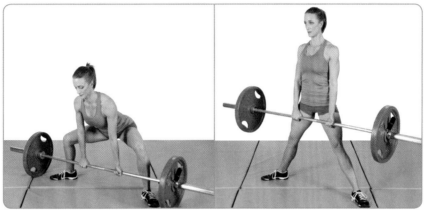

This deadlift variation places slightly less loading on your lower back and emphasizes the glutes and quads to a slightly greater degree than the conventional version. Many individuals prefer to deadlift sumo-style compared to the traditional way. The sumo version is more similar to a squat and requires slightly less hamstring flexibility.

What You Feel: Back, quads, glutes, hamstrings, adductors

Tips

- *Don't let the bar drift out in front of you. The bar should skim your body.*
- *The eccentric component (lowering) should be a mirror image of the concentric component (rising). Don't neglect eccentric technique.*
- *Be concerned with your neck position, and keep it neutral throughout the deadlift ROM.*
- *Line up with the shoulders slightly in front of the bar.*
- *Don't round your back down low or hyperextend your back up high. Keep your spine in a neutral position, and revolve around the hips.*

What to Do

1. Begin standing with a wide stance and your feet flared outward with your shins approximately 2-3 inches from the barbell.
2. Sit back and down, bend over, and grasp hold of the barbell, making sure to keep an even grip. (A double overhand grip can be used, or a mixed grip can be used if going heavy.)
3. Make sure you keep your chest up, and hold a strong lower back arch. If a mirror were in front of you, you should be able to read your shirt in the mirror.
4. From a side view, your hips should be higher than your knees, and your shoulders should be higher than your hips. Your shoulders should be positioned slightly in front of the bar.
5. Before the lift begins, look down so that your neck is in a neutral position. (Obviously, you'll no longer be able to read your shirt in the mirror.)
6. Take a deep breath, and raise the barbell, making sure that the bar skims your body throughout the entire repetition.
7. Force your knees out, and keep your trunk upright.
8. Your lower back will want to round (flex), and your pelvis will want to posteriorly tilt (roll rearward). Don't let this happen.
9. Rise to full extension, stand tall, and use the glutes to push your hips forward to lockout.
10. Begin the descent by sitting back as if performing an RDL. Keep a strong lower back arch, and keep the bar close to your body.
11. Once the bar descends lower than your knees, bend the knees, and keep lowering until you return to the starting position.

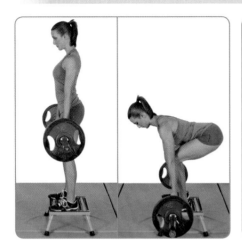
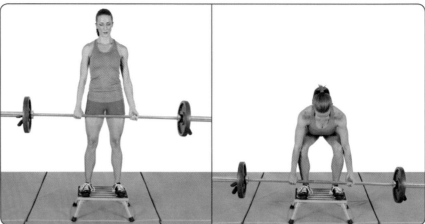

The deficit variation allows for greater hip and knee range of motion and makes for a more challenging movement. This exercise does require sufficient hamstring flexibility, so make sure you can perform the movement correctly before going heavy.

What You Feel: Back, hamstrings, glutes

Tips

- *The deadlift is not a squat; it's a hip hinge. The hips stay higher than they do in a squat.*
- *Don't let the bar drift out in front of you. The bar should skim the body.*
- *The eccentric component (lowering) should be a mirror image of the concentric component (rising). Don't neglect eccentric technique.*
- *Be concerned with your neck position, and keep it neutral throughout the deadlift ROM.*
- *Line up with your shoulders slightly in front of the bar.*
- *Don't round your back down low or hyperextend your back up high. Keep your spine in a neutral position, and revolve around the hips.*

What to Do

1. Begin by standing on a box with a narrow stance and your feet pointed straight ahead with your shins skimming the barbell.
2. Sit back and down, bend over, and grasp hold of the barbell, making sure to keep an even grip. (A double overhand grip can be used, or a mixed grip can be used if going heavy.)
3. Make sure you keep your chest up, and hold a strong lower back arch. If a mirror were in front of you, you should be able to read your shirt in the mirror.
4. From a side view, your hips should be higher than your knees, and your shoulders should be higher than your hips. Your shoulders should be positioned slightly in front of the bar.
5. Before the lift begins, look down so that your neck is in a neutral position. (Obviously, you'll no longer be able to read your shirt in the mirror.)
6. Take a deep breath, and raise the barbell, making sure that the bar skims your body throughout the entire repetition.
7. Your lower back will want to round (flex), and your pelvis will want to posteriorly tilt (roll rearward). Don't let this happen.
8. Rise to full extension, stand tall, and use the glutes to push your hips forward to lockout.
9. Begin the descent by sitting back as if performing an RDL. Keep a strong lower back arch, and keep the bar close to your body.
10. Once the bar descends lower than your knees, bend the knees, and keep lowering until you return to the starting position.

Deficit Deadlift from Plate

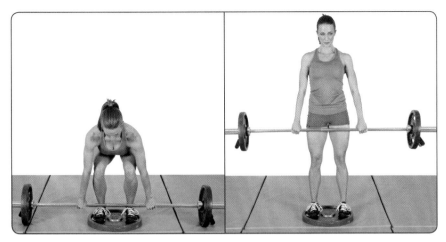 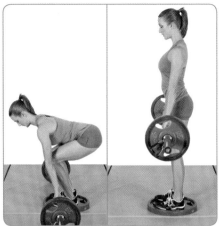

The deficit variation allows for greater hip and knee range of motion and makes for a more challenging movement. This exercise requires sufficient hamstring flexibility, however, so make sure you can perform the movement correctly before going heavy.

What You Feel: Back, hamstrings, glutes

Tips

- *The deadlift is not a squat; it's a hip hinge. The hips stay higher than they do in a squat.*
- *Don't let the bar drift out in front of you. The bar should skim the body.*
- *The eccentric component (lowering) should be a mirror image of the concentric component (rising). Don't neglect eccentric technique.*
- *Be concerned with your neck position, and keep it neutral throughout the deadlift ROM.*
- *Line up with your shoulders slightly in front of the bar.*
- *Don't round your back down low or hyperextend your back up high. Keep your spine in a neutral position, and revolve around the hips.*

What to Do

1. Begin by standing on a plate with a narrow stance and your feet pointed straight ahead with your shins approximately 2-3 inches from the barbell.
2. Sit back and down, bend over, and grasp hold of the barbell, making sure to keep an even grip. (A double overhand grip can be used, or a mixed grip can be used if going heavy.)
3. Make sure you keep your chest up, and hold a strong lower back arch. If a mirror were in front of you, you should be able to read your shirt in the mirror.
4. From a side view, your hips should be higher than your knees, and your shoulders should be higher than your hips. Your shoulders should be positioned slightly in front of the bar.
5. Before the lift begins, look down so that your neck is in a neutral position. (Obviously, you'll no longer be able to read your shirt in the mirror.)
6. Take a deep breath, and raise the barbell, making sure that the bar skims your body throughout the entire repetition.
7. Your lower back will want to round (flex), and your pelvis will want to posteriorly tilt (roll rearward). Don't let this happen.
8. Rise to full extension, stand tall, and use the glutes to push your hips forward to lockout.
9. Begin the descent by sitting back as if performing an RDL. Keep a strong lower back arch, and keep the bar close to your body.
10. Once the bar descends lower than your knees, bend them, and keep lowering until you return to the starting position.

Barbell Single-Leg Abducted RDL

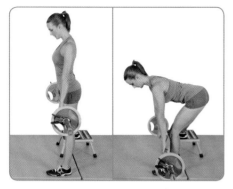
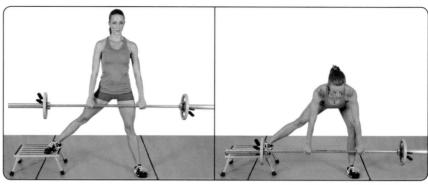

The single-leg abducted RDL is akin to the Bulgarian split squat. It isn't a "true" single-leg exercise since you're using the "non-working" leg for support. This variation provides increased balance and stability, which allows for heavier loads to be used. You can begin with the dumbbell variation, but as you gain strength, you might need to progress to this barbell version.

What You Feel: Hamstrings, glutes

Tips

- *Keep most of the load on your working leg, and just use the other leg for balance/stability.*
- *Try to mimic the traditional RDL form except that one leg will be out to the side.*
- *Sit back, and skim your body with the barbell.*

What to Do

1. Hold onto a barbell. Plant on the left leg, and place your right leg on top of a small box with the leg straight out to the side.
2. Bend at the hips while keeping your spine in a neutral position.
3. Squeeze the glutes to lockout, and lower the load under control.
4. Perform all of the reps on the left leg, and repeat on your right leg.

Barbell Single-Leg RDL

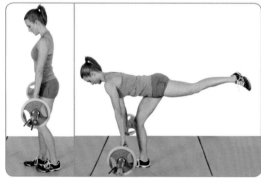
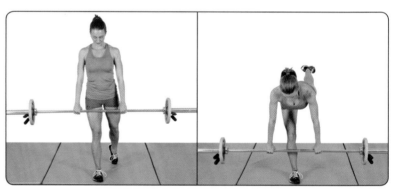

The single-leg RDL is an excellent movement for teaching balance and proprioception. This movement requires a tremendous blend of balance, coordination, hamstring flexibility, and core stability. Initially, it will feel awkward, and you will likely feel uncoordinated. But over time, it will feel more natural and comfortable.

What You Feel: Hamstrings, glutes

Tips

- *Keep your back leg in line with your torso as you bend over.*
- *At the top of the movement, your back leg should be pointed straight back.*
- *Sit back just as you would with a bilateral RDL.*
- *Focus intensively on your balance. If you screw up on a repetition, just reset and continue.*
- *Keep your core stable while hinging at the hips. Don't allow your back to round.*
- *Keep the bar close to your body.*

What to Do

1. Grab hold of a barbell, and begin in a standing position with the weight shifted to your right leg.
2. Squeeze the glute of your left leg, and lock it into position so that it stays in line with your torso as you bend over.
3. Hinge at the hips, lowing the weight toward the floor while keeping the bar close to your body. As you lower the weight, bring your back leg out behind you.
4. Lower the bar to, at, or slightly below the knee, aligning your rear leg with your spine.
5. From this position, raise back up slowly, lowering your back leg down to the floor while returning to starting position.
6. Repeat, and switch to the left leg.

Deadlift Mistakes and How to Fix Them

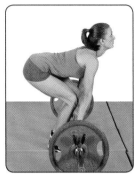 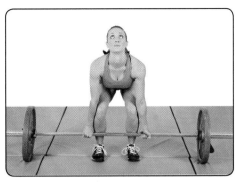

Improper Neck Alignment—As you can see in the picture, Kellie is hyperextending her cervical spine. You want to look down, and keep your head and neck in line with your torso.

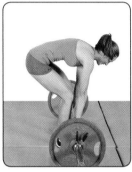 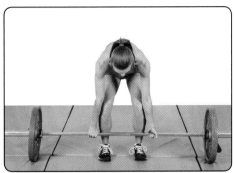

Rounded Back—This is the most common deadlifting error and is more prevalent at the bottom of a deadlift. Hamstring tightness and poor core stability can be the culprit, but quite often, your back is simply stronger when rounded. For this reason, you must build up the discipline to keep your core stable and your back in a neutral position while revolving around the hip joint. Practice makes perfect.

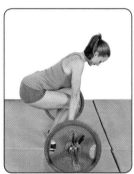 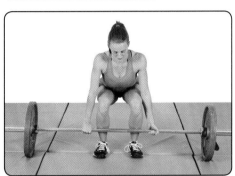

Squatting the Weight Up—The deadlift is not a squat, and many people set up with their hips too low. Your hips should be higher than your knees but lower you're your shoulders when you set up for a deadlift, and your hamstrings should be taut and ready to contribute to the pull.

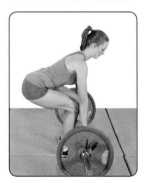 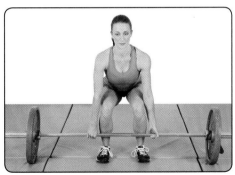

Shoulders Behind Bar—Your shoulders should be directly above or, better yet, slightly in front of the bar when initiating the pull. They should not be positioned behind the bar, which is a common beginner error.

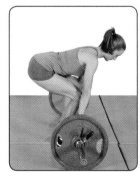 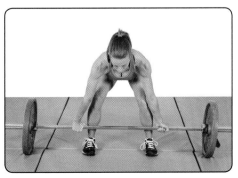

Stance and Hands Too Wide—The proper set up for a deadlift involves a narrow stance with your feet straight ahead and your arms positioned just outside the legs. Don't stand too wide or grip too far out on the barbell.

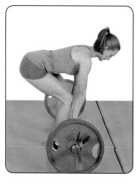 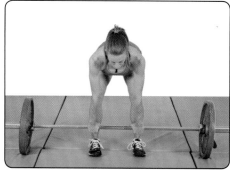

Arms Over the Legs—Proper arm position is just outside the legs in a conventional deadlift and just inside the legs in a sumo deadlift. Do not position your arms over your legs, or the bar won't skim your body. This will make the movement harder on your lower back.

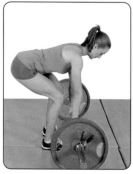 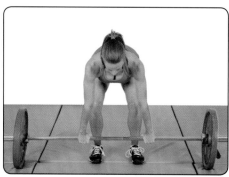

Bar Too Far Forward—The bar skims your body throughout the entire deadlift ROM. At no point should the bar be more than an inch away from your body.

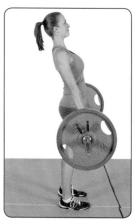 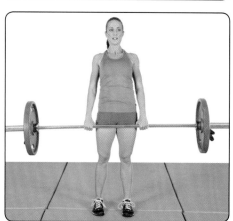

Hyperextended Back—This deadlifting error usually occurs at the top of a deadlift during the lockout. It happens because of weak glutes. Instead of the glutes pushing the hips forward into full hip extension, the spinal erectors pull the spine too far backward, leading to overarching and potential injury. Use the glutes up top, and push your hips forward while keeping your back in a neutral position.

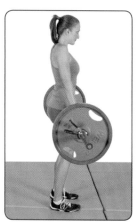 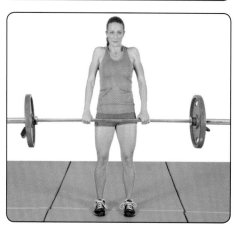

Shrugging—Beginners who have bodybuilding experience are accustomed to pulling too much with the arms. You'll see them bending the elbows or shrugging the shoulders during the deadlift. This is not efficient and will prevent you from getting stronger. Your arms are hooks, and the movement occurs at the hips, not the arms and scapulae.

Barbell Good Morning

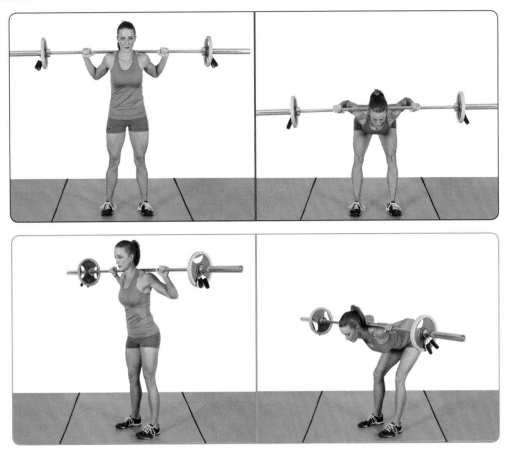

This exercise targets the hamstrings and works the hips incredibly well in a flexed position. It also builds tremendous core stability and transfers well to squat and deadlift strength. For this reason, it's a favorite of powerlifters.

What You Feel: **Back, hamstrings, glutes**

Tips

- *Sit back, and feel your hamstrings receiving the load, keeping your weight on your heels.*
- *Keep your spine in a neutral position, and don't allow your back to round.*
- *Don't be overly-concerned with loading on this exercise. If your form is strict, you can obtain an amazing workout without going too heavy on these.*

What to Do

1. Take the bar out of the rack, placing it in the "high bar" position just above the small bone in the scapulae called "the spine of the scapulae."
2. Step back, and set your feet in a shoulder-width stance.
3. Sit back, and bend over at the hips. Your knees will bend as you move your hips rearward. Try to feel the movement in your hamstrings as much as possible, and keep your core stable in a neutral position.
4. Reverse the movement, and squeeze the glutes to lockout.

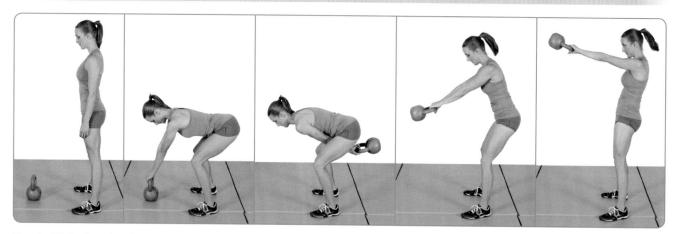

The kettlebell swing is a good glute-builder and an excellent metabolic driver due to the powerful repetitions combined with the considerable range of motion. Done properly, the kettlebell swing is one of the most important measures of proper lumbopelvic-hip complex mechanics. It forces you to keep your lumbar spine in a neutral position while swiveling at the hips and properly positioning the pelvis. The kettlebell swing is a favorite of many exercisers worldwide for good reason. Performed all alone, it's an incredibly efficient workout. Unfortunately, most kettlebellers don't use heavy enough kettlebells to significantly challenge the glutes. Using a heavy kettlebell increases glute activation and really challenges you metabolically. As you improve your strength, you may want to invest in a heavy kettlebell for this reason. Another alternative is to build a t-handle (as shown on Bret's YouTube channel).

What You Feel: Hamstrings, glutes

Tips

- *Think of the kettlebell swing as a combination of an explosive RDL and hip thrust.*
- *Your spine stays in a neutral position while the movement revolves around the hips.*
- *Make your hips do the work, not your arms.*

What to Do

1. Stand in front of a kettlebell. Bend over at the hips, and grab hold of the kettlebell, stretching the hamstrings, keeping your chest up, and activating the lats.

2. "Hike" the kettlebell rearward between the legs.

3. Forcefully contract your hips, and "push" the kettlebell forward with the glutes.

4. Keep your arms straight, and let the momentum drive the load upward. Don't use your arms to raise the kettlebell unnaturally high; just raise the kettlebell as high as your hips push it upward.

5. Let gravity reverse the motion, and as the kettlebell approaches your body, use the arms to accelerate the motion into your hips to accentuate the load on the glutes and hamstrings

6. Keep your chest tall, stretch the hamstrings, sit back, keep your spine and neck in a neutral position, and explode your hips forward, squeezing the glutes at endrange.

7. Repeat for the desired number of reps.

American Kettlebell Swing

The American kettlebell swing differs from the Russian version in that it's slightly less hip dominant, it requires more upper body involvement, and the kettlebell moves through a larger range of motion. Both variations are valuable.

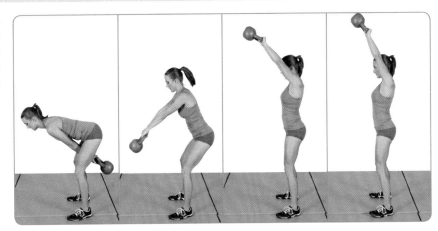

What You Feel: Hamstrings, glutes, upper back, shoulders

Tips

- *Your spine stays in a neutral position while the movement revolves around the hips.*
- *Your hips, quads, upper back, and shoulders all contribute to powering the kettlebell upward.*
- *You won't bend over at the hips quite as much in this variation compared to the Russian version.*

What to Do

1. Stand in front of a kettlebell. Bend over at the hips, and grab hold of the kettlebell, stretching the hamstrings, keeping your chest up, and activating the lats.
2. "Hike" the kettlebell rearward between your legs.
3. Forcefully contract your hips, and "push" the kettlebell forward with the glutes.
4. Keep your arms straight, and drive the kettlebell upward by using your upper body muscles. Raise the kettlebell straight overhead.
5. Let gravity reverse the motion, bend your knees, and try to absorb much of the load with the hips.
6. Repeat.

Pendulum Donkey Kick

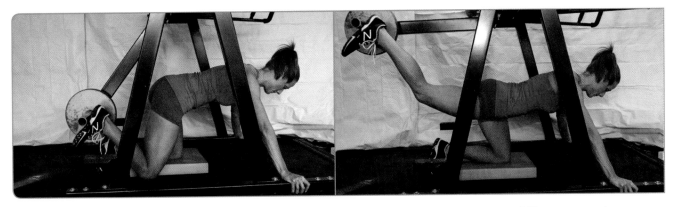

This exercise maintains constant tension on the glutes and requires considerable core stability to prevent your core from shifting or twisting. It works the thighs very well, too. Most gyms don't contain reverse hyper machines, but if you have access to one, make sure you perform this movement from time to time.

What You Feel: Glutes, quads, core

Tips

- *Maintain alignment without twisting your torso or shifting it left or right.*
- *Push through the middle of your foot.*
- *Hold the side rails for support.*
- *Control your core by keeping it tight.*

What to Do

1. Get on your hands and knees beneath a reverse hyper machine. Note where the hands grip the siderails.
2. Center your right foot onto the pendulum.
3. Push the weight upward while extending your hip and knee at the same time so that your leg is fully extended at lockout.
4. Squeeze the glute at the top of the lift.
5. Return to start position, repeat for reps, and switch legs.

Straight-leg Hip Dominant

Straight-leg hip dominant exercises are pretty self-explanatory. Your knees are straight, and the movement centers entirely around the hips. These exercises are great for producing simultaneous hamstring flexibility and strength. They actively stretch your hamstrings down low when the hips are flexed, and they activate the hamstrings very well as the movement rises and the hips extend.

As with each of the hip extension categories (glute dominant, quad dominant, hip dominant, and straight-leg hip dominant), it's imperative to learn how to move at the hips while preventing your lower back from overarching. When women learn how to perform back extensions with their glutes, the exercises become instant favorites because it's possible to feel the glutes contracting forcefully to raise the torso.

Just as in the case of bodyweight exercises like squats, bridges, and lunges, you must continue to push the envelope when bodyweight resistance becomes easy by holding onto dumbbells or placing a band around your neck during straight-leg hip extension movements. Since you won't be holding onto extremely heavy loads, the spinal extensor muscles won't activate quite as high as during hip dominant movements. Most lifters will never have access to a reverse hyper machine, but if you're lucky enough to train at a gym with one, you'll grow to like the reverse hyper. Even if you don't have access to the machine, you can always perform bodyweight reverse hyperextensions, which are very effective when performed correctly.

Even though I'm capable of holding onto very heavy dumbbells and/or placing bands around my neck, I sometimes just use my body weight and focus on using my glutes to their fullest potential during back extension movements, while keeping constant tension on the hip extensors and trying to incorporate a slight posterior pelvic tilt while extending the hips. This isn't easy to do, but it's highly effective. Just twenty bodyweight reps with good form provide your glutes with an incredible workout.

Cable Kickback

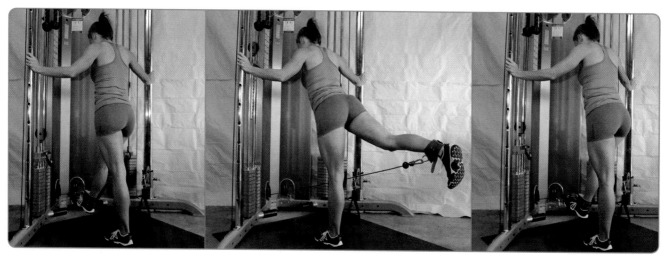

The cable kickback is not one of the best glute exercises, but I included it in the book because it fits well into a circuit along with cable hip flexion, hip abduction, and hip adduction work. Sometimes, it's nice to hit all four directions at once and receive a quick, well-rounded hip workout.

What You Feel: Glutes, quads, core

Tips

- *Keep your torso stable, and don't squirm too much during the movement.*

- *Don't utilize momentum; squeeze the glute, and control the load through the entire range of motion.*

What to Do

1. Attach the ankle cuff to a low pulley. Strap the cuff around your right ankle, and grasp the bar so that you are facing the pulley.

2. Keep your right leg straight while extending it behind your body by contracting your glutes.

3. Lower back to starting position, and repeat for reps on both sides.

Straight-leg Pull-through

The straight-leg pull-through is a decent glute and hamstring exercise that is occasionally employed by power-lifters and athletes. If you learn to stay stable, it's a good exercise.

What You Feel: Glutes, hamstrings

Tips

- *Concentrate very hard on maintaining balance, as it will become difficult as you gain strength in this exercise.*
- *Keep an arched back as you sit back and sink down into the lift.*
- *Use the glutes to push your hips all the way forward into full hip extension.*
- *Keep your neck in a neutral position.*

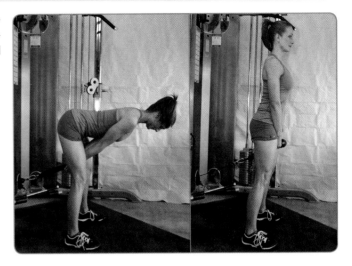

What to Do

1. Attach a rope to the low pulley. Stand facing away from the pulley, and bend forward to grasp the rope with both hands between your legs.
2. Walk forward to create tension on the rope.
3. With your feet slightly wider than your shoulders, your legs relatively straight with only a slight knee bend, and your arms straight, extend through your hips to an upright position while thrusting your hips forward.
4. Lower back to starting position, and repeat.

Swiss Ball Back Extension

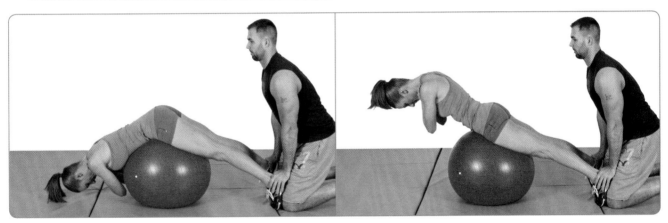

The Swiss ball back extension is not the best of exercises, but I have included it because it's a movement that can be performed at home or in a hotel-gym as long as you have a Swiss ball. If you learn to feel the glutes and hamstrings while raising your torso, you'll love this exercise.

What You Feel: Hamstrings, glutes

Tips

- *If you don't have a partner to secure your feet, press your feet against a wall for stability.*
- *Raise your torso using your hamstrings first and your glutes to finish off the movement.*
- *Learn to keep your core in a neutral position, and prevent lumbar hyperextension and anterior pelvic tilt.*
- *Keep your neck in a neutral position.*

What to Do

1. Lie face down on a ball with your feet pressed firmly into the floor and your torso draped over the ball. If you have a partner, have him or her secure your feet.
2. Place your hands behind your head or crossed over your chest.
3. Keeping your spine relaxed, raise up by contracting your glute and hamstring muscles.
4. Lower back down, and repeat.

Swiss Ball Reverse Hyper

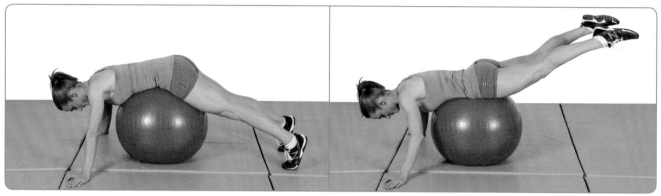

The Swiss ball reverse hyper is another movement that can be performed from home or a hotel gym as long as a Swiss ball is present. The reverse hyper is easier to pull off than the traditional back extension since it's easier to stabilize the upper body over the ball and move the legs up and down compared to stabilizing the legs over the ball and moving the torso up and down. This is an effective glute exercise when done with proper form for high reps.

What You Feel: Hamstrings, glutes, erectors

Tips

- *Don't allow your lower back to hyperextend or your pelvis to rotate anteriorly. Make sure that the movement centers around the hip joints and that your core is kept in a neutral position.*
- *Keep your upper body stable. It's easier if you have something to grasp hold of.*
- *Keep your neck in a neutral position.*

What to Do

1. Lie face down on a ball with your hands positioned out in front of you for support.
2. Raise your feet off of the floor slightly for the starting position.
3. Keeping your spine relaxed, raise your legs by contracting your glute muscles.
4. Lower back down, and repeat.

45-Degree Hyperextension

The 45-degree hyper is a staple in all of my exercise programs. When done properly, it effectively targets the hamstrings at the bottom of the movement and the glutes at the top of the movement. Many people perform it incorrectly and have a hard time learning how to keep their core in a neutral position, while moving entirely at the hips. I spend considerable time with new clients teaching them proper form on this exercise, but it's a great exercise for ingraining proper hip extension mechanics.

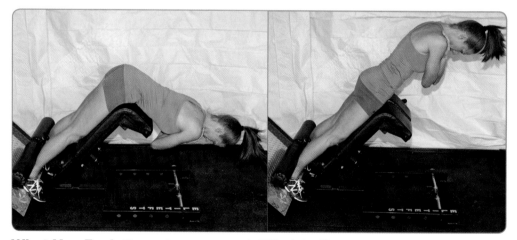

What You Feel: Hamstrings, glutes

Tips

- *Keep your spine relaxed during the movement, and pull up using your hamstrings and glutes.*
- *Feel the glutes "take over" at the top of the movement.*
- *Do not hyperextend your lower back; learn to revolve around the hip joints.*
- *Keep your neck in a neutral position.*

What to Do

1. Position your thighs on the padding, and hook your heels on the platform lip (or hook your Achilles heels on the available pads).
2. Cross your arms over your chest, and lower down into the starting position.
3. From the bottom, release the tension in your back muscles, and rise up by contracting your glute muscles until your hips are fully extended.
4. Lower back down, and repeat.

Prisoner 45-Degree Hyperextension

The prisoner 45-degree hyper is also a staple in all of my exercise programs. When done properly, it effectively targets the hamstrings at the bottom of the movement and the glutes at the top of the movement. Placing your hands in the prisoner position increases the lever arm and makes the movement surprisingly more challenging.

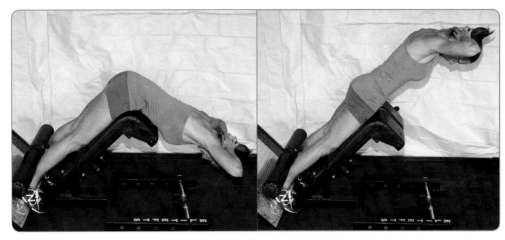

What You Feel: Hamstrings, glutes

Tips

- *Keep your spine relaxed during the movement, and pull up using your hamstrings and glutes.*
- *Feel the glutes "take over" at the top of the movement.*
- *Do not hyperextend your lower back; learn to revolve around the hip joints.*
- *Keep your neck in a neutral position.*

What to Do

1. Position your thighs on the padding, and hook your heels on the platform lip (or hook your Achilles heels on the available pads).
2. Place your hands behind your head, and lower down into the starting position.
3. From the bottom, release the tension in your back muscles, and rise up by contracting your glute muscles until your hips are fully extended.
4. Lower back down, and repeat.

Single-Leg 45-Degree Hyperextension

The single-leg 45-degree hyper is another staple in all of my exercise programs. When done properly, like the other 45-degree hypers, it effectively targets the hamstrings at the bottom of the movement and the glutes at the top of the movement. Performing the movement one leg at a time, however, dramatically increases glute and hamstring activation.

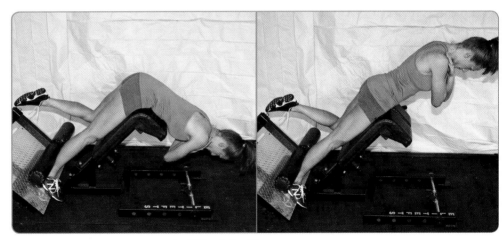

What You Feel: Hamstrings, glutes

Tips

- *Keep your spine relaxed during the movement, and pull up using your hamstrings and glutes.*
- *Feel the glutes "take over" at the top of the movement.*
- *Do not hyperextend your lower back; learn to revolve around the hip joints.*
- *Keep your neck in a neutral position.*

What to Do

1. Position your thighs on the padding, and hook your right heel on the platform lip (or hook your Achilles heels on the available pads). Keep your left foot free from the platform.
2. Cross your arms over your chest, and lower down into the starting position.
3. From the bottom, release the tension in your back muscles, and rise up by contracting your glute muscles until your hips are fully extended.
4. Lower back down, and repeat for reps on both sides.

Single-Leg Prisoner 45-Degree Hyperextension

The single-leg prisoner 45-degree hyper is yet another staple in all of my exercise programs. Like the other 45-degree hypers, it effectively targets the hamstrings at the bottom of the movement and the glutes at the top of the movement, if done properly. Performing the movement one leg at a time dramatically increases glute and hamstring activation, as does placing your hands in the prisoner position.

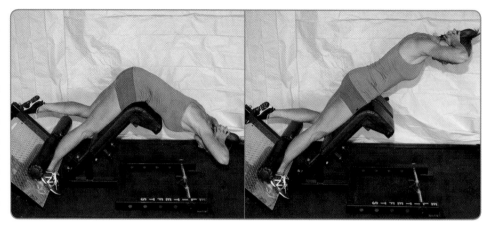

What You Feel: Hamstrings, glutes

Tips

- *Keep your spine relaxed during the movement, and pull up using your hamstrings and glutes.*
- *Feel the glutes "take over" at the top of the movement.*
- *Do not hyperextend your lower back; learn to revolve around the hip joints.*
- *Keep your neck in a neutral position.*

What to Do

1. Position your thighs on the padding, and hook your right heel on the platform lip (or hook your Achilles heels on the available pads). Keep your left foot free from the platform.
2. Place your hands behind your head, and lower down into the starting position.
3. From the bottom, release the tension in your back muscles, and rise up by contracting your glute muscles until your hips are fully extended.
4. Lower back down, and repeat for reps on both sides.

Dumbbell 45-Degree Hyperextension

The dumbbell 45-degree hyper is another staple in all of my exercise programs. When done properly, it also effectively targets the hamstrings at the bottom of the movement and the glutes at the top of the movement. Holding onto a dumbbell makes the exercise much more difficult, however.

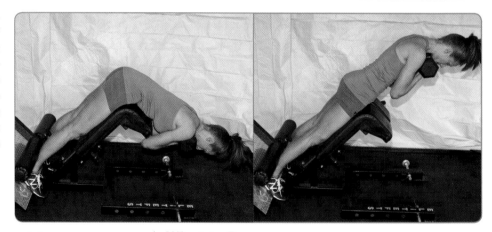

What You Feel: Hamstrings, glutes

Tips

- *Keep your spine relaxed during the movement, and pull up using your hamstrings and glutes.*
- *Feel the glutes "take over" at the top of the movement.*
- *Do not hyperextend your lower back; learn to revolve around the hip joints.*
- *Keep your neck in a neutral position.*

What to Do

1. Position your thighs on the padding, and hook your heels on the platform lip (or hook your Achilles heels on the available pads).
2. Lower to starting position, and grasp a single dumbbell by the handle with both hands, bringing it to the top of your chest with your hands facing toward you.
3. From the bottom, release the tension in your back muscles, and rise up by contracting your glute muscles until your hips are fully extended.
4. Lower back down, and repeat.

Band 45-Degree Hyperextension

Like the other 45-degree hypers, the band 45-degree hyper is a staple in all of my exercise programs. When done properly, it, too, effectively targets the hamstrings at the bottom of the movement and the glutes at the top of the movement. Utilizing a band, however, makes the exercise much more difficult.

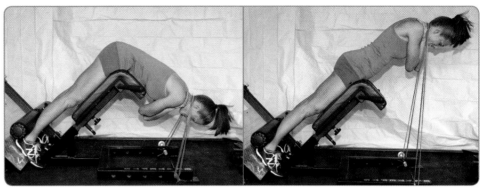

What You Feel: Hamstrings, glutes

Tips

- *Keep your spine relaxed during the movement, and pull up using your hamstrings and glutes.*
- *Feel the glutes "take over" at the top of the movement.*
- *Do not hyperextend your lower back; learn to revolve around the hip joints.*
- *Keep the neck in a neutral position.*

What to Do

1. Secure a loop band to the hyperextension by looping each end around the bottom of your legs.
2. Position your thighs on the padding, and hook your heels on the platform lip (or hook your Achilles heels on the available pads).
3. Lower to starting position, and secure the band behind your neck. You may feel more comfortable with a towel between your neck and the band.
4. From the bottom, release the tension in your back muscles, and rise up by contracting your glute muscles until your hips are fully extended.
5. Lower back down, and repeat.

Back Extension

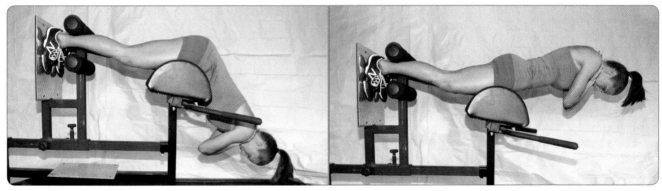

The back extension is one of my favorite posterior chain exercises. It leads to exceptionally high levels of hamstring and glute activation and develops end-range hip extension strength. At the bottom of the movement, the hamstrings receive a big stretch, and the glutes contract forcefully at the top of the movement to lock the hips and pelvis into place.

What You Feel: Hamstrings, glutes

Tips

- *Keep your spine relaxed during the movement, and pull up using your hamstrings and glutes.*
- *Feel the glutes "take over" at the top of the movement by envisioning that you're driving your hips into the bench.*
- *Do not hyperextend your lower back; learn to revolve around the hip joints.*
- *Keep your neck in a neutral position.*

What to Do

1. Using a hyperextension or glute/ham raise developer, position your thighs on the large pad so that you are lying face down. Secure your feet under the padded brace.
2. Lower to starting position, and cross your arms over your chest.
3. From the bottom, release the tension in your back muscles, and rise up by contracting your glute muscles until your hips are fully extended and you are parallel to the floor.
4. Lower back down, and repeat.

Prisoner Back Extension

The prisoner back extension also leads to exceptionally high levels of hamstring and glute activation and develops end-range hip extension strength. Unfortunately, the vast majority of exercisers fail to perform the movement optimally. At the bottom of the movement, the hamstrings receive a big stretch, and the glutes contract forcefully at the top of the movement to lock the hips and pelvis into place. Placing your hands in the prisoner position increases the lever arm and makes the movement more challenging.

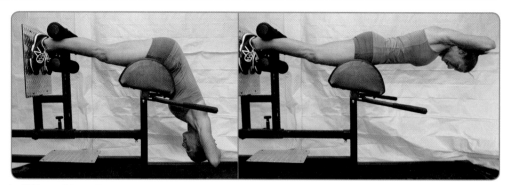

What You Feel: **Hamstrings, glutes**

Tips

- *Keep your spine relaxed during the movement, and pull up using your hamstrings and glutes.*
- *Feel the glutes "take over" at the top of the movement by envisioning that you're driving your hips into the bench.*
- *Do not hyperextend your lower back; learn to revolve around the hip joints.*
- *Keep your neck in a neutral position.*

What to Do

1. Using a hyperextension or glute/ham raise developer, position your thighs on the large pad so that you are lying face down. Secure your feet under the padded brace.
2. Lower to starting position, and place your hands behind your head.
3. From the bottom, release the tension in your back muscles, and rise up by contracting your glute muscles until your hips are fully extended and you are parallel to the floor.
4. Lower back down, and repeat.

Single-Leg Back Extension

The back extension movements are among my favorite posterior chain exercises. Again, they lead to exceptionally high levels of hamstring and glute activation and develop end-range hip extension strength. At the bottom of the movement, the hamstrings receive a big stretch, and the glutes contract forcefully at the top of the movement to lock the hips and pelvis into place. Performing the movement one leg at a time is much more challenging than the bilateral variation.

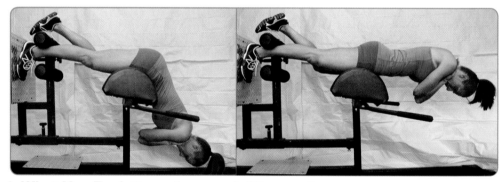

What You Feel: **Hamstrings, glutes**

Tips

- *Keep your spine relaxed during the movement, and pull up using your hamstrings and glutes.*
- *Feel the glutes "take over" at the top of the movement by envisioning that you're driving your hips into the bench.*
- *Do not hyperextend your lower back; learn to revolve around the hip joints.*
- *Keep your neck in a neutral position.*

What to Do

1. Using a hyperextension or glute/ham raise developer, position your thighs on the large pad so that you are lying face down. Secure your right foot under the padded brace, and leave your left foot free.
2. Lower to starting position, and cross your arms over your chest.
3. From the bottom, release the tension in your back muscles, and rise up by contracting your right glute muscle until your hips are fully extended and you are parallel to the floor.
4. Lower back down, and repeat for reps on both sides.

The single-leg prisoner back extension provides very high levels of hamstring and glute activation and develops end-range hip extension strength. At the bottom of the movement, the hamstrings receive a big stretch, and the glutes contract forcefully at the top of the movement to lock the hips and pelvis into place. This version is an advanced movement, however. Performing the movement one leg at a time is much more challenging than the bilateral variation, and placing your hands in the prisoner position makes the movement even more difficult.

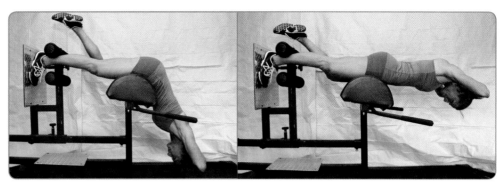

What You Feel: Hamstrings, glutes

Tips

- *Keep your spine relaxed during the movement, and pull up using your hamstrings and glutes.*
- *Feel the glutes "take over" at the top of the movement by envisioning that you're driving your hips into the bench.*
- *Do not hyperextend your lower back; learn to revolve around the hip joints.*
- *Keep your neck in a neutral position.*

What to Do

1. Using a hyperextension or glute/ham raise developer, position your thighs on the large pad so that you are lying face down. Secure your right foot under the padded brace, and leave your left foot free.
2. Lower to starting position, and place your hands behind your head.
3. From the bottom, release the tension in your back muscles, and rise up by contracting your right glute muscle until your hips are fully extended and you are parallel to the floor.
4. Lower back down, and repeat for reps on both sides.

Dumbbell Back Extension

Another of my favorite posterior chain exercises, the dumbbell back extension, leads to exceptionally high levels of hamstring and glute activation and develops end-range hip extension strength. At the bottom of the movement, the hamstrings receive a big stretch, and the glutes contract forcefully at the top of the movement to lock the hips and pelvis into place. Using a dumbbell makes the movement much more difficult, however.

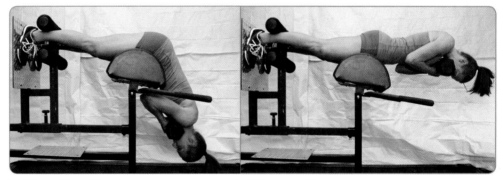

What You Feel: Hamstrings, glutes

Tips

- *Keep your spine relaxed during the movement, and pull up using your hamstrings and glutes.*
- *Feel the glutes "take over" at the top of the movement by envisioning that you're driving your hips into the bench.*
- *Do not hyperextend your lower back; learn to revolve around the hip joints.*
- *Keep your neck in a neutral position.*

What to Do

1. Using a hyperextension or glute/ham raise developer, position your thighs on the large pad so that you are lying face down. Secure your feet under the padded brace.
2. Lower to starting position, and grasp a single dumbbell by the handle with both hands, bringing it to the top of your chest with your hands facing toward you.
3. From the bottom, release the tension in your back muscles, and rise up by contracting your glute muscles until your hips are fully extended and you are parallel to the floor.
4. Lower back down, and repeat.

Band Back Extension

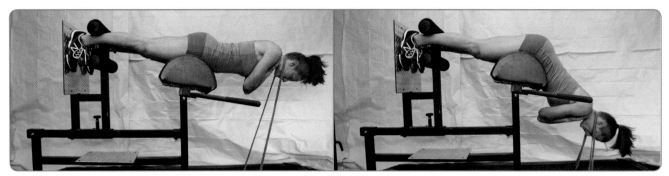

The band back extension is another of my favorite posterior chain exercises. It leads to exceptionally high levels of hamstring and glute activation and develops end-range hip extension strength. At the bottom of the movement, the hamstrings receive a big stretch, and the glutes contract forcefully at the top of the movement to lock the hips and pelvis into place. Utilizing a band makes the movement much more difficult.

What You Feel: Hamstrings, glutes

Tips

- *Keep your spine relaxed during the movement, and pull up using your hamstrings and glutes.*
- *Feel the glutes "take over" at the top of the movement by envisioning that you're driving your hips into the bench.*
- *Do not hyperextend your lower back; learn to revolve around the hip joints.*
- *Keep your neck in a neutral position.*

What to Do

1. Secure a loop band to the hyperextension or glute/ham developer by looping each end around the bottom of your legs.
2. Using a hyperextension or glute/ham raise developer, position your thighs on the large pad so that you are lying face down. Secure your feet under the padded brace.
3. Lower to starting position, and secure the band behind your neck. You may feel more comfortable with a towel between your neck and the band.
4. From the bottom, release the tension in your back muscles, and rise up by contracting your glute muscles until your hips are fully extended and you are parallel to the floor.
5. Lower back down, and repeat.

Bodyweight Reverse Hyper on Pendulum

The reverse hyper is another staple in my programs, but clients must first master their body weight before adding additional loading. If you perform the movement properly and don't rely too heavily on momentum, you'll realize that it's a great glute exercise in addition to being a good exercise for the core. If you feel this movement irritates your lower back, causes pain to radiate down your legs, or just feels "off," try to slow it down and perform it with optimal mechanics. If it still doesn't feel right, omit it from your workouts entirely.

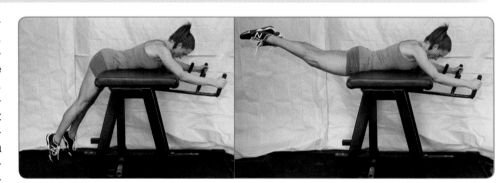

What You Feel: Glutes, hamstrings

Tips

- *Feel your glute muscles raising your legs.*
- *Avoid rounding your lower back as you lower your legs; keep a slight anterior tilt in the pelvis, and put your hamstrings on stretch down low during the movement.*
- *Avoid overarching your lower back as you raise your legs; keep a slight posterior pelvic tilt by squeezing the glutes up high during the movement.*
- *Keep your neck in a neutral position.*

What to Do

1. Lie face down with your torso on the bench up to your waist.
2. Grasp the handles for support, and lower your legs to a 90-degree angle.
3. From this position, raise your legs behind you by contracting your glute muscles.
4. Raise your legs until they're fully extended and parallel to the ground.
5. Lower back down, and repeat.

Weighted Reverse Hyper on Pendulum

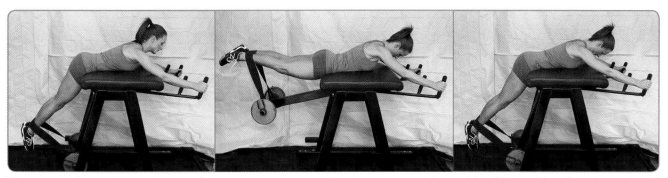

The reverse hyper is another staple in my programs, and using the pendulum with additional loading dramatically increases the challenge of the exercise compared to the bodyweight version. The reverse hyper is an excellent core, hamstring, and glute exercise, but most gyms don't contain a reverse hyper machine. If you're lucky enough to have access to one, definitely perform this movement from time to time.

What You Feel: Glutes, hamstrings

Tips

- *Feel your glute muscles raising your legs.*
- *Avoid rounding your lower back as you lower your legs; keep a slight anterior tilt in the pelvis and put your hamstrings on stretch down low during the movement.*
- *Avoid overarching your lower back as you raise your legs; keep a slight posterior pelvic tilt by squeezing the glutes up high during the movement.*
- *Keep your neck in a neutral position.*

What to Do

1. Secure your feet in the pendulum straps or behind the padded levers, making sure you've attached the proper amount of weight to the pendulum.
2. Lie face down with your torso on the bench up to your waist. Grasp the handles for support, and lower your legs to a 90-degree angle.
3. From this position, raise your legs behind you, pulling the weight up by contracting your glute muscles.
4. Raise your legs until they're fully extended and parallel to the ground.
5. Lower back down, and repeat.

Single-Leg Weighted Reverse Hyper

Many people find that they prefer the single-leg reverse hyper because it's easier on the core but still hammers the hamstrings and glutes. Those who find the reverse hyper to be problematic are usually able to safely employ the single-leg variation.

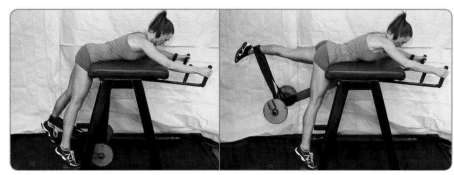

What You Feel: Hamstrings, glutes

Tips

- *Feel your glute muscles raising your legs.*
- *Avoid rounding your lower back as you lower your legs; keep a slight anterior tilt in the pelvis, and put your hamstrings on stretch down low during the movement.*
- *Avoid overarching your lower back as you raise your legs; keep a slight posterior pelvic tilt by squeezing the glutes up high during the movement.*
- *Keep your neck in a neutral position.*

What to Do

1. Secure your right foot in the pendulum straps or behind the padded levers, making sure you've attached the proper amount of weight to the pendulum. The left leg will plant on the side rail and needs to be out of the way of the pendulum as it rises.
2. Lie face down with your torso on the bench up to your waist. Grasp the handles for support, and lower your legs to a 90-degree angle.
3. From this position, raise your right leg behind you, pulling the weight up by contracting your glute muscles.
4. Raise your leg until it's fully extended and parallel to the ground.
5. Lower back down, and repeat for reps on both sides.

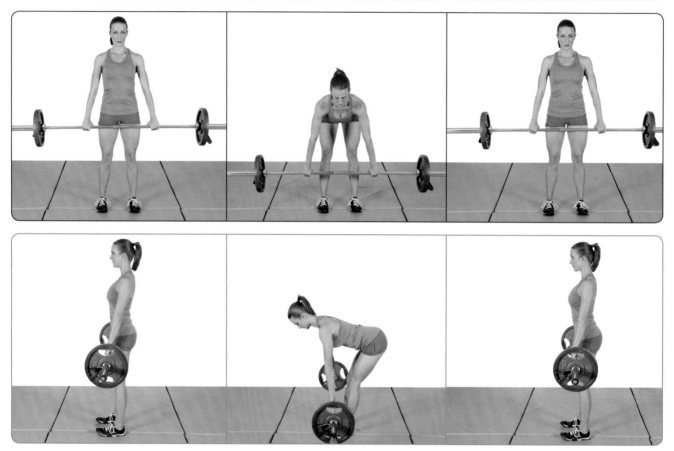

The straight-leg deadlift puts the greatest stretch load on the hamstrings and can build strength and flexibility simultaneously. The straight-leg deadlift differs from the Romanian deadlift in that you don't sit back as much, your knees don't bend, and you don't skim your body with the barbell.

What You Feel: Back, hamstrings, glutes

Tips

- *Keep your spine in a neutral position throughout the movement, and do not round your back while lowering the weight.*
- *Range of motion will depend on your hamstring flexibility.*
- *Keep your neck in a neutral position.*

What to Do

1. Remove the barbell from the rack using a double overhand or mixed grip.
2. With your feet shoulder-width apart and your arms and legs straight, bend at the hips, and lower the bar. Allow the bar to drift away from your body.
3. Descend until you feel a big stretch in your hamstrings.
4. Rise back up to top position, and repeat.

Hamstring Dominant

While I feel that hamstring strength is important, I'm always focused on the glutes, of course, when I train women. Sculpting amazing glutes is not easy, and most of the workout should be concentrated on glute strengthening. Shapely thighs are appealing to most women, however, and as women become lean, it really helps to reveal a hard-earned pair of legs. Nevertheless, the quads are usually easy to shape, and the hamstrings are often difficult to sculpt.

Many women are weak in this category of exercise. Again, I'm much more concerned with hip thrust strength, squat strength, and deadlift strength than knee flexion strength, but the benefit to the exercises included in this category is that they do work the glutes a bit while training the hamstrings efficiently.

Hamstring dominant movements require that the glutes (and hamstrings) hold the hips in an extended position while the hamstrings bend the knee. In this manner, hamstring dominant movements strengthen the hamstrings as both hip extensors and knee flexors.

I provided many exercises in this category, but consider it a fair warning that these are not for the faint of heart. Even a sliding leg curl is too hard for many who are new to strength training or these types of movements. Remember, however, that the *Strong Curves* plan was written as a template that can be followed for many years to come. Eventually, your hamstrings will strengthen and allow for the performance of many of these movements.

I've never trained a woman who could do a Russian leg curl with no assistance from the upper body or a glute/ham raise with extra loading, though. I'm certain that some of my female fitness colleagues could do so, however, especially if they focused on these movements for a couple of months.

The hamstrings are crucial in sports, especially sprint running. I feel the hamstrings are the most critical speed muscle due to their excellent leverage for hip extension during the sprint and their dual requirements as anti-knee extensors and hip extensors during the stance phase of running. This becomes more important as speed increases.

The exercises in this category are performed from time to time for their excellent levels of hamstring activation, but their level of glute activation is not very impressive. Just keep that in mind, and don't prioritize them over glute dominant, quad dominant, or hip dominant exercises.

Swiss Ball Leg Curl

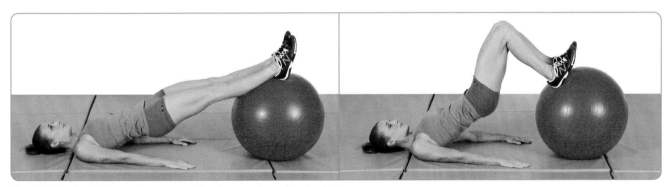

The Swiss ball leg curl targets the hamstrings in dual roles as hip extensors and as knee flexors. It's a great exercise for beginners.

What You Feel: Hamstrings

Tips

- *Make sure you get your hips up as high as possible; don't let them sag as you're flexing your knees.*

What to Do

1. Lie on your back with your lower legs positioned over a Swiss ball. Extend your arms to your sides for support.
2. Raise your hips off the floor, and maintain a neutral spine.
3. Bending at the knees, pull the ball toward your hips by rolling it with your heels.
4. Lower to starting position, and repeat.

Sliding Leg Curl with Gliders

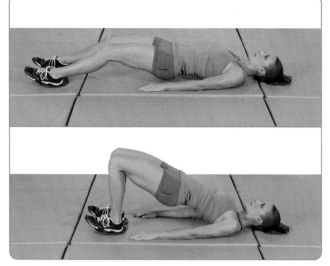

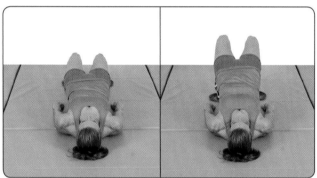

The sliding leg curl works the glutes while targeting the hamstrings in dual roles as hip extensors and as knee flexors. It's surprisingly challenging, so make sure you've mastered the Swiss ball leg curl before attempting this variation. (Note: Sliders won't work on a rubber floor).

What You Feel: Hamstrings, glutes

Tips

- *Make sure you get your hips up as high as possible; don't let them sag as you're flexing your knees.*

What to Do

1. Lie face up on the floor with a Glider, towel, or Valslide positioned under each heel.
2. Bend your knees to a 90-degree angle so that your feet are flat on the Gliders.
3. Raise your hips off of the floor in a bridge position, and place your arms to your sides for support.
4. Slide your heels away from your body until your legs fully extend without letting your hips touch the floor.
5. Move your legs back toward your body until you reach starting position. Repeat.

Gliding Leg Curl

The gliding leg curl is a creative and effective hamstring exercise designed to work the hamstrings as hip extensors and knee flexors. Don't let this exercise fool you; it looks easy but done properly, it will challenge the hamstrings.

What You Feel:

Hamstrings, glutes, erectors, grip

Tips

- *Make sure you get your hips up as high as possible; don't let them sag as you're flexing your knees.*
- *Pull your body all the way forward with the hamstrings; don't stop half way.*

What to Do

1. Lying supine, grasp hold of a racked barbell or a suspension system, and elevate your feet onto a bench or box. Make sure your legs are straight.
2. Raise your hips up into the air, and straighten your hips, forming a straight line from head to toes. Your arms don't bend, but serve as "hooks" throughout the movement.
3. Keeping your hips high and elevated, curl your body forward via knee flexion.
4. Reverse the movement, sinking back to starting position. Repeat for reps.

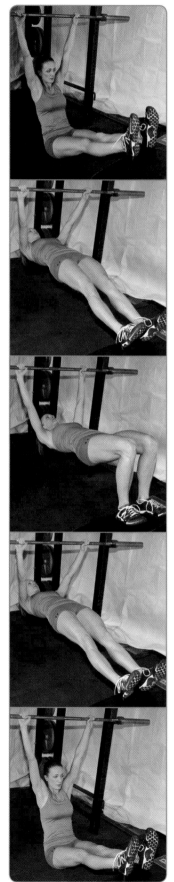

Russian Leg Curl

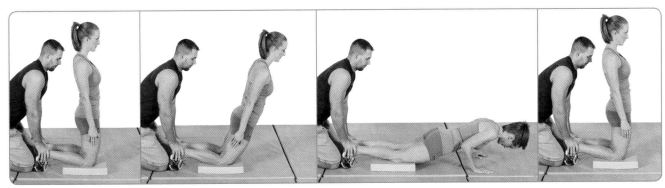

The Russian leg curl is popular with strength coaches due to its forceful eccentric requirements in the hamstrings. This is a highly challenging movement that takes some practice until it feels right.

What You Feel: Hamstrings

Tips

- *Keep your glutes and abs tight as you lower down.*
- *Avoid hyperextending your lower back or rotating your pelvis anteriorly.*
- *Don't bend over at the hips; keep your torso in line with your thighs throughout the movement.*
- *As you progress through the movement, make it a goal to rely on your hands less and less. Ultimately, you want to lower and rise without touching the floor.*

What to Do

1. Get into a kneeling position facing away from your partner. You can use a pad beneath your knees. If no partner is available, you may use a lat pulldown bench or secure your feet under a stable surface (not shown).
2. With your partner securing your feet, lower your torso toward the floor while maintaining alignment from your neck to your knees.
3. Lower down as far as possible, and rise back up. You may assist your upward movement by pressing on the floor with your hands. Repeat.

Glute/Ham Raise

The glute/ham raise is a classic hamstring exercise that is popular with powerlifters, sprinters, and football players. It's akin to a "bodyweight leg curl," and done properly, it dramatically strengthens the hamstrings and calves, as well as the glutes and erectors.

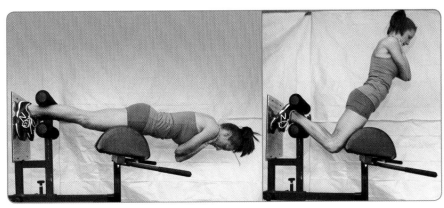

What You Feel: Hamstrings, calves, glutes, erectors

Tips

- *Keep your glutes and abs tight as you lower down.*
- *Avoid hyperextending your lower back or rotating your pelvis anteriorly.*
- *Don't bend over at the hips; keep your torso in line with your thighs throughout the movement.*

What to Do

1. Secure your ankles between the roll pads on the glute/ham developer, and place your feet on the back platform.
2. Position your lower thighs on top of the pad.
3. Lower your torso by straightening your legs until your body is in a straight line, parallel with the ground.
4. From this position, keeping your glutes and core tight, bend your knees and raise your body until your torso is in an upright position.
5. Lower back down by straightening your knees until your body is horizontal. Then, repeat for reps.

Dumbbell Glute/Ham Raise

The glute/ham raise is a classic hamstring exercise that is popular with powerlifters, sprinters, and football players. It's akin to a "bodyweight leg curl," and when done properly, it dramatically strengthens the hamstrings and calves, as well as the glutes and erectors. Holding onto a dumbbell increases the difficulty of the exercise considerably.

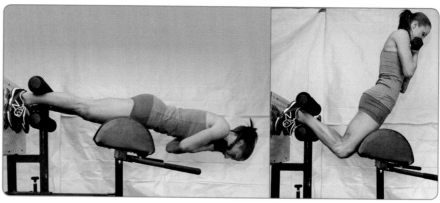

What You Feel: Hamstrings, calves, glutes, erectors

Tips

- *Keep your glutes and abs tight as you lower down.*
- *Avoid hyperextending your lower back or rotating your pelvis anteriorly.*
- *Don't bend over at the hips; keep your torso in line with your thighs throughout the movement.*

What to Do

1. Secure your ankles between the roll pads on the glute/ham developer, and place your feet on the back platform.
2. Position your lower thighs on top of the pad.
3. Lower your torso by straightening your legs until your body is in a straight line parallel with the ground.
4. Grasp a single dumbbell by the handle with both hands, bringing it to the top of your chest with your hands facing toward you.
5. From this position, keeping your glutes and core tight, bend your knees, and raise your body until your torso is in an upright position.
6. Lower back down by straightening your knees until your body is horizontal. Then, repeat for reps.

Band Glute/Ham Raise

The glute/ham raise is a classic hamstring exercise that is popular with powerlifters, sprinters, and football players. It's akin to a "bodyweight leg curl," and when done properly, it dramatically strengthens the hamstrings and calves, as well as the glutes and erectors. Using band resistance greatly increases the difficulty of the exercise.

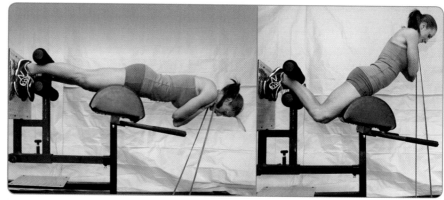

What You Feel: Hamstrings, calves, glutes, erectors

Tips

- *Keep your glutes and abs tight as you lower down.*
- *Avoid hyperextending your lower back or rotating your pelvis anteriorly.*
- *Don't bend over at the hips; keep your torso in line with your thighs throughout the movement.*

What to Do

1. Place each end of a loop band under the glute/ham developer legs to secure.
2. Secure your ankles between the roll pads on the glute/ham developer, and place your feet on the back platform.
3. Position your lower thighs on top of the pad.
4. Lower your torso by straightening your legs until your body is in a straight line parallel with the ground.
5. Position the center of the band over the back of your neck. You may feel more comfortable with a towel between the band and your skin.
6. From this position, keeping your glutes and core tight, bend your knees, and raise your body until your torso is in an upright position.
7. Lower back down by straightening your knees until your body is horizontal. Then, repeat for reps.

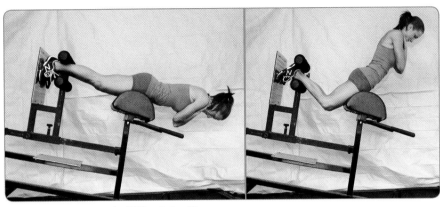

The glute/ham raise is a classic hamstring exercise that is popular with powerlifters, sprinters, and football players. Performing the movement from a rear-elevated position increases the exercise's challenge and keeps more constant tension on the hamstrings. Like the other glute/ham raises, it's akin to a "bodyweight leg curl." Done properly, it dramatically strengthens the hamstrings and calves and also works the glutes and erectors.

What You Feel: Hamstrings, calves, glutes, erectors

Tips

- *Keep your glutes and abs tight as you lower down.*
- *Avoid hyperextending your lower back or rotating your pelvisanteriorly.*
- *Don't bend over at the hips; keep your torso in line with your thighs throughout the movement.*

What to Do

1. Position the back of the glute/ham developer on a low bench so that it's slanted downward at about a 30-degree angle.
2. Secure your ankles between the roll pads on the glute/ham developer, and place your feet on the back platform.
3. Position your lower thighs on top of the pad.
4. Lower your torso by straightening your legs until your body is in a straight line parallel with the ground.
5. From this position, keeping your glutes and core tight, bend your knees, and raise your body until your torso is in an upright position.
6. Lower back down by straightening your knees until your body is horizontal. Then, repeat for reps.

Horizontal Pull

The horizontal pulling category exercises resemble rowing motions. You start out with your arms in front of your body and pull your hands toward your body (or your body toward your hands as in the case of the inverted row). Horizontal pulling works the traps, especially the mid and lower fibers, the rhomboids, the lats, the biceps, and the brachialis.

Many women appreciate a strong mid-back because they feel it makes them look sexier in a strapless dress or a bikini, and horizontal pulling is your quickest route to that goal. But horizontal pulling isn't just for show. Rowing motions strengthen the scapular retractors (muscles responsible for pulling the shoulder blades toward each other), and this strength is essential for optimal shoulder health and functioning. Many male lifters tend to focus on horizontal pressing while ignoring horizontal pulling strength, and this tends to create negative postural adaptations over time by adducting the scapulae (spreading them apart) and internally rotating the shoulders (twisting the shoulders inward). Horizontal pulls prevent these negative postural adaptations, so you don't have to worry about exhibiting poor posture over time.

Dumbbell One-Arm Row

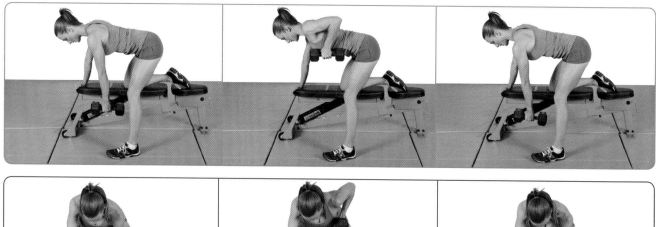

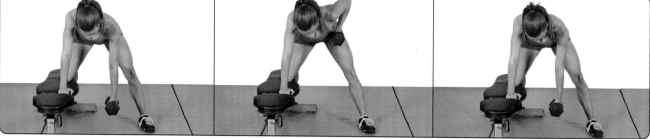

The one-arm row is an amazing exercise that builds grip strength and works the lats, rhomboids, traps, and rear delts in a safe manner.

What You Feel: Upper back, biceps

Tips

- *Pull the weight through your back muscles. Don't rely on excessive momentum, and don't twist/contort your body.*
- *Use a full range of motion, starting from a full stretch and pulling your upper arm up slightly past horizontal.*
- *It's important to keep good posture. Be athletic in appearance. Maintain a neutral spine, get a stretch in your hamstrings, keep your neck in a neutral position, get a strong brace with the grounded arm, and have a wide enough step to allow for ideal stability.*

What to Do

1. Place your left knee on the bench and lean forward, supporting your weight on your left hand.
2. Position your right foot on the floor away from the bench, and grasp the dumbbell from the floor with your right hand (palm facing in). Lift it off the ground to put tension on the back muscles.
3. Pull the dumbbell up your side by extending your shoulder and bending at the elbow until it reaches your ribs.
4. Lower the weight until your arm is fully stretched.
5. Repeat for reps on both sides.

Dumbbell Chest Supported Row

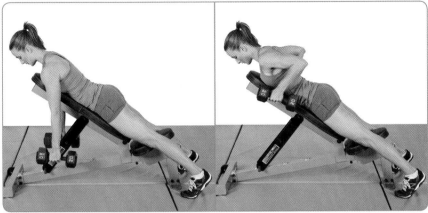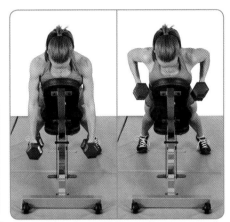

The dumbbell chest supported row is an amazing back exercise that works the upper back and biceps in a very safe manner.

What You Feel: Upper back, biceps

Tips

- *Make sure you keep your neck relatively neutral and don't allow it to hyperextend too much.*
- *Don't rely on momentum; squeeze the dumbbells through a full range of motion.*

What to Do

1. Lie chest down on an incline bench. Grasp a dumbbell in each hand with your palms facing each other.
2. Pull the dumbbells toward your sides until your hands align with your ribs.
3. Lower the weight back down, fully extending your arms and stretching your shoulders forward. Repeat.

Standing One-Arm Cable Row

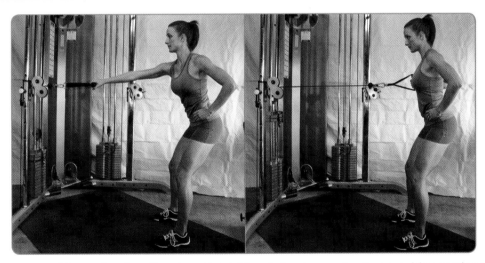

The standing one-arm cable row is a functional and joint-friendly back exercise that provides a unique training stimulus. For this reason, it should be performed from time to time for variety's sake.

What You Feel: Upper back, biceps

Tips

- *Stand in an athletic, functional position.*
- *Get a stretch in your back muscles when the weight is out in front, and pull your shoulder blade in when the weight is close to your body. Achieve a full ROM.*

What to Do

1. Position your body facing a medium-height cable pulley. Grasp the handle with your right hand, allowing your shoulder to stretch forward, and step back from the pulley to create tension on the cable.
2. Pull the cable handle toward your right side until it reaches your chest, contracting your back muscles.
3. Return arm to starting position, and repeat on both sides.

Seated Cable Row

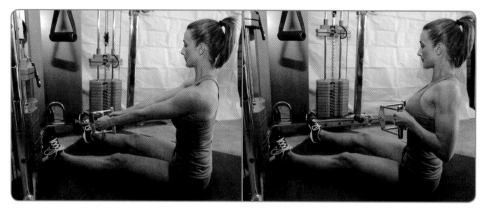

The seated cable row is a classic back exercise and a favorite of many seasoned lifters. This exercise allows you to squeeze your shoulder blades together and feel the scapular retractors working efficiently.

What You Feel: Upper back, biceps

Tips

- *Do not round your back during the movement. Keep your chest tall, and stay mostly upright throughout the set.*

- *Don't rely on excessive momentum. It's okay to use slight momentum, but keep in mind that this is an upper back exercise, not a lower back movement.*

What to Do

1. Sit down on a seat or bench with your knees bent. Grasp the cable attachment, placing your feet on the vertical platform (not shown in photo).
2. Allow the cable to pull your shoulders forward to stretch your back muscles.
3. Retract your scapulae, and pull the cable toward your torso, pushing your chest out while squeezing your back muscles together.
4. Return to the starting position, and repeat for reps.

Seated Face Pull

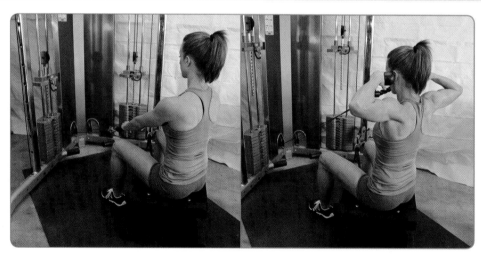

The face pull is a unique upper back movement that strengthens the scapular retractors (mid traps and rhomboids) along with the shoulder external rotators.

What You Feel: Upper back, rear shoulders

Tips

- *Keep your head and neck in neutral position; don't let your head jut forward.*

- *Don't go too heavy to where it limits your range of motion.*

What to Do

1. Sit on a bench or box facing the low pulley with a rope attachment.
2. Grasp the rope attachment with your palms facing out, allowing the weight to pull your shoulders forward to a full stretch.
3. Pull the weight toward your forehead, separating the rope on each side of your face until your upper arms align with your shoulders.
4. Return to the starting position, and repeat.

JC Band Row

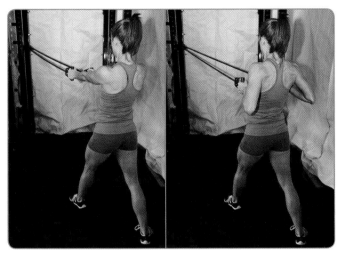

Sometimes, you have to train from home, or you're traveling and don't have access to a gym. This is where suspension systems and bands become important. They allow for a good training effect without weights. The JC Band row is a decent back exercise that requires a good squeeze at the end-range of the movement.

What You Feel: Upper back, biceps

Tips

* *Stand in an athletic, functional position.*
* *Get a stretch in your back muscles when the weight is out in front, and pull your shoulder blade in when the weight is close to your body. Achieve a full ROM.*

What to Do

1. Attach the band to a support so that each side of the band is of equal length. This is automatic if using JC Bands.
2. Grasp each handle with your arms fully extended and your hands facing in.
3. From a split stance, pull the bands toward your torso by contracting your back muscles until your forearms reach your ribs.
4. Slowly release the bands back to starting position, and repeat.

Modified Inverted Row with Suspension System

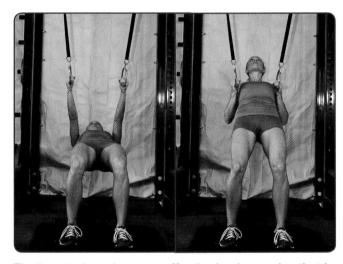 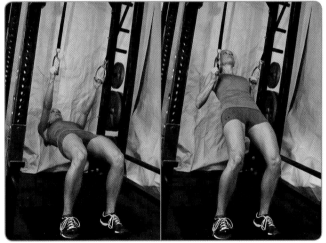

The inverted row is a very effective back exercise that is easy on the joints. It can also be performed at home if you own a suspension system. Bending the knees makes the exercise easier, which is ideal for beginners.

What You Feel: Upper back, biceps

Tips

* *Inverted row intensity can be adjusted by simply changing your angle. The lower you are to the floor, the more intense the exercise.*
* *Remember to squeeze your shoulder blades together at the top of the movement.*
* *Too often, individuals let their form deteriorate at the end of a set. Stop yourself before form erodes, and maintain good body position throughout the duration of the set.*

What to Do

1. Grasp the handles in each hand with your palms facing down and your arms fully extended.
2. Walk your body forward and down into a top bridge position, keeping your knees bent at a 90-degree angle.
3. Keeping your core and glutes tight, pull your torso toward the handles while rotating your palms in.
4. Return to the starting position, and repeat.

Inverted Row with Suspension System

The inverted row is a very effective back exercise that is easy on the joints and can be performed at home if you own a suspension system.

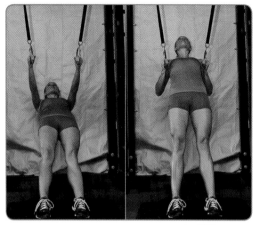 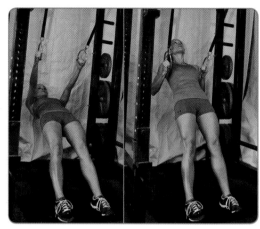

What You Feel: Upper back, biceps

Tips

- *Inverted row intensity can be adjusted by simply changing your angle. The lower you are to the floor, the more intense the exercise.*
- *Remember to squeeze your shoulder blades together at the top of the movement.*
- *Too often, individuals let their form deteriorate at the end of a set. Stop yourself before form erodes, and maintain good body position throughout the duration of the set.*

What to Do

1. Grasp the handles in each hand with your palms facing down and your arms fully extended.
2. Walk your body forward and down until you reach about a 45-degree angle.
3. Keeping your core and glutes tight, pull your torso toward the handles while rotating your palms in.
4. Return to the starting position, and repeat.

Modified Inverted Row with Bar

The inverted row is another very effective back exercise that is easy on the joints. Bending your knees makes the exercise easier, which is ideal for beginners.

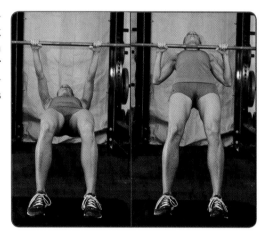 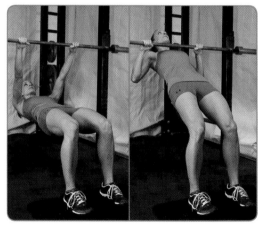

What You Feel: Upper back, biceps

Tips

- *Inverted row intensity can be adjusted by simply changing your angle. The lower you are to the floor, the more intense the exercise.*
- *Remember to squeeze your shoulder blades together at the top of the movement.*
- *Too often, individuals let their form deteriorate at the end of a set. Stop yourself before form erodes, and maintain good body position throughout the duration of the set.*

What to Do

1. Adjust the barbell on a rack or Smith machine to a comfortable height for your fitness level. High bar rows are easier for beginners.
2. Grasp the bar with an overhand grip slightly wider than your shoulders.
3. Walk your body forward and down into a top bridge position, keeping your knees bent at a 90-degree angle.
4. With your core and glutes tight, pull your torso toward the bar until it reaches the middle of your chest.
5. Return to the starting position, and repeat.

Inverted Row with Bar

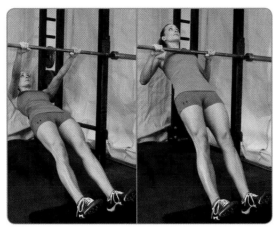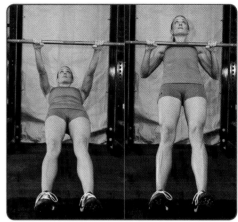

Another very effective back exercise that is easy on the joints, the inverted row can also be performed at home iby using a broomstick and two chairs.

What You Feel: Upper back, biceps

Tips

- *Inverted row intensity can be adjusted by simply changing your angle. The lower you are to the floor, the more intense the exercise.*
- *Remember to squeeze your shoulder blades together at the top of the movement.*
- *Too often, individuals let their form deteriorate at the end of a set. Stop yourself before form erodes, and maintain good body position throughout the duration of the set.*

What to Do

1. Adjust the barbell on a rack or Smith machine to a comfortable height for your fitness level. High bar rows are easier for beginners.
2. Grasp the bar with an overhand grip slightly wider than your shoulders.
3. Walk your feet out until the middle of your chest is positioned below the bar.
4. Lower down until your arms and legs are fully extended.
5. Keeping your core and glutes tight, pull your torso toward the bar.
6. Return to the starting position, and repeat.

Feet-Elevated Inverted Row with Suspension System

This inverted row exercise is also very effective and easy on the joints. It can be performed at home as well if you own a suspension system. Elevating the feet makes the exercise more difficult, which is ideal for more advanced lifters.

What You Feel: Upper back, biceps

Tips

- *Inverted row intensity can be adjusted by simply changing your angle. The lower you are to the floor, the more intense the exercise.*
- *Remember to squeeze your shoulder blades together at the top of the movement.*
- *Too often, individuals let their form deteriorate at the end of a set. Stop yourself before form erodes, and maintain good body position throughout the duration of the set.*

What to Do

1. Grasp the handles in each hand with your palms facing down and your arms fully extended.
2. Place your feet on a bench positioned in front of you. The bench should be far enough out that you can fully extend your legs.
3. Keeping your core and glutes tight, pull your torso toward the handles while rotating your palms in.
4. Return to the starting position, and repeat.

Feet-elevated Inverted Row with Bar

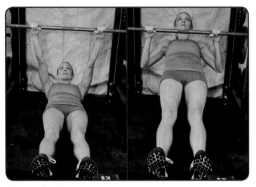 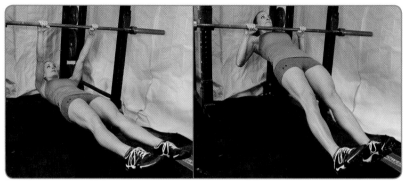

This inverted row exercise is also a very effective back exercise that is easy on the joints. Elevating the feet makes the exercise more difficult, which is ideal for more advanced lifters.

What You Feel: Upper back, biceps

Tips

- *Inverted row intensity can be adjusted by simply changing your angle. The lower you are to the floor, the more intense the exercise.*

- *Remember to squeeze your shoulder blades together at the top of the movement.*

- *Too often, individuals let their form deteriorate at the end of a set. Stop yourself before form erodes, and maintain good body position throughout the duration of the set.*

What to Do

1. Adjust the barbell on a rack or Smith machine to a comfortable height.
2. Grasp the bar with an overhand grip slightly wider than your shoulders, and fully extend your arms.
3. Place your feet on a bench positioned in front of you. The bench should be far enough out that you can fully extend your legs.
4. Keeping your core and glutes tight, pull your torso toward the bar until your middle chest touches.
5. Return to the starting position, and repeat.

Dumbbell Bent Over Row

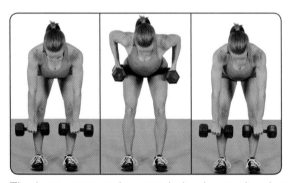 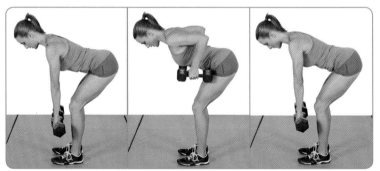

The bent over row is a staple back exercise that has stood the test of time. The movement requires considerable core stability and hamstring flexibility in order to maintain proper position throughout the duration of the set. Using dumbbells allows for slightly increased range of motion.

What You Feel: Upper back, lower back, hamstrings, glutes, biceps, grip

Tips

- *Maintaining a horizontal torso requires good hamstring flexibility. If your back begins to round due to poor hamstring flexibility, you may bend your knees more or raise your torso to a higher position.*

- *Avoid relying on momentum to move the weight. Do not jerk the weight up to the top position.*

- *Use a full range of motion, fully extending your arms at the bottom and bringing the bar to your torso at the top.*

What to Do

1. Bending at the knees, pick up the dumbbells with an overhand grip.
2. With a straight back and slightly bent knees, pull the dumbbells toward your sides, squeezing the shoulder blades together up top.
3. Lower the weight down to starting position, fully extending your arms. Repeat.

Barbell Bent-over Row

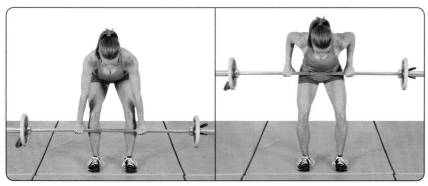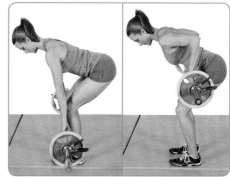

The barbell row is a staple back exercise that has stood the test of time. The movement requires considerable core stability and hamstring flexibility in order to properly maintain position throughout the duration of the set.

What You Feel: Upper back, lower back, hamstrings, glutes, biceps, grip

Tips

- *Maintaining a horizontal torso requires good hamstring flexibility. If your back begins to round due to poor hamstring flexibility, you may bend your knees more or raise your torso to a higher position.*

- *Avoid relying on momentum to move the weight. Do not jerk the weight up to the top position.*

- *Use a full range of motion, fully extending your arms at the bottom and bringing the bar to your torso at the top.*

What to Do

1. Remove the weighted barbell from the rack, positioning your hands on the outside of your hips with an overhand grip.
2. Bend slightly at your knees, and bend forward at the hips until your torso is parallel to the floor.
3. Pull the bar to your upper abdomen, contracting your back muscles as you bring the weight closer to your body.
4. Return to the starting position until your arms fully extend and your shoulders stretch downward. Repeat.

T-bar Row

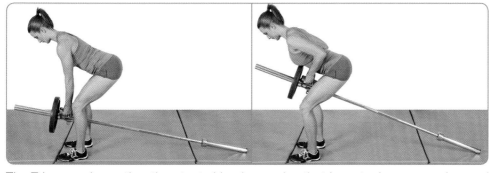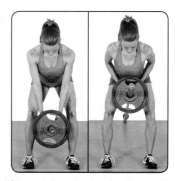

The T-bar row is another time-tested back exercise that is a staple among advanced lifters. Like the barbell row, it requires good hamstring flexibility and posterior chain strength and endurance to hold proper positioning.

What You Feel: Upper back, lower back, hamstrings, glutes, biceps, grip

Tips

- *You may either use a lever T-bar found at some gyms or set up your own T-bar row with a barbell and an attachment handle (usually found from a cable pulley machine). This second suggestion is shown in the photos.*

- *If you find that you are raising your body higher than a 45-degree angle to pull the weight, lessen the load, and lower the torso angle.*

What to Do

1. Stand over the barbell or lever with the weighted plate positioned in front of you.
2. Grasp the handles, bending slightly at the knees and considerably at the hips.
3. Keeping your back in a neutral position, pull the barbell or lever toward your torso while contracting your back muscles.
4. Return to the starting position with your arms fully extended and your shoulders stretched down. Repeat.

Horizontal Press

Horizontal presses are the most popular exercises with men because they build a strong chest, but they don't just work the pectorals. They also work the front delts and the triceps considerably. For this reason, many women like performing horizontal presses because the triceps tend to be a weak area of muscle development in women.

Horizontal presses begin with your hands near the torso and end with your hands away from the torso out in front of your body. This can involve pressing dumbbells or barbells away from the body while lying on a bench or pushing your body away from the floor as in the case of a push-up.

Many women feel empowered when they're able to finally perform push-ups with good technical form. It's important to balance horizontal pressing with horizontal pulling to ensure proper structural balance and posture.

Torso Elevated Push-up

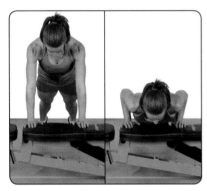 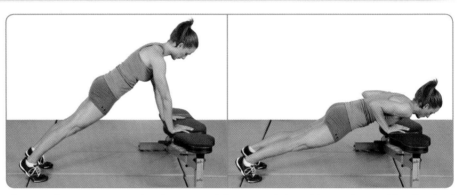

The push-up is a legendary upper body pressing movement that has stood the test of time. It's performed in physical education classes, army workouts, and sports training sessions around the world day in and day out. Done properly, the push-up builds upper body pressing strength, while also strengthening the scapular stabilizers and teaching proper lumbopelvic stability. Elevating the torso makes the movement easier, which makes this variation ideal for beginners.

What You Feel: Chest, triceps

Tips

- *Keep your spine neutral to create a straight line from the top of your shoulders to your ankles. Do not allow your middle back to sag or your glutes to hike upward.*
- *Keep your abs and glutes tight throughout the duration of the movement.*
- *Avoid moving like a snake, pushing your chest up prior to the rest of your torso. Maintain a rigid spine so that your entire body moves in one fluid motion.*
- *Do not place your hands out in front of your head. They should be placed out to the sides of your body so that your arms form about a 45-degree angle relative to your torso when at the bottom of the movement.*
- *Use a full range of motion, bringing your chest to the floor.*

What to Do

1. Stand facing a bench, platform, or an elevated barbell secured on a rack.
2. Place your hands on the edge of the bench slightly wider than your shoulders and assume a push-up position.
3. Keeping your body straight, lower your body back down to the bench until your chest touches, then press the body upward. Repeat for the desired number of repetitions.

Knee Push-up

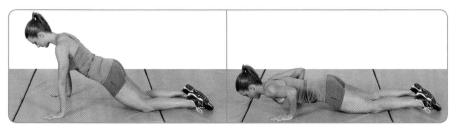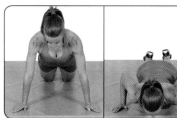

The knee push-up is a variation of the traditional push-up, which is a legendary upper body pressing movement that has stood the test of time. The push-up is performed in physical education classes, army workouts, and sports training sessions around the world day in and day out. Done properly, the push-up builds upper body pressing strength, while also strengthening the scapular stabilizers and teaching proper lumbopelvic stability. Performing push-ups from the knees is easier than the standard version, which makes this variation ideal for beginners.

What You Feel: Chest, triceps

Tips

- *Keep your spine neutral to create a straight line from the top of your shoulders to your ankles. Do not allow your middle back to sag or your glutes to hike upward.*
- *Keep your abs and glutes tight throughout the duration of the movement.*
- *Avoid moving like a snake, pushing your chest up prior to the rest of your torso. Maintain a rigid spine so that your entire body moves in one fluid motion.*
- *Do not place your hands out in front of your head. They should be placed out to the sides of your body so that your arms form about a 45-degree angle relative to your torso when at the bottom of the movement.*
- *Use a full range of motion, bringing your chest to the floor.*

What to Do

1. Lie face down on the floor on your knees with your hands positioned on the sides of your body.
2. Bend your knees. You may feel most comfortable crossing your feet behind you.
3. Keeping your body straight, raise your torso off of the floor by pressing up.
4. Lower your body back down to the floor until your chest almost touches the ground. Repeat.

Close-Width Knee Push-up

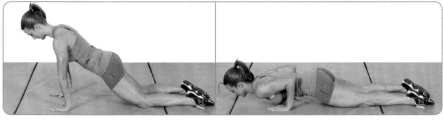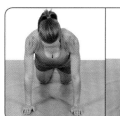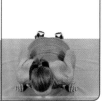

The close-width knee push-up is a variation on the legendary upper body pressing movement that has stood the test of time. Push-ups are performed in physical education classes, army workouts, and sports training sessions around the world day in and day out. Done properly, the push-up builds upper body pressing strength, while also strengthening the scapular stabilizers and teaching proper lumbopelvic stability. While performing push-ups from the knees is easier than the standard version, keeping your arms tucked makes the movement more difficult, so this variation is surprisingly challenging.

What You Feel: Chest, triceps

Tips

- *Keep your spine neutral to create a straight line from the top of your shoulders to your ankles. Do not allow your middle back to sag or your glutes to hike upward.*
- *Keep your abs and glutes tight throughout the duration of the movement.*
- *Avoid moving like a snake, pushing your chest up prior to the rest of your torso. Maintain a rigid spine so that your entire body moves in one fluid motion.*
- *Do not place your hands out in front of your head.*
- *Use a full range of motion, bringing your chest to the floor.*

What to Do

1. Lie face down on the floor on your knees with your hands positioned to your sides so that your upper arms are tucked in close to your body while performing the movement.
2. Bend your knees. You may feel most comfortable crossing your feet behind you.
3. Keeping your body straight, raise your torso off of the floor by pressing up.
4. Lower your body back down to the floor until your chest touches. Repeat.

Push-up

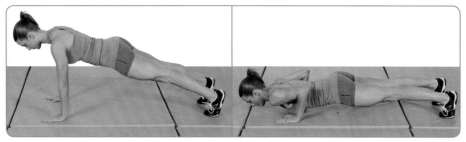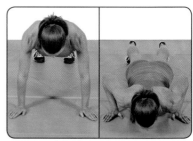

The push-up is a legendary upper body pressing movement that has stood the test of time. It's performed in physical education classes, army workouts, and sports training sessions around the world day in and day out. Done properly, the push-up builds upper body pressing strength, while also strengthening the scapular stabilizers and teaching proper lumbopelvic stability.

What You Feel: Chest, triceps

Tips

- *Keep your spine neutral to create a straight line from the top of your shoulders to your ankles. Do not allow your middle back to sag or your glutes to hike upward.*
- *Keep your abs and glutes tight throughout the duration of the movement.*
- *Avoid moving like a snake, pushing your chest up prior to the rest of your torso. Maintain a rigid spine so that your entire body moves in one fluid motion.*
- *Do not place your hands out in front of your head. They should be placed out to the sides of your body so that your arms form about a 45-degree angle relative to your torso when at the bottom of the movement.*
- *Use a full range of motion, bringing your chest to the floor.*

What to Do

1. Lie face down on the floor with your hands positioned on the sides of your body.
2. Keeping your body straight, raise your torso off of the floor by pressing up.
3. Lower your body back down to the floor until your chest almost touches the ground. Repeat.

Close-Width Push-up

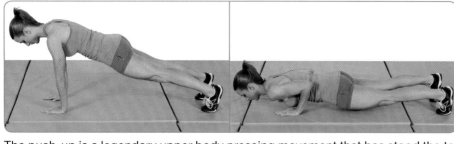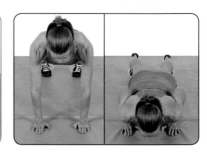

The push-up is a legendary upper body pressing movement that has stood the test of time. It's performed in physical education classes, army workouts, and sports training sessions around the world day in and day out. Done properly, the push-up builds upper body pressing strength, while also strengthening the scapular stabilizers and teaching proper lumbopelvic stability. Keeping the arms tucked makes the movement more difficult. This variation is quite challenging, and may take a bit longer to master than a standard push-up.

What You Feel: Chest, triceps

Tips

- *Keep your spine neutral to create a straight line from the top of your shoulders to your ankles. Do not allow your middle back to sag or your glutes to hike upward.*
- *Keep your abs and glutes tight throughout the duration of the movement.*
- *Avoid moving like a snake, pushing your chest up prior to the rest of your torso. Maintain a rigid spine so that your entire body moves in one fluid motion.*
- *Do not place your hands out in front of your head.*
- *Use a full range of motion, bringing your chest to the floor.*

What to Do

1. Lie face down on the floor with your hands positioned to your sides so that your upper arms are tucked in close to your body while performing the movement.
2. Keeping your body straight, raise your torso off of the floor by pressing up.
3. Lower your body back down to the floor until your chest touches. Repeat.

Feet Elevated Push-up

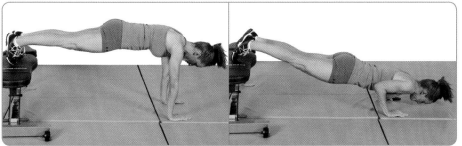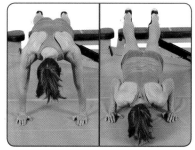

The push-up is a legendary upper body pressing movement that has stood the test of time. It's performed in physical education classes, army workouts, and sports training sessions around the world day in and day out. Done properly, the push-up builds upper body pressing strength, while also strengthening the scapular stabilizers and teaching proper lumbopelvic stability. Elevating the feet increases the difficulty of the movement, making it ideal for more advanced lifters.

What You Feel: Chest, triceps

Tips

- *Keep your spine neutral to create a straight line from the top of your shoulders to your ankles. Do not allow your middle back to sag or your glutes to hike upward.*
- *Keep your abs and glutes tight throughout the duration of the movement.*
- *Avoid moving like a snake, pushing your chest up prior to the rest of your torso. Maintain a rigid spine so that your entire body moves in one fluid motion.*
- *Do not place your hands out in front of your head. They should be placed out to the sides of your body so that the arms form about a 45-degree angle relative to your torso when at the bottom of the movement.*
- *Use a full range of motion, bringing your chest to the floor.*

What to Do

1. Lie face down on the floor with your forefeet positioned on a bench or platform.
2. Raise your torso into a plank position.
3. Keeping your body straight, lower your body down to the floor, and raise your torso off of the floor by pressing up. Repeat.

Band Chest Press

The JC Band chest press is a great chest and triceps exercise that is convenient when training without access to a gym. JC Bands are portable and can be used to train the upper body when on vacation or training at home. This movement requires considerable stability in the shoulders and hips for proper performance.

What You Feel: Chest, triceps

Tips

- *Fine-tune the perfect distance to allow for optimal performance. You may have to walk further out or in during the set to get the right feel.*
- *Remain stable during the exercise. Don't squirm, shift, or twist.*
- *Alternate foot position from one set to the next for balance purposes. On the first set, put the right foot forward, and on the next set, put the left foot forward, etc.*

What to Do

1. Hold band handles in each hand positioned away from the anchor point of the bands with your palms facing each other.
2. Position your hands on the outer sides of your chest, bending your arms so that your wrists align with your elbows.
3. Stand with both feet facing forward in a split stance. Lunge forward slightly while contracting your abdominals and locking the rear glute in place.
4. Press the bands outward until your elbows are fully extended while rotating your arms so that your palms are facing downward at the exercise's lockout.
5. Flex your elbows back until your arms reach the starting position, and repeat.

Dumbbell Bench Press

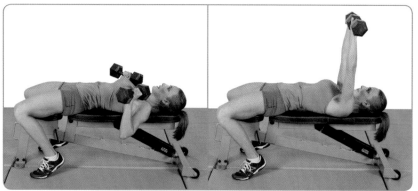 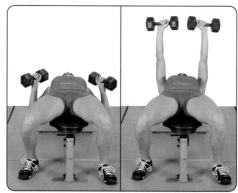

The dumbbell bench press is an excellent pressing exercise that allows for greater range of motion at the bottom of the movement and, therefore, a greater stretch on the pectorals. Dumbbells require increased stabilizer muscle recruitment, which makes it a worthy exercise in and of itself.

What You Feel: Chest, triceps

Tips

- *Keep your feet on the floor; don't place your feet on top of the bench.*
- *Using a full range of motion, bring the dumbbells down to the sides of your chest, and press it back up until your arms fully extend.*
- *Keep your butt on the bench, and do not lift it as you press the weight up.*

What to Do

1. Lie face up on a flat bench. Grasp a dumbbell in each hand, and position them at mid-chest level.
2. Press upward until your arms fully extend overhead.
3. Lower the weight back down to starting position, and repeat.

Dumbbell One-Arm Bench Press

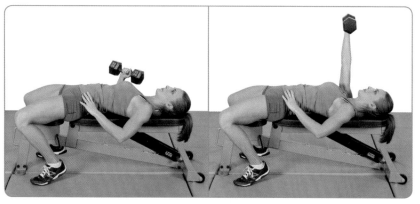 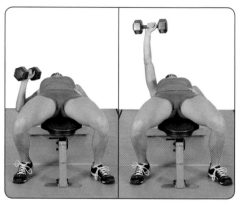

The one-arm dumbbell bench press is incredibly effective for two main reasons. First, it hammers the chest, shoulders, and triceps. Second, it's highly challenging in terms of core stability, especially as you gain strength and coordination. The obliques must work very hard to stabilize the midsection and prevent rotation during this movement.

What You Feel: Chest, triceps

Tips

- *Keep your feet on the floor; don't place your feet on top of the bench.*
- *Use a full range of motion, bring the dumbbells down to the sides of your chest, and press it back up until your arms fully extend.*
- *Keep your butt on the bench, and do not lift it as you press the weight up.*

What to Do

1. Lie face up on a flat bench. Grasp a dumbbell in your right hand, and position it at mid-chest level. Keep your left hand on your left hip.
2. Press upward until your arm fully extends overhead.
3. Lower the weight back down to starting position, and repeat for all reps on this side.
4. Switch and repeat on the other side.

Dumbbell Incline Press

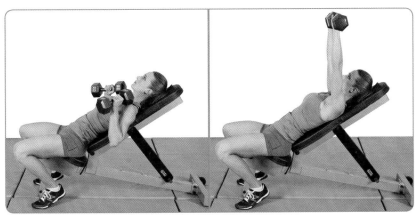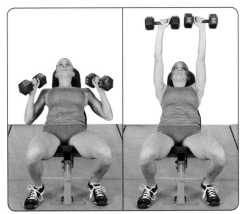

The dumbbell incline press is my favorite upper body pressing movement for women. The dumbbells allow for an increased range of motion and increased stretch on the chest muscles compared to the barbell version. Furthermore, light dumbbells can be used for beginners who are unable to perform push-ups or barbell pressing.

What You Feel: Chest, triceps

Tips

- *Keep your feet on the floor, and remain stable.*
- *Use a full range of motion, bring the dumbbells down to the sides of your chest, and press them back up until your arms fully extend.*
- *Keep your butt on the bench, and do not lift it as you press the weight up.*

What to Do

1. Lie face up on a bench positioned at a 45-degree incline.
2. Grasp a dumbbell in each hand, and position them near the tops of your shoulders.
3. Press upward until your arms fully extend overhead.
4. Lower the weight back down to starting position, and repeat.

Dumbbell One-Arm Incline Press

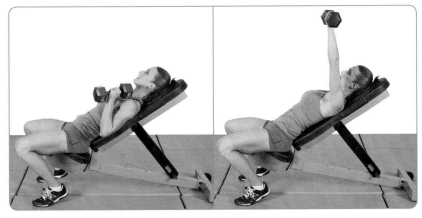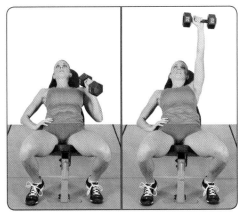

The one-arm incline press is a nice variation that introduces an element of core stability to the equation while still thoroughly working the chest muscles, shoulders, and triceps.

What You Feel: Chest, triceps

Tips

- *Keep your feet on the floor, and remain stable.*
- *Use a full range of motion, bring the dumbbell down to the side of your chest, and press it back up until your arms fully extend.*
- *Keep your butt on the bench, and do not lift it as you press the weight up.*

What to Do

1. Lie face up on a bench positioned at a 45-degree incline. Grasp a dumbbell in your right hand, and position it near the top of your shoulders.
2. Press upward until your arm fully extends overhead.
3. Lower the weight back down to starting position, and repeat for all reps on this side.
4. Switch, and repeat on the other side.

The barbell floor press is an excellent exercise for several reasons. First, it allows for heavier loads to be lifted due to the shortened range of motion. This provides a novel stimulus and should be utilized from time to time. Second, it can be performed in the absence of a bench; all you need is a loaded barbell and a floor. Third, the shortened ROM is sometimes good for those who are experiencing shoulder problems and feel pain when using a full range of motion.

What You Feel: Chest, triceps

Tips

- *If you don't have a rack or a spotter, you can simply "bridge" the barbell into place by performing a glute bridge and transitioning into a floor press.*
- *Pause for a brief moment when your elbows touch the ground before rising up into the next repetition.*
- *Keep your elbows at about a 45-degree angle relative to your torso.*

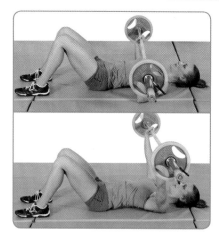
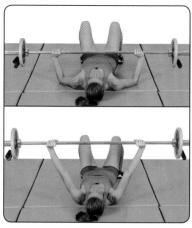

What to Do

1. Lie with your back on the floor. You may either use a power rack with the barbell racked on pins or have a partner hand you the bar once you are in position.
2. Position your hands slightly wider than your shoulders and the bar directly over your shoulders.
3. Lower the weight down until your upper arms touch the floor.
4. Press the weight back up straight overhead. Repeat.

Barbell Bench Press

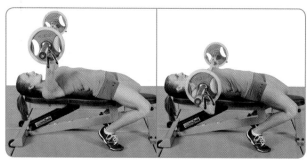

The bench press is the most popular exercise in the entire world, mostly because men want nice chest muscles, and the bench press is a good measure of chest strength and development. For women, however, it isn't quite as important, though it's an excellent triceps exercise, which shouldn't be ignored. For pectoral development, I like the incline press for women more than the standard bench press. The bench press is better for the triceps, though, so it's worth performing regularly.

What You Feel: Chest, triceps

Tips

- *Keep your feet on the floor, and do not place them on top of the bench.*
- *Use a full range of motion, bring the barbell down to your chest, and press it back up until your arms fully extend.*
- *Keep your butt on the bench, and do not lift it as you press the weight upward.*
- *Don't squirm; stay tight and stable.*
- *Keep your arms at about a 45-degree angle relative to your torso.*

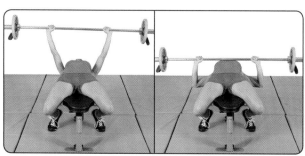

What to Do

1. Lie face up on the bench. Position yourself so that your forehead is directly under the bar.
2. Grasp the bar wider than shoulder width with an overhand grip.
3. Dismount the bar from the rack, and position it directly over your upper chest.
4. Lower the weight down to the middle of your chest.
5. Press upward until your arms fully extend. Repeat.

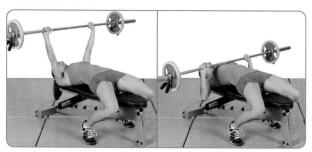

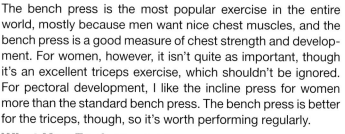

Barbell Close Grip Bench Press

Performing the bench press with a narrow grip increases the emphasis on the triceps and decreases the emphasis on the chest, making it even better for the triceps. For this reason, the close grip bench press is particularly effective and is a staple in my training routines for women desiring increased upper body shape.

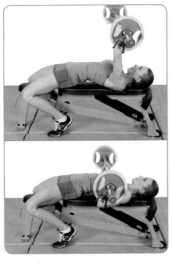
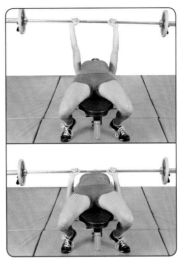
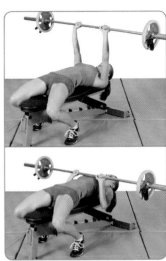

What You Feel: Chest, triceps

Tips

- *Keep your feet on the floor, and do not place them on top of the bench.*
- *Use a full range of motion, bring the barbell down to your chest, and press it back up until your arms fully extend.*
- *Keep your butt on the bench, and do not lift it as you press the weight upward.*
- *Don't squirm; stay tight and stable.*
- *Keep your arms at about a 45-degree angle relative to your torso.*

What to Do

1. Lie face up on the bench. Position yourself so that your forehead is directly under the bar.
2. Grasp the bar at shoulder width with an overhand grip.
3. Dismount the bar from the rack, and position it directly over your upper chest.
4. Lower the weight down to the middle of your chest.
5. Press upward until your arms fully extend. Repeat.

Barbell Incline Press

The barbell incline press is one of my favorite upper body exercises for women. Since women have breasts, it makes more sense to focus on upper pectoral development so that the results will be more evident, as mid/lower chest development will be concealed. Contrary to popular belief, a slightly narrower grip works the upper chest muscles better than a wide grip during this exercise.

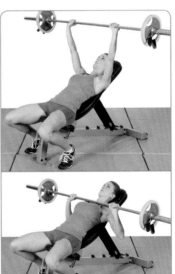
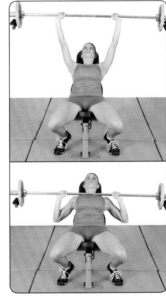

What You Feel: Chest, triceps

Tips

- *Keep your feet on the floor, and remain stable.*
- *Use a full range of motion, bring the barbell down to your upper chest, and press it back up until your arms fully extend.*
- *Keep your butt on the bench, and do not lift it as you press the weight up.*

What to Do

1. Lie face up on an incline bench. Position yourself so that your forehead is directly under the bar.
2. Grasp the bar wide with an overhand grip.
3. Dismount the bar from the rack, and position it directly over your upper chest.
4. Lower the weight down to the top of your chest.
5. Press upward until your arms fully extend. Repeat.

Vertical Pull

Vertical pulling resembles a pull-up. The arms start out overhead and end up next to the body. There are many types of grips and widths that can be employed during vertical pulls, and vertical pulls can involve pulling a cable toward your body or pulling your body toward a stationery bar.

Many women have a strong desire to perform a bodyweight chin-up. It's always great to witness my clients perform their first chin-up, and many have done so while working with me. With proper progression, you may eventually build up the strength to perform a chin-up without assistance, but not every body type is well suited for chins.

Vertical pulls work the lats very well, in addition to strengthening the traps, rhomboids, biceps, and brachialis muscles.

Front Lat Pulldown

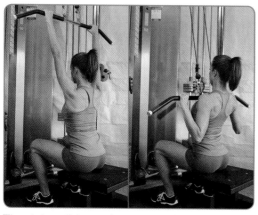

The lat pulldown is an excellent alternative to pull-ups, especially for people who are unable to perform pull-ups or find them problematic for the shoulder joints. Lat pulldowns are highly effective and joint-friendly.

What You Feel: Back, biceps

Tips

- *At the top position, fully extend your arms, but avoid shrugging your shoulders up by your ears.*
- *Pull the weight down by squeezing your upper back muscles together. The bar should come down to your clavicle, not to your mid-chest.*
- *Don't lean back too far or use excessive momentum.*

What to Do

1. Grasp the bar overhead at shoulder-width with your palms facing away from you.
2. Keeping your arms straight overhead, sit down on the bench, securing your knees under the padding (not shown in photo).
3. Pull the cable bar down by squeezing your back muscles and bending your elbows until the bar reaches the top of your chest.
4. Return to the starting position until your arms are fully extended and your back and arms are vertical. Repeat.

Wide Grip Lat Pulldown

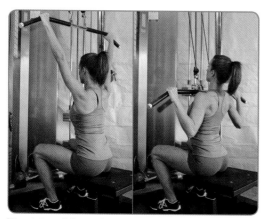

The lat pulldown is an excellent alternative to pull-ups, especially for people who are unable to perform pull-ups or find them problematic for the shoulder joints. Lat pulldowns are highly effective and joint-friendly. The wide grip variation is well-suited for targeting the lats.

What You Feel: Back, biceps

Tips

- *At the top position, fully extend your arms, but avoid shrugging your shoulders up by your ears.*
- *Pull the weight down by squeezing your upper back muscles together. The bar should come down to your clavicle, not to your mid-chest.*
- *Don't lean back too far or use excessive momentum.*
- *Gripping too wide may compromise your range of motion.*

What to Do

1. Grasp the bar overhead at twice the width of your shoulders with your palms facing away from you.
2. Keeping your arms straight overhead, sit down on the bench, securing your knees under the padding (not shown in photo).
3. Pull the cable bar down by squeezing your back muscles and bending your elbows until the bar reaches the top of your chest.
4. Return to the starting position until your arms are fully extended and your back is vertical. Repeat.

Underhand Grip Lat Pulldown

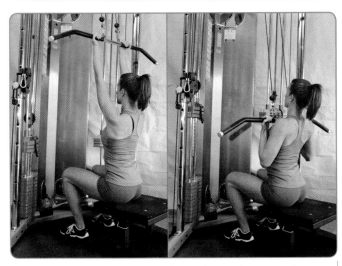

The lat pulldown is an excellent alternative to pull-ups, especially for people who are unable to perform pull-ups or find them problematic for the shoulder joints. Lat pulldowns are highly effective and joint-friendly. The underhand version is my favorite variation because it stretches the lats and targets the biceps.

What You Feel: Back, biceps

Tips

- *At the top position, fully extend your arms, but avoid shrugging your shoulders up by your ears.*
- *Pull the weight down by squeezing your upper back muscles together. The bar should come down to your clavicle, not to your mid-chest.*
- *Don't lean back too far or use excessive momentum.*

What to Do

1. Grasp the bar overhead at shoulder-width with your palms facing toward you.
2. Keeping your arms straight overhead, sit down on the bench, securing your knees under the padding (not shown in photo).
3. Pull the cable bar down by squeezing your back muscles and bending your elbows until the bar reaches the top of your chest.
4. Return to the starting position until your arms are fully extended and your back and arms are vertical. Repeat.

D-Handle Lat Pulldown

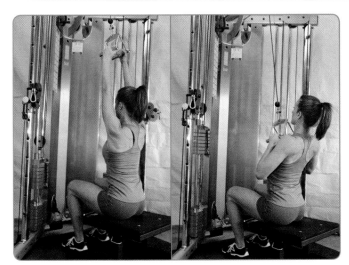

The lat pulldown is an excellent alternative to pull-ups, especially for people who are unable to perform pull-ups or find them problematic for the shoulder joints. Lat pulldowns are highly effective and joint-friendly. The D-handle variation is the most comfortable and the easiest on the joints, in my opinion.

What You Feel: Back, biceps

Tips

- *At the top position, fully extend your arms, but avoid shrugging your shoulders up by your ears.*
- *Pull the weight down by squeezing your upper back muscles together. The bar should come down to your clavicle, not to your mid-chest.*
- *Don't lean back too far or use excessive momentum.*

What to Do

1. Grasp the D-handle overhead with your palms facing each other.
2. Keeping your arms straight overhead, sit down on the bench, securing your knees under the padding (not shown in photo).
3. Pull the cable bar down by squeezing your back muscles and bending your elbows until the bar reaches the top of your chest.
4. Return to the starting position until your arms are fully extended and your back and arms are vertical. Repeat.

Band-Assisted Parallel Grip Pull-up

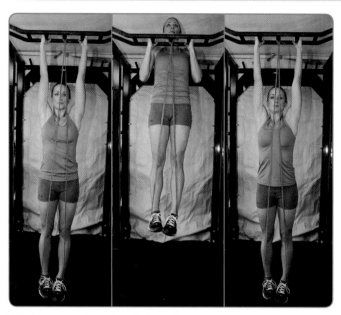

What You Feel: Back, core, biceps

Tips

- *Complete the movement with a full range of motion, pulling your sternum up to the bar and lowering down until your arms straighten.*
- *Keep your abdominal muscles tight throughout the movement to avoid arching your back as you pull up.*
- *Resistance bands only help you at the bottom position. You will do most of the work at the top.*
- *Stronger resistance bands are best for beginners. You may find the movement easier when using two resistance bands at first. You can gradually take away one band or reduce the strength of the bands as you progress.*

What to Do

1. Place the loop band over the bar, and secure it by pulling one end through the other.
2. Pull the single band end to the floor, and step inside with both feet. This may be tricky and require a partner's assistance.
3. Once your feet are secured in the band, grasp the bars at shoulder-width with your palms facing each other. From this position, your arms should be fully extended to keep the band in place.
4. Pull your body upward until the top of your chest reaches the height of the bar.
5. Lower, and repeat.

The band-assisted variation of the pull-up is an excellent way for beginners to build up necessary pulling strength to eventually be able to perform an unassisted body-weight pull-up.

Moderate Grip Chin-Up

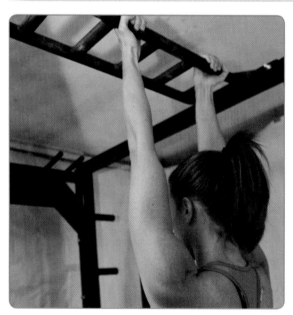

What You Feel: Back, core, biceps

Tips

- *Complete the movement with a full range of motion, pulling your sternum up to the bar and lowering down until your arms straighten.*
- *Keep your abdominal muscles tight throughout the movement to avoid arching your back as you pull up.*
- *Avoid swinging your body up and relying on excessive momentum from the legs.*

What to Do

1. Grasp the bar at shoulder-width with your palms facing toward you. From this position, your arms should be fully extended and your legs either straight or slightly bent at the knees.
2. Pull your body upward until the top of your chest reaches the height of the bar.
3. Lower, and repeat.

The moderate grip chin-up is my favorite pull-up variation because I feel it works the back very well through a full range of motion, while also significantly targeting the biceps.

Narrow Grip Chin-Up

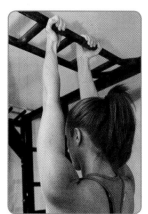

Some lifters find the narrow grip chin-up to be easiest on their shoulders, elbows, and wrists.

What You Feel: Back, core, biceps

Tips

- *Complete the movement with a full range of motion, pulling your sternum up to the bar and lowering down until your arms straighten.*
- *Keep your abdominal muscles tight throughout the movement to avoid arching your back as you pull up.*
- *Avoid swinging your body up and relying on excessive momentum from the legs.*

What to Do

1. Grasp the bar directly overhead with your palms facing toward you, taking a very narrow grip. From this position, your arms should be fully extended and your legs either straight or slightly bent at the knees.
2. Pull your body upward until the top of your chest reaches the height of the bar.
3. Lower, and repeat.

Wide Grip Chin-up

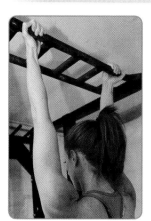

Personally, I prefer the moderate and narrow grip chin-up variations, but some people (usually heavily muscled males) prefer the wider grip variation. This is not a very joint-friendly variation, as it requires considerable supination of the elbow joints.

What You Feel: Back, core, biceps

Tips

- *Complete the movement with a full range of motion, pulling your sternum up to the bar and lowering down until your arms straighten.*
- *Keep your abdominal muscles tight throughout the movement to avoid arching your back as you pull up.*
- *Avoid swinging your body up and relying on excessive momentum from the legs.*

What to Do

1. Grasp the bar at slightly wider than your shoulders with your palms facing toward you. From this position, your arms should be fully extended and your legs either straight or slightly bent at the knees.
2. Pull your body upward until the top of your chest reaches the height of the bar.
3. Lower, and repeat.

Moderate Parallel Grip Pull-up

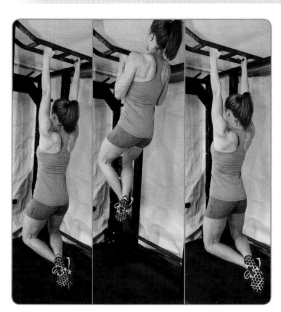

I believe this variation of the pull-up to be the safest and easiest on your joints. This should be your preferred pull-up variation if you have access to equipment that allows for this grip.

What You Feel: Back, core, biceps

Tips

- *Complete the movement with a full range of motion, pulling your sternum up to the bar and lowering down until your arms straighten.*
- *Keep your abdominal muscles tight throughout the movement to avoid arching your back as you pull up.*
- *Avoid swinging your body up and relying on excessive momentum from the legs.*

What to Do

1. Grasp the bars at slightly wider than your shoulders with your palms facing each other. From this position, your arms should be fully extended and your legs either straight or slightly bent at the knees.
2. Pull your body upward until the top of your chest reaches the height of the bar.
3. Lower, and repeat.

Narrow Parallel Grip Pull-up

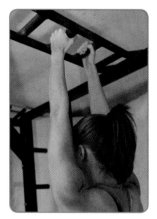

The narrow parallel grip pull-up is another joint-friendly pull-up variation, and it works the arms a bit more while slightly decreasing the contribution of the back muscles. Nevertheless, it's worth performing from time to time if you have access to narrow parallel handles.

What You Feel: Back, core, biceps

Tips

- *Complete the movement with a full range of motion, pulling your sternum up to the bar and lowering down until your arms straighten.*
- *Keep your abdominal muscles tight throughout the movement to avoid arching your back as you pull up.*
- *Avoid swinging your body up and relying on excessive momentum from the legs.*

What to Do

1. Grasp the bars directly overhead with your palms facing each other and a very narrow grip. From this position, your arms should be fully extended and your legs either straight or slightly bent at the knees.
2. Pull your body upward until the top of your chest reaches the height of the bar.
3. Lower, and repeat.

Wide Parallel Grip Pull-up

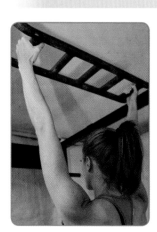

I like this variation better than the traditional wide grip pull-up because the parallel hand position seems to be easier on the joints and is more conducive to achieving proper range of motion during the movement.

What You Feel: Back, core, biceps

Tips

- *Complete the movement with a full range of motion, pulling your sternum up to the bar and lowering down until your arms straighten.*
- *Keep your abdominal muscles tight throughout the movement to avoid arching your back as you pull up.*
- *Avoid swinging your body up and relying on excessive momentum from the legs.*
- *If you grip the bar too wide, you may not get the right range of motion.*

What to Do

1. Grasp the bars at about twice the width of your shoulders with your palms facing each other. From this position, your arms should be fully extended in a Y formation and your legs either straight or slightly bent at the knees.
2. Pull your body upward until the top of your chest reaches the height of the bar.
3. Lower, and repeat.

Moderate Grip Pull-up

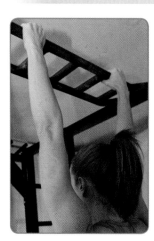

The pull-up is a classic back exercise that works the lats very well. In my experience, there aren't many feats in the gym that women are more proud of than performing their first pull-up. Rowing exercises, lat pulldowns, negative pull-ups, and band-assisted pull-ups can be used to develop the strength to eventually perform a full range pull-up. Body weight must be reasonable, however, in order for the feat to occur. Within several months of hard training, women can usually perform a proper pull-up on their own with no assistance.

What You Feel: Back, core, biceps

Tips

- *Complete the movement with a full range of motion, pulling your sternum up to the bar and lowering down until your arms straighten.*
- *Keep your abdominal muscles tight throughout the movement to avoid arching your back as you pull up.*
- *Avoid swinging your body up and relying on excessive momentum from the legs.*

What to Do

1. Grasp the bar at slightly wider than your shoulders with your palms facing away from you. From this position, your arms should be fully extended and your legs either straight or slightly bent at the knees.
2. Pull your body upward until the top of your chest reaches the height of the bar.
3. Lower, and repeat.

Wide Grip Pull-up

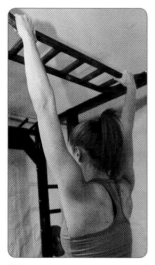
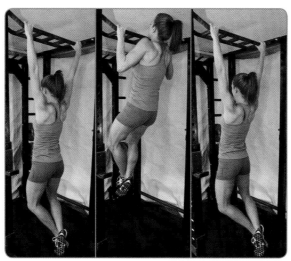

The wide grip pull-up is a staple among bodybuilders, who feel that the wider grip variation works the lats best. I'm not a huge fan of the wider variation; I believe it can be problematic for some people over the long haul. I see nothing wrong with performing this variation occasionally, however, for the sake of variety. I haven't trained many women who were capable of performing multiple reps in the wide grip pull-up, though.

What You Feel: Back, core, biceps

Tips

- *Complete the movement with a full range of motion, pulling your sternum up to the bar and lowering down until your arms straighten.*
- *Keep your abdominal muscles tight throughout the movement to avoid arching your back as you pull up.*
- *Avoid swinging your body up and relying on excessive momentum from the legs.*
- *If you grip the bar too wide, you may not be able to achieve optimal range of motion.*

What to Do

1. Grasp the bar at about twice the width of your shoulders with your palms facing away from you. From this position, your arms should be fully extended in a Y formation and your legs either straight or slightly bent at the knees.
2. Pull your body upward until the top of your chest reaches the height of the bar.
3. Lower, and repeat.

Weighted Parallel Pull-up with Belt

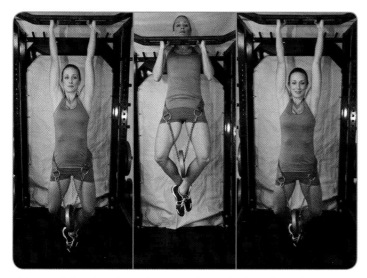

The weighted pull-up is the crème de la crème for upper body pulling strength. Some of my colleagues have trained women who could perform three reps with 45 additional pounds, but these were high-level pro athletes. I've trained a few women who could do a rep with 25 extra pounds. Once you're able to perform five bodyweight reps, you may opt for weighted pull-ups from time to time, starting with five extra pounds and gradually working your way upward in weight.

What You Feel: Back, core, biceps

Tips

- *Complete the movement with a full range of motion, pulling your sternum up to the bar and lowering down until your arms straighten.*
- *Keep your abdominal muscles tight throughout the movement to avoid arching your back as you pull up.*
- *Don't choose a weight that is too heavy because it will reduce your range of motion.*

What to Do

1. Secure the weight belt around your waist with an appropriate amount of weight.
2. Grasp the bars at slightly wider than your shoulders with your palms facing away from you. From this position, your arms should be fully extended and your legs either straight or slightly bent at the knees.
3. Pull your body upward until the top of your chest reaches the height of the bar.
4. Lower, and repeat.

Weighted Parallel Pull-up with Dumbbell

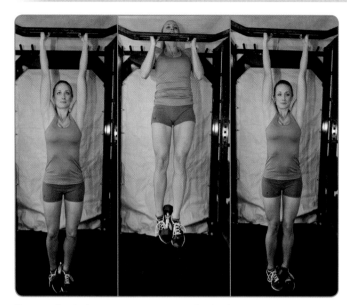

If you don't have access to a dip belt, you can simply place a dumbbell between crossed legs in order to add load to the pull-up and increase its difficulty.

What You Feel: Back, core, biceps

Tips

- *Complete the movement with a full range of motion, pulling your sternum up to the bar and lowering down until your arms straighten.*
- *Keep your abdominal muscles tight throughout the movement to avoid arching your back as you pull up.*
- *Don't choose a weight that is too heavy, as it will reduce your range of motion.*
- *You may find it easier to have a partner position the weight between your legs once you are in starting position.*

What to Do

1. Position a dumbbell between your crossed legs slightly above your ankles.
2. Grasp the bars at slightly wider than your shoulders with your palms facing away from you. From this position, your arms should be fully extended and your legs either straight or slightly bent at the knees.
3. Pull your body upward until the top of your chest reaches the height of the bar.
4. Lower, and repeat.

Vertical Press

Strong shoulder muscles are appealing to many women, as they feel it helps add symmetry to their shape. Vertical presses are the best exercises for shoulder development. Always start these presses with your arms near your body and end with your arms overhead.

The overwhelming majority of women can safely employ vertical pressing, which might not be the case for men who quite often have banged up shoulders from poor training practices. Women tend to have good mo-bility in the shoulders and T-spine, which allows for proper form. If you are new to this type of exercise, you may initially lack shoulder and scapular stability, so ease into this section, and build up strength gradually.

Barbell Push Press

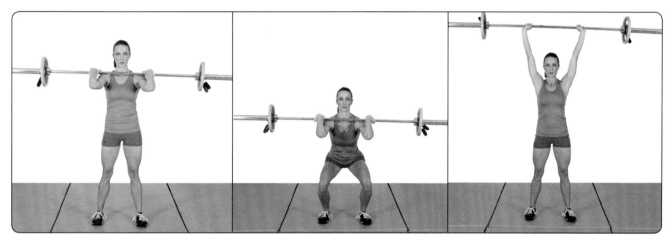

The push press is an effective shoulder exercise that allows you to use more weight, providing a novel training stimulus. Since the legs are helping out, this variation is more of a full body exercise compared to the standard military press.

What You Feel: Shoulders and legs

Tips

- *Do not fully squat the weight down before driving up. Just dip down slightly.*
- *Push the weight up explosively, and catch the bar overhead in a locked-out position; don't push the weight halfway up to finish off with a slow, grinding military press.*
- *Avoid leaning back as you hoist the weight overhead. This becomes more difficult as you move up in weight. Squeeze your glutes and abs to help keep a neutral core.*
- *After the bar passes your head, move your head forward so that the bar travels directly overhead and your upper back is fully extended.*
- *Keep a somewhat narrow grip, and feel tension in the lats at the bottom of the movement.*

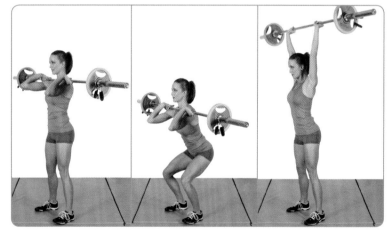

What to Do

1. Grasp the barbell from the rack slightly wider than shoulder-width. Position the bar at chest height, and step back from the rack.
2. Staying upright, dip down at the knees and hips, and explosively drive the weight upward, extending your arms overhead.
3. Lower the bar down, and catch it at your upper chest while dipping down to absorb the load.
4. Return to the starting position, and repeat.

Dumbbell Push Press

The push press is an effective shoulder exercise that allows you to use more weight, providing a novel training stimulus. Since the legs are helping out, this variation is more of a full body exercise compared to the standard military press. Dumbbells are ideal for beginners who are unable to use the barbell, and these weights require more stability, making them worthwhile for any lifter. Furthermore, your head doesn't interfere with the bar path like it does when using a barbell, allowing for a more natural range of motion.

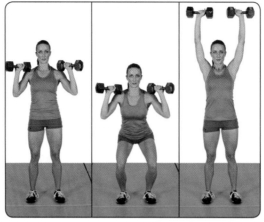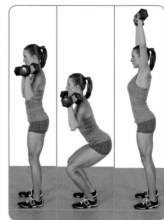

What You Feel: Shoulders and legs

Tips

- *Do not fully squat the weight down before driving up; just dip down slightly.*
- *Push the weight up explosively, and catch the dumbbells overhead in a locked-out position; don't push the weight halfway up to finish off with a slow, grinding military press.*
- *Avoid leaning back as you hoist the weight overhead. This becomes more difficult as you move up in weight. Squeeze your glutes and abs to help keep a neutral core.*

What to Do

1. Position a dumbbell on each side of your shoulders with your palms facing in.
2. Stand with your feet slightly wider than your shoulders or in a split stance.
3. Staying upright, dip down at the knees and hips, and explosively drive the weight upward, extending your arms overhead.
4. Lower the dumbbells down to your shoulders, dipping down at the knees with the catch to absorb some of the load with the legs.
5. Return to the starting position, and repeat.

Dumbbell Standing Overhead Press

The dumbbell overhead press is a classic shoulder exercise that has stood the test of time. It not only targets the shoulders and triceps, but also ensures ideal shoulder health and function when performed properly. Dumbbells are ideal for beginners who are unable to use the barbell, and these weights require more stability, making them worthwhile for any lifter. Furthermore, your head doesn't interfere with the bar path like it does when using a barbell, allowing for a more natural range of motion.

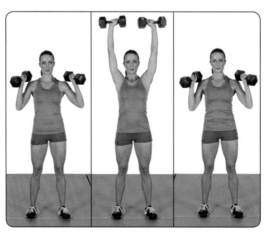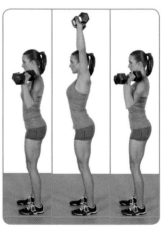

What You Feel: Shoulders

Tips

- *Use a full range of motion, raising the dumbbells until your arms are fully extended. Stand tall at the top of the motion.*
- *Avoid leaning back as you hoist the weight overhead. This becomes more difficult as you move up in weight. Squeeze your glutes and abs to help keep a neutral core.*

What to Do

1. Position a dumbbell on each side of your shoulders with your palms facing in.
2. Stand with your feet slightly wider than your shoulders or in a split stance.
3. Press the weight upward, rotating your forearms outward while fully extending your arms overhead.
4. Lower the weight back down to your shoulders, rotating your forearms in. Repeat.

Dumbbell One-Arm Shoulder Press

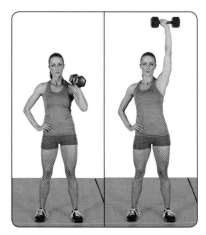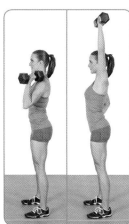

The one-arm shoulder press is a unique variation that increases the core stability requirements and can allow for slightly heavier loads to be used with some lifters. This is an excellent shoulder exercise that is easy on the joints.

What You Feel: Shoulders

Tips

- *Use a full range of motion, raising the dumbbell until your arm is fully extended. Stand tall at the top of the motion.*
- *Avoid leaning back as you hoist the weight overhead. This becomes more difficult as you move up in weight. Squeeze your glutes and abs to help keep a neutral core.*

What to Do

1. Position a dumbbell at your right shoulder with your thumb touching the middle of your front deltoids and your forearm facing in.
2. Stand with your feet slightly wider than your shoulders or in a split stance.
3. Press the weight upward, rotating your forearm outward while fully extending your arm overhead.
4. Lower the weight back down to your shoulder, rotating your forearms in.
5. Repeat on both sides.

Seated Dumbbell Shoulder Press

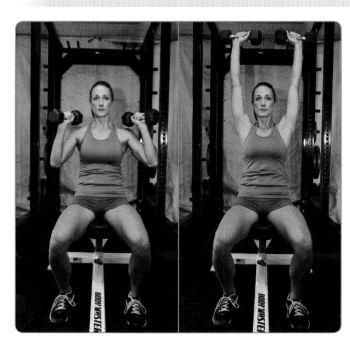

The seated shoulder press is one of my favorite upper body exercises. Many lifters who find the standing military press problematic for their low back can safely and effectively train their shoulders with the seated shoulder press, and most people can lift heavier loads with this variation compared to the standing counterpart.

What You Feel: Shoulders

Tips

- *Use a full range of motion, raising the weights until your arms are fully extended and lowering the weights down to your shoulders.*
- *When using heavier weight, you can mount the weight by resting the dumbbells on your thighs and using your legs to help push the weight up into the starting position.*

What to Do

1. Sit on a bench with a back support, planting your feet on the ground.
2. Position a dumbbell at each shoulder with your forearms facing in.
3. Press the dumbbells upward while rotating your arms outward until your arms fully extend overhead.
4. Lower the weight to the starting position, and repeat.

Military Press

The military press is a classic shoulder exercise that has stood the test of time. It not only targets the shoulders and triceps, but also ensures ideal shoulder health and function when performed properly.

What You Feel: Shoulders

Tips

- *Use a full range of motion, raising the bar until your arms are fully extended and lowering the bar down to your upper chest region.*

- *Avoid leaning back as you hoist the weight overhead. This becomes more difficult as you move up in weight. Squeeze your glutes and abs to help keep a neutral core.*

- *After the bar passes your head, move your head forward so that the bar travels directly overhead and the upper back is fully extended.*

- *Keep a somewhat narrow grip, and feel tension in the lats at the bottom of the movement.*

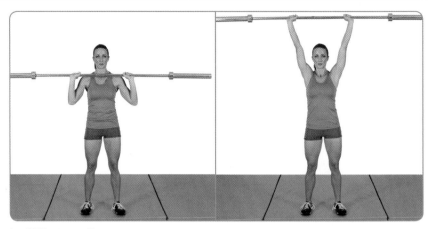

What to Do

1. Grasp the bar from the rack just outside shoulder-width. Step away from the rack, and position the bar at the top of the chest.
2. Stand with your feet slightly wider than your shoulders or in a split stance.
3. Press the bar upward, fully extending your arms overhead.
4. Lower the bar back down to your upper chest region, and repeat.

Dip

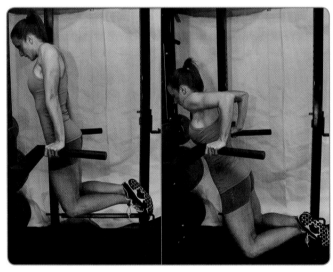

The dip is a great chest, shoulder, and triceps exercise that has stood the test of time. If you find the exercise problematic for your shoulder joints, assess your technique to see what the issue may be. This is a challenging movement, so make sure you're proficient in push-ups prior to attempting dips.

What You Feel: Chest, front shoulders, triceps

Tips

- *Don't try to stay perfectly upright during the movement; lean forward a bit to absorb more loading with the pectorals.*

- *Lower until you feel a stretch in your chest and front shoulders, and rise up all the way into a complete lockout. Don't sink down too far to where it's painful.*

- *Don't use too wide a grip, as this is not safe for the shoulder joint; a narrower dip is ideal for long-term shoulder health. Keep your elbows directly over your wrists, and don't let them flare outward during the movement.*

- *Don't allow the shoulders to shrug at the top of the movement. Keep your shoulder blades depressed to prevent your shoulders from rising toward your ears.*

What to Do

1. Mount the dip bar with your palms facing your sides. Your arms should be straight, and your shoulders should be positioned over your hands.
2. Bend your knees and hips slightly.
3. Lower your body by bending at the shoulders and elbows while leaning your torso forward.
4. Push back up, straightening your arms, and repeat.

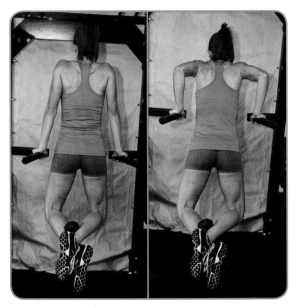

What You Feel: **Chest, front shoulders, triceps**

Tips

- *Don't try to stay perfectly upright during the movement; lean forward a bit to absorb more loading with the pectorals.*
- *Lower until you feel a stretch in your chest and front shoulders, and rise up all the way into a complete lockout. Don't sink down too far to where it's painful.*
- *Don't use too wide a grip, as this is not safe for the shoulder joint; a narrower dip is ideal for long-term shoulder health. Keep your elbows directly over your wrists, and don't let them flare outward during the movement.*
- *Don't allow your shoulders to shrug at the top of the movement. Keep your shoulder blades depressed to prevent your shoulders from rising toward your ears.*

What to Do

1. Position the weight belt around your waist, or place a dumbbell between your lower legs slightly above your feet.
2. Mount the dip bar with your palms facing your sides. Your arms should be straight, and your shoulders should be positioned over your hands.
3. Bend your knees and hips slightly.
4. Lower your body by bending at the shoulders and elbows while leaning your torso forward.
5. Push back up, straightening your arms, and repeat.

The dip is a great chest, shoulder, and triceps exercise that has stood the test of time. If you find the exercise problematic for your shoulder joints, assess your technique to see what the issue might be. This is a challenging movement, so make sure you're proficient in push-ups prior to attempting dips. Adding extra weight is challenging, but it can be done by advanced lifters.

Pike Push-up

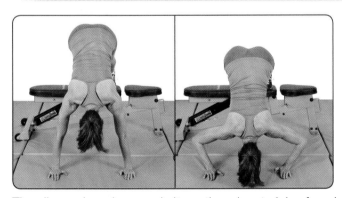

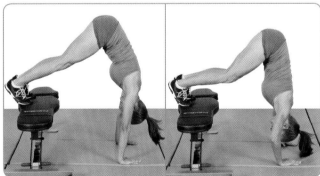

The pike push-up is a good alternative when training from home or when it isn't possible to access a gym. It effectively targets the delts while building shoulder stability and coordination.

What You Feel: **Shoulders, triceps**

Tips

- *This is an advanced shoulder exercise. You can make it easier by placing your feet on the floor rather than on a bench.*

What to Do

1. Get in push-up position with your feet on a flat bench.
2. Walk your hands back while hiking your hips upward until your upper body is relatively vertical. Make sure your hands are wider than your shoulders.
3. Lower your body down by bending at your shoulders and elbows until your head touches the floor.
4. Push back up, and repeat.

Linear Core

Concentrated abdominal work is talked about often with regard to training programs. Over the years, I've realized something as a personal trainer—a client will never question you when you prescribe abdominal exercises. There have been times when I spent five minutes discussing the myth of spot reduction (abs exercises don't selectively burn fat off of the midsection) and preaching the merits of proper nutrition and high intensity full body exercise for fat loss and a lean physique, only to have the client ask me at the end of the session why I didn't prescribe any core exercises. It's quite comical.

So, even though I don't feel that core training is necessary for physique training purposes, I always want my clients to enjoy their workout. For this reason, I often meet them in the middle and prescribe a couple of core exercises.

The truth is that the core will be worked during full body exercise. The spinal erectors (low back muscles) get worked hard during squats, deadlifts, back extensions, and hip thrusts; the obliques get worked hard during band hip rotations, squats, and deadlifts; and the abdominals get worked during chin-ups. If you get down in body weight and body fat and reach impressive strength levels on the big lifts, you'll be very happy with the way your midsection/abdominals look. Neverthe-

less, it's always good to have strong abs for functional strength and postural purposes, so a couple of sets of targeted core exercises can be beneficial as long as you don't overdo it.

Linear core exercises primarily work the abdominals and secondarily work the obliques. The word "linear" implies forward and backward, and this category of exercise involves performing movements in these directions. Exercises like planks, sit-ups, and crunches are "linear" in that they work the core from front to back and target the abdominals. My favorite linear core exercise is the RKC plank because it requires glute endurance and works the glutes through its role as a posterior pelvic tilter.

Crunch

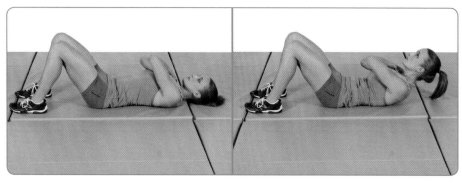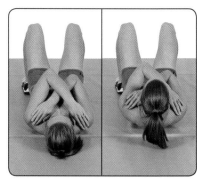

The crunch is a beginner exercise that targets the rectus abdominis.

What You Feel: Abdominals

Tips

- *Do not pull your neck toward your chest with your hands when you contract your abdominals. Keep your neck in a neutral position.*
- *Limit the range of motion; 30 degrees of flexion from the horizontal is sufficient.*

What to Do

1. Lie on your back with your knees bent and feet positioned slightly out from your glutes.
2. Place your hands next to your ears or across your chest.
3. Flex the waist to raise your upper torso to a 30-degree angle by moving your ribcage toward your hips.
4. Lower, and repeat.

Swiss Ball Crunch

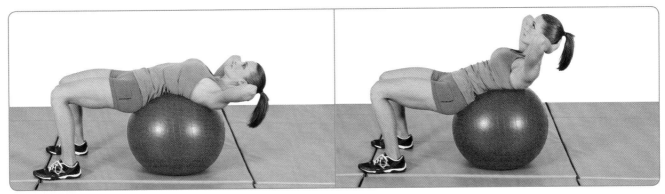

The Swiss ball crunch is a very effective abdominal exercise that works the upper abs.

What You Feel: Abdominals

Tips

- *Focus on contracting the abdominal muscles rather than trying to sit up on the ball and/or use your hip flexors too much.*
- *Keep your neck aligned with your spine, and avoid pulling your neck toward your chest with your hands.*

What to Do

1. Sit on the exercise ball. Walk forward on the ball until your lower back rests across the ball and your head and shoulders hang off.
2. Your knees will be bent with your feet flat on the floor.
3. Gently extend your back over the contour of the ball to put the abdominals on stretch. Place your hands next to your ears or across your chest.
4. Squeeze your abdominals, pulling your ribs toward your hips. Don't raise your torso too high; 30 degrees of trunk flexion relative to the horizontal is sufficient.
5. Lower back down, and repeat.

Dumbbell Swiss Ball Crunch

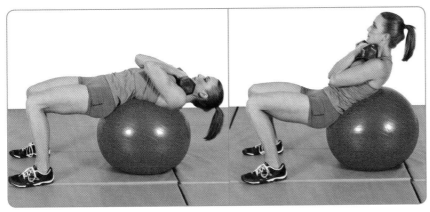
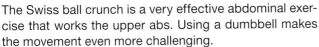
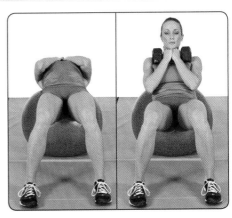

The Swiss ball crunch is a very effective abdominal exercise that works the upper abs. Using a dumbbell makes the movement even more challenging.

What You Feel: Abdominals

Tips

- *Focus on contracting the abdominal muscles rather than trying to sit up on the ball and/or use your hip flexors too much.*
- *Keep your neck aligned with your spine, and avoid pulling your neck toward your chest with your hands.*

What to Do

1. Grasp a dumbbell by the handle with both hands with your palms out. Place the dumbbell directly under your chin.
2. Sit on the exercise ball. Walk forward on the ball until your lower back rests across the ball and your head and shoulders hang off.
3. Your knees will be bent with your feet flat on the floor.
4. Raise your head, shoulders, and neck in a forward lean by contracting your abdominal muscles. Focus on pulling your ribs toward your hip bones as you come up.
5. Slowly lower back to starting position and repeat for reps.

Straight-leg Sit-up

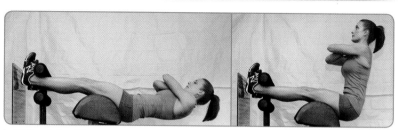

The straight-leg sit-up is a favorite of many clients because it trains the abdominals and hip flexors simultaneously. If performed properly, it's an amazing anterior chain movement.

What You Feel: Abdominals

Tips

- *You may perform this exercise lying on the floor if you do not have access to the glute/ham developer, but it's best when you can anchor your feet under something secure.*
- *Keep your chest up, and use your abdominals and hip flexors to raise your body.*
- *Don't descend too far and hyperextend the lumbar spine, and don't round your back too far up top to limit the amount of lumbar flexion.*

What to Do

1. Adjust the glute/ham developer so that when seated, your feet are secured between the rollers, and your butt is resting on the far end of the pad.
2. Straighten your legs, and position your trunk vertically with your hands across your chest for the starting position.
3. Slowly lower your trunk until your body reaches a horizontal position.
4. Curl back up, straightening your back as you move beyond a 45-degree angle.
5. Return to an upright position. Repeat.

Kneeling Front Plank

This plank variation is perfect for those who are not quite ready to do a front plank. By bracing your torso from the knees, you reduce the total amount of body weight you're supporting, which makes the movement easier.

What You Feel: Abdominals

Tips

- *Squeeze your glutes and quads along with your abdominals to prevent your lower back from sagging.*
- *It's easy to bend at the neck and push your hips up into a pike while performing these. Keep your neck and spine in neutral alignment.*
- *It's better to maintain good form for a shorter period of time than to allow your form to break down just to add seconds to the clock.*

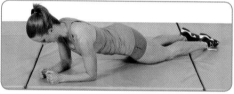
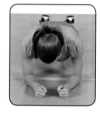

What to Do

1. Lie facedown on a mat. Pushup onto your forearms and knees, placing your elbows under your shoulders.
2. Raise your body upward, creating a straight line from your head to your knees.
3. Contract your abdominals, glutes, and quads throughout the duration of the exercise.
4. Hold isometrically for as long as possible, and release. This is performed in a single rep with an isometric hold.

Front Plank

The front plank trains your core for linear stability, specifically the lumbar spine to resist being pulled into hyperextension.

What You Feel: Abdominals

Tips

- *Squeeze your glutes and quads along with your abdominals to prevent your lower back from sagging.*
- *It's easy to bend at the neck and push your hips up into a pike while performing these. Keep your neck and spine in neutral alignment.*
- *It's better to maintain good form for a shorter period of time than to allow your form to break down just to add seconds to the clock.*

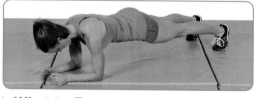
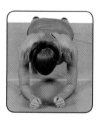

What to Do

1. Lie facedown on a mat. Pushup onto your forearms, placing your elbows under your shoulders.
2. Place your feet together with your shins resting on the floor.
3. Raise your body upward, creating a straight line from your head to your feet.
4. Contract your abdominals, glutes, and quads throughout the duration of the exercise.
5. Hold for as long as possible, and release.

Use this exercise to increase the difficulty of a front plank by moving your arms farther out from your torso.

What You Feel: Abdominals

Tips

- *Squeeze your glutes and quads along with your abdominals to prevent your lower back from sagging.*
- *It's easy to bend at the neck and push your hips up into a pike while performing these. Keep your neck and spine in neutral alignment.*
- *It's better to maintain good form for a shorter period of time than to allow your form to break down just to add seconds to the clock..*

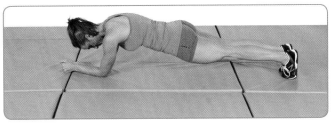

What to Do

1. Lie facedown on a mat. Pushup onto your forearms, positioning your elbows near your forehead.
2. Raise your body upward, creating a straight line from your head to your toes.
3. Contract your abdominals, glutes, and quads throughout the duration of the exercise.
4. Hold for as long as possible, and release.

RKC Plank

This plank variation trains the lumbar spine to resist hyperextension while simultaneously training the glutes to work as posterior pelvic tilters and building glute endurance. Many people struggle to activate their glutes in this position. If you are one of these people, I recommend performing the RKC plank every single day for two months until it becomes natural. Just perform one or two sets of 10 to 30 seconds. The RKC plank is also a valuable exercise for increasing the effectiveness of other glute exercises. Perform a 10 second hold immediately before or after sets of hip thrusts or kettlebell swings and you'll put the glutes on overdrive. This is a good strategy to experiment with from time to time.

What You Feel: Abdominals, glutes, quads

Tips

- *The RKC plank turns on every muscle in the body. It's a great way to fully exert your muscles for a very short duration.*
- *It's easy to bend at the neck and push your hips up into a pike while performing these. Keep your neck and spine in neutral alignment.*
- *It's better to maintain good form for a shorter period of time than to allow your form to break down just to add seconds to the clock.*

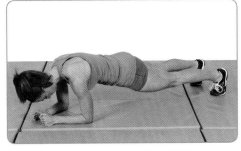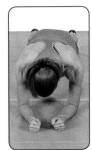

What to Do

1. Lie facedown on a mat. Pushup onto your forearms, positioning your elbows directly under your shoulders. Tighten your shoulders into place, and squeeze your fists.
2. Raise your body upward, creating a straight line from your head to your toes.
3. Squeeze your glutes as hard as possible into a posterior pelvic tilt. Don't lose this contraction.
4. Pull your elbows toward your toes and your toes toward your elbows as hard as you can.
5. Hold for as long as possible, and release.

Feet-Elevated RKC Plank

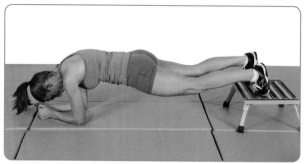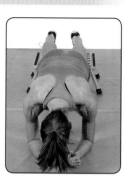

This plank variation trains the lumbar spine to resist hyperextension while simultaneously training the glutes to work as posterior pelvic tilters and building glute endurance. Elevating the feet increases the challenge slightly.

What You Feel: Abdominals, glutes, quads

Tips

- *The RKC plank turns on every muscle in the body. It's a great way to fully exert your muscles for a short duration.*
- *It's easy to bend at the neck and push your hips up into a pike while performing these. Keep your neck and spine in neutral alignment.*
- *It's better to maintain good form for a shorter period of time than to allow your form to break down just to add seconds to the clock.*

What to Do

1. Lie facedown on a mat. Pushup onto your forearms, positioning your elbows directly under your shoulders. Tighten your shoulders into place, and squeeze your fists. Place the feet on top of a step or box.
2. Raise your body upward, creating a straight line from your head to your toes.
3. Squeeze your glutes as hard as possible into a posterior pelvic tilt. Don't lose this contraction.
4. Pull your elbows toward your toes and your toes toward your elbows as hard as you can.
5. Hold for as long as possible, and release.

Body Saw

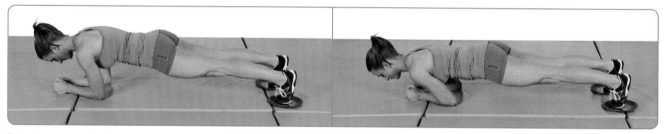

The body saw builds anti-extension capacity in the lumbar spine, thereby increasing core stability while working the abdominals efficiently. (Note: Sliders won't work on a rubber floor).

What You Feel: Abdominals

Tips

- *Squeeze your glutes and quads along with your abdominals to prevent your lower back from sagging.*
- *It's easy to bend at the neck and push your hips up into a pike while performing these. Keep your neck and spine in neutral alignment.*
- *You do not have to move forward and backward too much for this exercise to be effective.*

What to Do

1. Place your feet in the center of the Gliders or Valslides. Get down in plank position, placing your elbows under your shoulders.
2. Pull your torso forward without moving your forearms.
3. Push your torso back, creating longer levers with your arms.
4. Repeat for reps.

Ab Wheel Roll Out

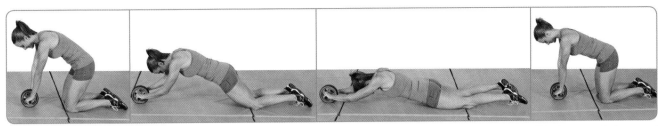

This exercise builds core stability and improves your body's ability to resist lumbar extension. This is one of the most challenging and effective abdominal exercises in this program.

What You Feel: Abdominals

Tips

- *Keep your spine in neutral throughout the duration of the exercise to make sure you avoid arching your lower back or tilting your pelvis anteriorly as you roll out.*
- *You may not be able to fully extend your arms in front of your body when you begin this exercise. If this is the case, just roll out to a comfortable position, and progress to full range over time.*

What to Do

1. Kneel on an exercise mat, grasping the handle of the ab wheel with an overhand grip.
2. Position the wheel near your knees so that your shoulders are directly over the top of it.
3. Keeping your arms straight, roll the wheel out as far as possible, lowering your torso toward the floor.
4. Raise your body back up, returning the wheel to the starting position and repeat for reps.

Hanging Leg Raise

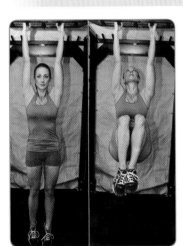

The hanging leg raise is a fantastic abdominal exercise that trains the lower abdominal musculature.

What You Feel: Abdominals

Tips

- *Concentrate on pulling your knees toward your chest in a controlled manner. Don't rely on momentum.*
- *Avoid swinging as you lower your legs.*

What to Do

1. Grasp and hang from the high bar with your hands positioned slightly wider than your shoulders in an overhand grip.
2. Raise your legs toward your chest, bending at the knees and flexing at the hips.
3. Pull up with your abdominals until your knees are well above your hips.
4. Return to the starting position, fully extending your knees and hips down and repeat for reps.

Kettlebell Farmer's Walk

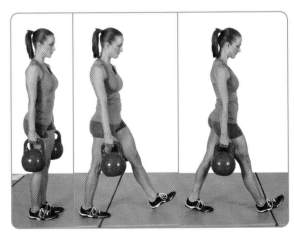

This exercise builds grip strength, shoulder and hip stability, and stamina.

What You Feel: Erectors, forearm muscles, traps, quads, upper glutes

Tips

- *Avoid shrugging the weight up as you walk.*

What to Do

1. Position a kettlebell by the outside of each foot. Bend straight down in a deadlift position, picking the weights up.
2. Hold the weights down at your sides, and walk straight forward with a normal gate.
3. Walk for a predetermined distance, and set the weight down.

This introduction exercise to the Turkish get-up builds full body stability, mobility, and coordination.

What You Feel:
Erectors, forearm muscles, traps, quads, upper glutes

Tips

- *Using a shoe or other flat object will help you maintain the correct posture and hand position throughout the movement.*

- *Learn this movement one sequence at a time; it takes practice to get it right. Be patient.*

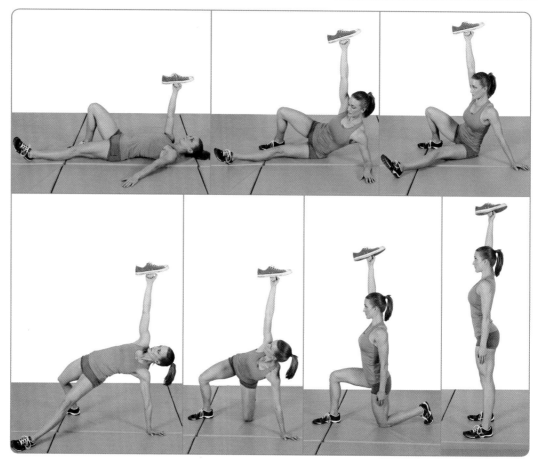

What to Do

1. Lie on your back on the floor. Position your right arm straight overhead with an object balanced on your knuckles and your left arm straight out at your side at a 45-degree angle.

2. Flex your right knee so that your foot is flat on the floor. Your left leg should remain straight out in front of you.

3. Leading with your chest, come up onto your left elbow. Your right foot should now be positioned away from your glutes as you turn up onto your side.

4. From this position, rise up onto your left hand. Your torso should now be facing forward.

5. Drive through your heels into a high bridge position. Focus on extending through the hips rather than the lumbar spine, keeping your chest up. Squeeze your glute and hamstrings to keep your hips up.

6. From here, sweep the left leg under the bent leg (threading the needle) so that your left knee is positioned on the ground underneath your body in a kneeling position.

7. Rotate your left lower leg (windshield wiper the shin outward), and raise your torso so that you end up in a tall half-kneeling position.

8. Stand up from this split squat position, bringing your feet next to each other and keeping your chest tall and arm straight up. The top position is the halfway point. Now, lower back down, repeating the steps in reverse.

9. Step backward with your left leg, lowering down into a reverse lunge, positioning your right knee on the floor.

10. From a half-kneeling position, lower down toward your left side, turning your left foot out while placing your hand back down on the floor.

11. Sweep your left leg out from under your body until it is straight out in front of you. Maintain a high bridge position with your hips, focusing on squeezing your glutes.

12. Drop your hips down to the ground, supporting your weight on your left hand.

13. With controlled movement, lower back down to your elbow.

14. Keeping your right knee up and left leg straight, slowly lower your torso down until your back is flat on the floor.

15. Repeat for reps. Then, switch to the other side.

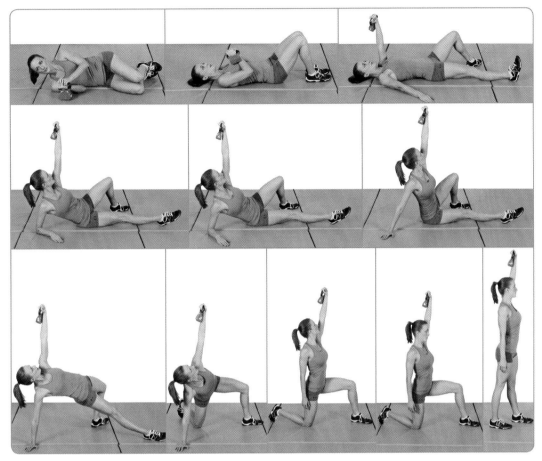

What You Feel:

What You Feel:

Glutes, hamstrings, quads, abdominals, obliques, erectors

Tips

- *Master the naked get-up before moving to the Turkish get up. Don't go too heavy to where you can't use proper form.*

The Turkish getup usually generates a few sideways heads when performed. It's definitely not your run-of-the-mill exercise and is far more challenging than it appears. Mastery takes a while, so start off with the naked getup. This exercise works well to build full body stability, mobility, and coordination.

What to Do

1. Lie on your back on the floor. Position your right arm straight overhead with an object in your right hand (preferably a kettlebell) and your left arm straight out at your side at a 45-degree angle.

2. Flex your right knee so that your foot is flat on the floor. Your left leg should remain straight out in front of you.

3. Leading with your chest, come up onto your left elbow. Your right foot should now be positioned away from your glutes as your turn up onto your side.

4. From this position, rise up onto your left hand. Your torso should now be facing forward.

5. Drive through your heels into a high bridge position. Focus on extending through the hips rather than the lumbar spine, keeping your chest up. Squeeze your glute and hamstrings to keep your hips up.

6. From here, sweep your left leg under the bent leg (threading the needle) so that your left knee is positioned on the ground underneath your body in a kneeling position.

7. Rotate your left lower leg (windshield wiper the shin outward), and raise your torso so that you end up in a tall half-kneeling position.

8. Stand up from this split squat position, bringing your feet next to each other and keeping your chest tall and arm straight up. The top position is the halfway point. Now, lower back down, repeating the steps in reverse.

9. Step backward with your left leg, lowering down into a reverse lunge, positioning your right knee on the floor.

10. From a half-kneeling position, lower down toward your left side, turning your left foot out while placing your hand back down on the floor.

11. Sweep your left leg out from under your body until it is straight out in front of you. Maintain a high bridge position with your hips, focusing on squeezing your glutes.

12. Drop your hips down to the ground, supporting your weight on your left hand.

13. With controlled movement, lower back down to your elbow.

14. Keeping your right knee up and left leg straight, slowly lower your torso down until your back is flat on the floor.

15. Repeat for reps. Then, switch to the other side.

Lateral/Rotary Core

In contrast to linear core exercises, which work the core from front to back, lateral/rotary core exercises work the core from side to side or in a twisting fashion (lateral meaning side to side and rotary meaning twisting). For this reason, they primarily work the obliques and work other core muscles such as the abdominals and spinal erectors secondarily.

From a functional standpoint, the obliques are very important. In fact, the obliques create much of the twisting torque used in sporting actions that involve twisting, throwing, swinging, and striking. As far as your physique goes, building oblique muscles is overrated, however. Overdeveloped obliques diminish your curves and give you a "blocky" appearance.

Don't fear the occasional lateral/rotary core exercise, but just don't go overboard. As I previously mentioned, the core (including the obliques) get worked during full body exercises, though not to the same degree as they do during more targeted exercises such as those included in this category.

I like to perform lateral/rotary core exercises that also work the glutes, such as side planks, anti-rotation holds, and half-kneeling cable anti-rotation presses. (The form takes some getting used to on this lift, but it's well worth the effort.)

Side Crunch

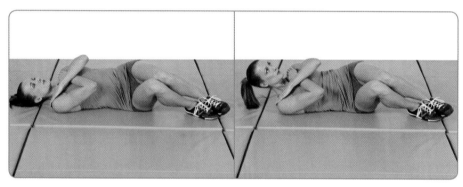 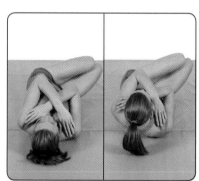

The side crunch is a beginner exercise that strengthens the obliques.

What You Feel: Obliques

Tips

- *This is not a twisting crunch; it's a side crunch. Lie on your side, and crunch straight upward with the obliques.*
- *Don't feel the need to crunch upward too high; 30 degrees of trunk lateral flexion is sufficient.*

What to Do

1. Lie on an exercise mat with your left side on the floor. Bend your knees at a 90-degree angle, positioning your top leg over your bottom leg. Lift your knees slightly off the floor.
2. Place your hands across your chest, and position your upper back so that it rests on the floor.
3. Pull upward, contracting your obliques so that your rib cage moves toward your hips.
4. Lower, and repeat for reps on both sides.

Swiss Ball Side Crunch

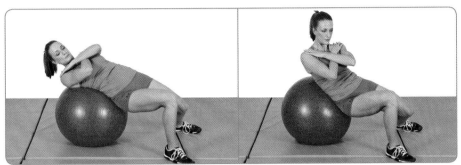

This exercise is the next level up from the side crunch, targeting the obliques.

What You Feel: Obliques

Tips

- *Focus on contracting the oblique muscles rather than trying to sit up on the ball.*
- *Keep your neck aligned with your spine, and avoid pulling your neck toward your chest with your hands.*
- *Don't feel the need to crunch upward too high; 30 degrees of trunk lateral flexion is sufficient.*

What to Do

1. Sit on the exercise ball. Walk forward on the ball until your mid-back rests across the ball and your head and shoulders hang off.
2. Bend your knees, positioning your feet flat on the floor. Cross your arms over your chest.
3. Roll forward and onto your left side so that the ball is positioned against your left ribs. Make sure that the right obliques are receiving a good stretch. Keep your feet planted firmly on the ground.
4. Contract your right side, pulling your ribs into your hips.
5. Lower, and repeat on both sides.

Dumbbell Side Bend

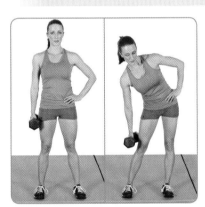

This is a basic core exercise that targets the obliques and the upper glutes.

What You Feel:

Obliques, upper glutes, forearms, traps

Tips

- *Don't bend down too far or shift the hips sideways to increase the demand on the upper glutes.*

What to Do

1. Grasp a dumbbell in your right hand, and hold it straight down by your side with your palm facing in.
2. Lean toward your right side by bending at the waist and the hips.
3. Rise back up, and repeat for reps on both sides.

45-Degree Side Bend

This exercise targets the obliques.

What You Feel: Obliques, upper glutes, forearms, traps

Tips

- *Many people tend to rely on momentum for this movement. Concentrate on getting a good oblique contraction; you don't need much range of motion for this exercise.*

What to Do

1. Adjust the 45-degree back extension so that the top of the pad is positioned at the top of your hip.
2. Grasp a dumbbell in your right hand, and place the side of your right thigh on the padding. Position your feet on the platform.
3. With the dumbbell straight down toward the floor, lower your torso by bending downward at the waist and hips.

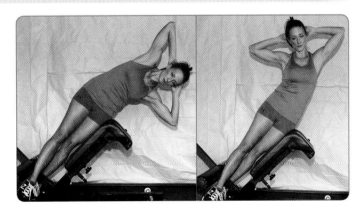

4. Rise back up, laterally flexing your waist in the opposite direction, while also feeling the upper glutes working to pull your body upward at the hips.
5. Repeat for reps on both sides.

Landmine

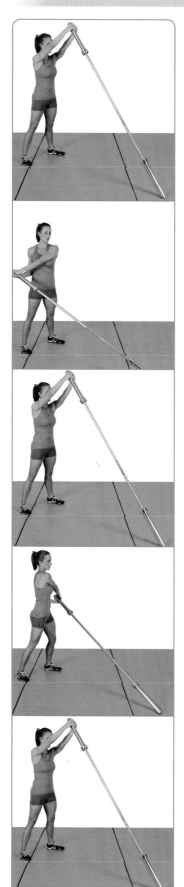

The landmine targets the obliques, upper glutes, and erectors, while building rotary strength and power and improving your core's ability to stabilize the spine and prevent unwanted rotational movement.

What You Feel:

Obliques, upper glutes, shoulders

Tips

- *Maintain a neutral spine, and avoid rotating your waist. Concentrate on moving the weight from side to side without twisting your torso.*

- *Perform the movement in a controlled manner; don't rely on too much momentum.*

- *If you do not have access to a landmine unit, you can position the barbell in a corner for stability.*

What to Do

1. Position one end of the barbell on the floor. Pick up the other end, and create a 90-degree angle from your arms to the top of the barbell.

2. Stand in an athletic stance, and move the barbell in a rainbow pattern from side to side.

3. Repeat for the desired number of reps.

Kneeling Side Plank

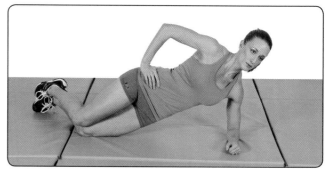

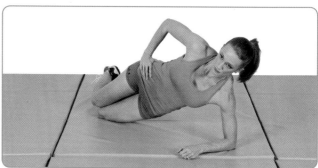

The side plank works the obliques and glute medius, while building lateral spinal stability so that your spine is able to resist being forced into lateral flexion. Performing the movement from the knees shortens the lever and makes the movement easier.

What You Feel: Obliques, upper glutes

Tips

- *Avoid leaning back or forward.*
- *Make sure your body is in a straight line from head to toe and that your neck is aligned with your spine.*

What to Do

1. Lie on an exercise mat with your right side down. Place your right forearm on the mat, positioning your elbow under your shoulder.

2. Bend your knees to a right angle, placing your upper leg directly on top of your lower leg.

3. Raise your torso upward, straightening your spine so that your hips are aligned with your torso. Contract your abdominals to hold this position.

4. Hold for as long as possible. Repeat on the left side.

Side Plank

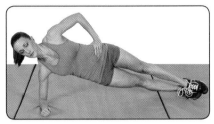

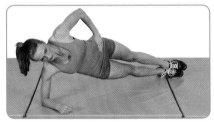

The side plank works the obliques and glute medius, while building lateral spinal stability so that your spine is able to resist being forced into lateral flexion.

What You Feel: Obliques, upper glutes

Tips

- *Avoid leaning back or forward.*
- *Make sure your body is in a straight line from head to toe and that your neck is aligned with your spine.*

What to Do

1. Lie on an exercise mat with your right side down. Place your right forearm on the mat, positioning your elbow under your shoulder.
2. Extend your legs straight out, placing your upper leg directly on top of your lower leg.
3. Raise your torso upward, straightening your spine so that your hips are aligned with your torso. Contract your abdominals to hold this position.
4. Hold for as long as possible. Repeat on the left side.

Side Plank with Abduction

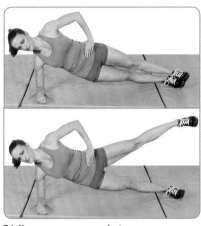

The side plank works the obliques and glute medius, while building lateral spinal stability so that your spine is able to resist being forced into lateral flexion. The movement is more difficult with top-leg abduction.

What You Feel: Obliques, upper glutes

Tips

- *Avoid leaning back or forward.*
- *Make sure your body is in a straight line from head to toe and that your neck is aligned with your spine.*

What to Do

1. Lie on an exercise mat with your right side down. Place your right forearm on the mat, positioning your elbow under your shoulder.
2. Extend your legs straight out, placing your upper leg directly on top of your lower leg.
3. Raise your torso upward, straightening your spine so that your hips and waist are aligned. Contract your abdominals to hold this position. As you rise up, lift your top leg, contracting the glutes in a hips-abducted position.
4. Holding this top-side plank position, lower and lift your top leg for reps. Repeat on the left side.

Feet-Elevated Side Plank with Abduction

The side plank works the obliques and glute medius, while building lateral spinal stability so that your spine is able to resist being forced into lateral flexion. Elevating your feet makes the movement more difficult, as does combining the plank with top-leg abduction.

What You Feel: Obliques, upper glutes

Tips

- *Avoid leaning back or forward.*
- *Make sure your body is in a straight line from head to toe and that your neck is aligned with your spine.*

What to Do

1. Lie on an exercise mat with your right side down. Place your right forearm on the mat, positioning your elbow under your shoulder.
2. Place your feet on a box or platform for elevation. Extend your legs straight out, placing your upper leg directly on top of your lower leg.
3. Raise your torso upward, straightening your spine so that your hips and waist are aligned. Contract your abdominals to hold this position. As you rise up, lift your top leg, contracting the glutes in a hips-abducted position.
4. Holding this top-side plank position, lower and lift your top leg for reps. Repeat on the left side.

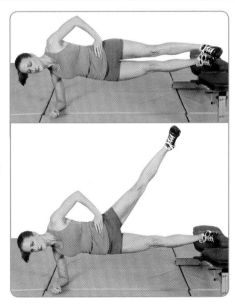

Feet-Elevated Side Plank with Clam

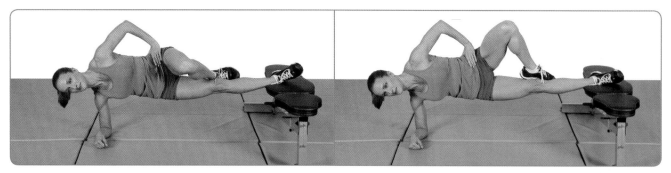

The side plank works the obliques and glute medius, while building lateral spinal stability so that your spine is able to resist being forced into lateral flexion. Elevating your feet makes the movement more difficult, as does combining the plank with a clam motion (hip external rotation) with the top leg.

What You Feel: Obliques, upper glutes

Tips

- *Avoid leaning back or forward.*
- *Make sure your body is in a straight line from head to toe and that your neck is aligned with your spine.*

What to Do

1. Lie on an exercise mat with your right side down. Place your right forearm on the mat, positioning your elbow under your shoulder.
2. Place your feet on a box or platform for elevation. Extend your legs straight out, placing your upper leg directly on top of your lower leg.
3. Raise your torso upward, straightening your spine so that your hips and waist are aligned. Contract your abdominals to hold this position. Rise up, and bend the knee of your top leg so that the ankle of the top leg is positioned just behind the knee of the bottom leg.
4. Holding this top-side plank position, lift and lower your top leg in a clam motion for reps. Repeat on the left side.

Band Anti-Rotation Hold

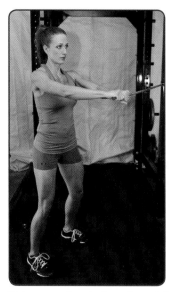 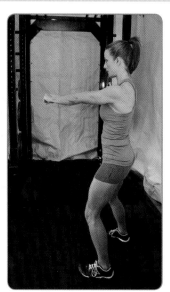

This exercise trains the obliques and the glutes, while building tremendous core stability, particularly from an anti-rotation perspective. In other words, your core will improve in its ability to resist being twisted.

What You Feel: Obliques

Tips

- *Keep your arms straight out in front of your chest throughout the duration of the exercise.*
- *Get in an athletic stance for better stability.*
- *The only thing moving should be your arms. Your torso, hips, and legs should remain motionless.*

What to Do

1. Secure a band to a rack or other stationary device.
2. Grasp the free end of the band, and walk away from the rack to create tension on the band.
3. With your arms slightly bent, pull the band straight out with your palms down until the band aligns with your chest. If you are using a tube band rather than a loop band, grasp both handles with your palms facing in.
4. Hold this position for a count, concentrating on contracting your obliques and abdominals to maintain the position. Repeat on both sides.

Cable Chop Variations   Rope Lift

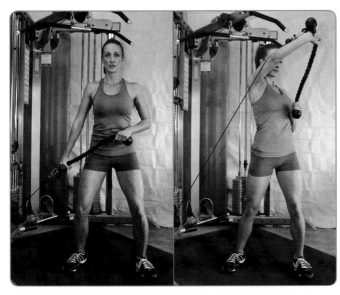

The rope lift is a challenging whole body rotary movement that works many different core muscles from a functional, athletic position.

What You Feel: Obliques, erectors, glutes

Tips

- *Make sure you have good posture and set up in proper position.*
- *Rotate mostly in the hips and upper back; don't twist too much in the lumbar spine.*
- *Don't go too heavy; make sure your form is smooth and coordinated.*
- *Don't stress so much about achieving perfect position and angles. Just make sure there is tension on the targeted muscles throughout the entire range of motion.*

What to Do

1. Grasp the rope from a low pulley position with both hands on each end of the rope.
2. Rotate to one side so that your body is positioned away from the pulley and your arms are extended down. Step away from the pulley to create tension on the cable, and get in an athletic stance.
3. Pull the rope diagonally across your body toward the ceiling with the arm closest to the pulley. This occurs while rotating at the hips.
4. Lower back down to the starting position, and repeat on both sides for reps.

Cable Chop Variations   Rope Horizontal Chop

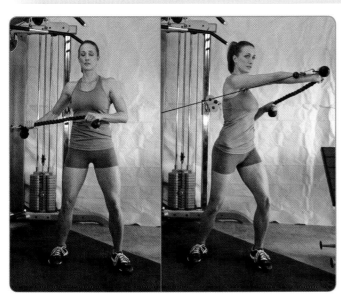

The rope horizontal chop is a challenging whole body rotary movement that works many core muscles from a functional, athletic position.

What You Feel: Obliques, erectors, glutes

Tips

- *Make sure you have good posture and set up in proper position.*
- *Rotate mostly in the hips and upper back; don't twist too much in the lumbar spine.*
- *Don't go too heavy; make sure your form is smooth and coordinated.*
- *Don't stress so much about achieving perfect position and angles. Just make sure there is tension on the targeted muscles throughout the entire range of motion.*

What to Do

1. Grasp the rope from a mid-pulley position with both hands on each end of the rope.
2. Rotate to one side so that your body is positioned away from the pulley and your arms are extended out toward the pulley. Step away from the pulley to create tension on the cable, and get in an athletic stance.
3. Pull the rope across your body with the arm closest to the pulley. This occurs while rotating at the hips.
4. Rotate back to the starting position, and repeat on both sides for reps.

Cable Chop Variations   Rope Chop

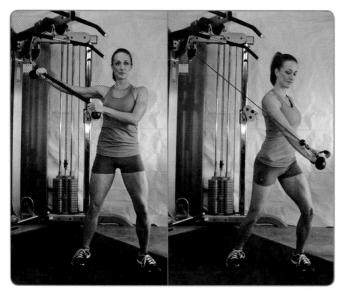

The rope chop is a challenging whole body rotary movement that works many core muscles from a functional, athletic position.

What You Feel: Obliques

Tips

- *Make sure you have good posture and set up in proper position.*
- *Rotate mostly in the hips and upper back; don't twist too much in the lumbar spine.*
- *Don't go too heavy; make sure your form is smooth and coordinated.*
- *Don't stress so much about achieving perfect position and angles. Just make sure there is tension on the targeted muscles throughout the entire range of motion.*

What to Do

1. Grasp the rope from a high pulley position with both hands on each end of the rope.
2. Rotate to one side so that your body is positioned away from the pulley and your arms are extended up. Step away from the pulley to create tension on the cable, and get in an athletic stance.
3. Pull the rope diagonally across your body toward the floor with the arm closest to the pulley. This occurs while rotating at the hips.
4. Rise back to the starting position, and repeat on both sides for reps.

Cable Chop Variations   Rope Half-Kneeling Horizontal Chop

The rope half-kneeling horizontal chop is a challenging whole body rotary movement that works many different core muscles, and the half-kneeling position works the glutes on the rear leg surprisingly well. This is one of my favorite core exercises.

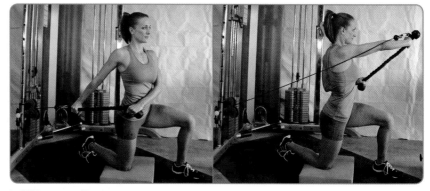

What You Feel: Obliques, erectors, glutes

Tips

- *Make sure you have good posture and set up in proper position.*
- *Rotate mostly in the hips and upper back; don't twist too much in the lumbar spine.*
- *Don't go too heavy; make sure your form is smooth and coordinated.*
- *Don't stress so much about achieving perfect position and angles. Just make sure there is tension on the targeted muscles throughout the entire range of motion.*

What to Do

1. Position the rope on a low pulley. You can choose to position a pad under your knee.
2. Get in a half-kneeling position with your right knee down facing away from the cable column. Grasp the rope on each end in both hands, extending your right arm directly behind you while crossing your left arm over your abdomen.
3. From this position, pull the rope straight out in front of your torso with your right arm until it fully extends, aligning with your right shoulder. At the same time, rotate your torso so that it faces forward, moving your left arm back by your left oblique.
4. Return to the starting position in a controlled fashion, and repeat for reps on both sides.

Cable Chop Variations Bar Half-Kneeling Horizontal Chop

The bar half-kneeling horizontal chop is a challenging whole body rotary movement that works many different core muscles, and the half-kneeling position works the glutes on the rear leg surprisingly well. This is one of my favorite core exercises, and the Cook bar makes the movement much more effective, in my opinion.

What You Feel: Obliques, erectors, glutes

Tips

- *Make sure you have good posture and set up in proper position.*
- *Rotate mostly in the hips and upper back; don't twist too much in the lumbar spine.*
- *Don't go too heavy; make sure your form is smooth and coordinated.*
- *Don't stress so much about achieving perfect position and angles. Just make sure there is tension on the targeted muscles throughout the entire range of motion.*

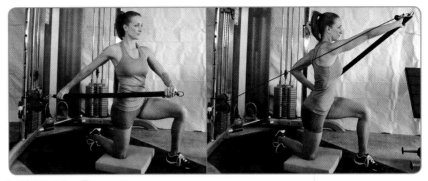

What to Do

1. Position the cook bar on a low pulley. You can choose to position a pad under your knee.
2. Get in a half-kneeling position with your right knee down facing away from the cable column. Grasp the bar on each end in both hands, extending your right arm directly behind you while crossing your left arm over your abdomen.
3. From this position, pull the bar straight out in front of your torso with your right arm until it fully extends, aligning with your right shoulder. At the same time, rotate your torso so that it faces forward, moving your left arm back by your left oblique.
4. Return to the starting position in a controlled fashion, and repeat for reps on both sides.

Cable Chop Variations Bar Horizontal Chop

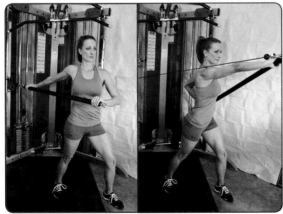

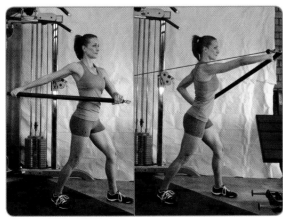

The bar horizontal chop is a challenging whole body rotary movement that works many different core muscles from a functional, athletic position. Most gyms don't have Cook bars, and the rope certainly suffices. But if you have access to a Cook bar, I prefer this variation over the rope version.

What You Feel: Obliques, erectors, glutes

Tips

- *Make sure you have good posture and set up in proper position.*
- *Rotate mostly in the hips and upper back; don't twist too much in the lumbar spine.*
- *Don't go too heavy; make sure your form is smooth and coordinated.*
- *Don't stress so much about achieving perfect position and angles. Just make sure there is tension on the targeted muscles throughout the entire range of motion.*

What to Do

1. Position the Cook bar on a mid-pulley. Stand with a slightly forward lean, facing away from the cable column. Grasp the bar on each end in both hands, extending your right arm directly behind you while crossing your left arm over your abdomen.
2. From this position, pull the bar straight out in front of your torso with your right arm until it fully extends, aligning with your right shoulder. At the same time, rotate your torso so that it faces forward, moving your left arm back by your left oblique.
3. Return to the starting position in a controlled fashion, and repeat for reps on both sides.

Isolation

Everyone in the world these days seems to bash isolation training, yet everyone secretly does the exercises. Before I elaborate, I'd like to mention that there's really no such thing as "isolation" training because it's impossible to truly isolate a muscle. Lots of muscles will contract even when performing a simple exercise such as a lateral raise. A better term for these exercises might be "targeted exercises," but this is just semantics. We'll stick to the term "isolation" for convenience.

Usually, compound movements refer to exercises that work multiple joints at a time, while isolation lifts refer to exercises that work one joint at a time. Isolation movements do not typically ramp up the metabolism like compound movements, but it isn't always a good idea to classify a movement based on how many joints move. For instance, a squat involves hip and knee flexion and extension, so it's a compound movement. A concentration curl involves elbow flexion and extension, so it's an isolation movement.

Compound movements are, therefore, clearly better than isolation movements because they involve much more muscle mass, right? Well, not exactly. Think of an upright row. It involves shoulder abduction and adduction, along with elbow flexion and extension, making it a compound movement that works the deltoids and biceps. A hip thrust, on the other hand, involves hip extension and flexion, making it an isolation lift since it only involves a single joint. Yet, the exercise dynamically works the glutes and hamstrings and requires considerable muscle contractions in the quads and erectors for stability purposes. The hip thrust involves a ton of muscle mass, which is not so much the case for the upright row.

Now that I've made my point, I'll say that there are benefits to isolation lifts. They can strengthen weak muscles, they can provide a novel training stimulus that sets the stage for further adaptation, and they can provide an excellent psychological advantage since everyone wants to really feel the muscle they wish to strengthen working hard. We all have our weaker body parts. For most, it's the glutes (hence, the considerable focus on the glutes in the *Strong Curves Program*), although some were shortchanged in the calf department, and others might have weak back or shoulder muscles.

It's wise to perform specific exercises targeting the weaker parts, but don't get carried away. In this program, you want to make sure you're consistently getting stronger at big glute movements like hip thrusts, squats, and deadlifts. These are the big rocks. Triceps kickbacks or rear delt raises are not going to reshape your entire body. But exercises like those can help round out a physique and add detail to important areas.

For these reasons, I'm giving you five minutes at the end of each workout where you can perform all the isolation exercises your heart desires. Want to blast the arms? Alternate between a few sets of curls and triceps extensions. Seeking more delt definition? Bust out a set of front raises, lateral raises, and rear delt raises. Not happy with your calves? Do some single-leg calf raises. Just don't exceed the five total minutes allotted.

Swiss Ball Adductor Squeeze

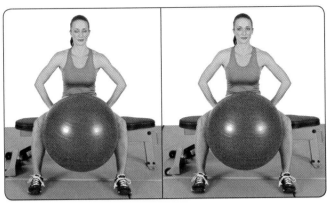 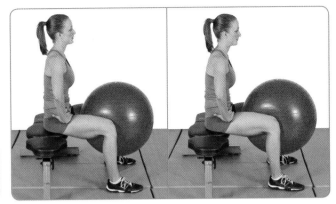

This exercise strengthens the inner thighs, which are important hip muscles for both movement and stability. The inner thigh region is a primary area of concern for women. Remember, however, that spot reduction is a myth and that to burn fat off of a particular area, you need to lose fat all over. Some targeted training can improve the appearance of a region by simply building muscular shape in that area, however.

What You Feel: Adductors (inner thighs)

Tips

- *Keep your feet flat on the ground, and don't come up onto your toes.*
- *For a better workout, squeeze the ball for 2 to 3 seconds.*
- *Keep your chest tall, and don't slouch.*

What to Do

1. Sit on a flat bench, positioning an exercise ball between your knees.
2. Place your hands on your hips, sit tall, and push your knees together.
3. Squeeze the ball and release. Repeat for reps.

Standing Cable Adduction

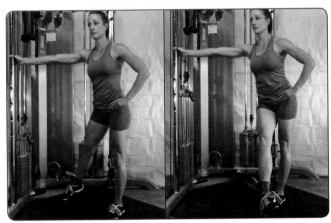 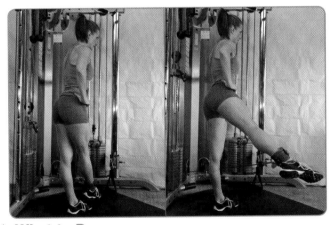

This exercise strengthens the inner thighs, which are important hip muscles for both movement and stability. The inner thigh region is a primary area of concern for women. Remember, however, that spot reduction is a myth and that to burn fat off of a particular area, you need to lose fat all over. Some targeted training can improve the appearance of a region by simply building muscular shape in that area, however.

What You Feel: Hip adductors (inner thighs)

Tips

- *Hold onto a support to maintain balance.*
- *Keep your spine in a neutral position, and stay upright.*
- *Contract your glutes throughout the movement.*

What to Do

1. Adjust the weight on the cable machine.
2. Place the ankle strap around your ankle closest to the machine.
3. Step away from the rack to create tension on the cable.
4. Place your weight on the outer foot, lifting your inner foot slightly off of the floor.
5. Pull your inner leg toward your outer leg until your raised foot is directly over the planted foot, getting a good contraction with your adductors (inner thigh).
6. Return to the starting position, and continue for the entire set.
7. Repeat on other side.

Cable Hip Flexion

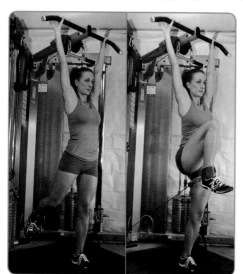

The cable hip flexion strengthens the hip flexors, which are important for hip stability and running. We do a ton of hip extensor strengthening, so it makes sense to perform some hip flexion exercise every once in a while.

What You Feel: Hip flexors

Tips

* *Remain in an upright position, and avoiding thrusting the weight up or coming up on your toes.*

What to Do

1. Stand away from the low pulley. Place an ankle strap around one ankle, and adjust the weight. Grab hold of a prop for support.
2. Stand forward, supporting the weight on the free leg.
3. Raise the working leg up toward your chest as high as it can go without moving your torso.
4. Lower the leg down in a controlled fashion, and repeat for reps.
5. Switch legs, and repeat.

Band Lying Hip Flexion

This exercise strengthens the hip flexors, which are important for hip stability and running. We do a ton of hip extensor strengthening, so it makes sense to perform some hip flexion exercise every once in a while.

What You Feel: Hip flexors

Tips

* *Press the spine and shoulders into the floor to maintain good posture throughout the movement.*

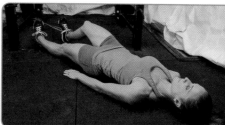 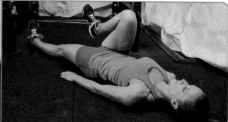

What to Do

1. Secure a band on a rack or support.
2. Lie on your back, wrapping the free end of the band over the top of one foot.
3. Pull your foot toward your hips as far as you can comfortably go.
4. Return to the starting position, and repeat for the prescribed number of reps.
5. Switch legs, and repeat.

Band Seated Leg Curl

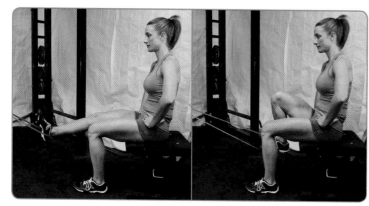

What You Feel: Hamstrings

Tips

* *Maintain good posture with tight abs throughout the exercise.*

What to Do

1. Secure a band around a rack or post.
2. Sit on a flat bench, and wrap the free end of the band around the back of your ankle.
3. Raise the working leg slightly off of the floor so that your foot hovers, keeping the other foot planted.
4. Bring your foot toward the bench.
5. Return to the starting position, and repeat for the prescribed number of reps before switching legs.

This exercise strengthens the hamstrings, which are very important in running and sprinting.

Single-Leg Calf Raise

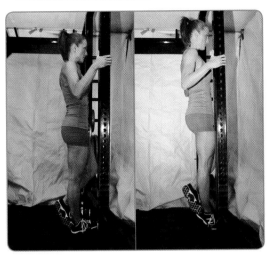

This exercise strengthens the calves, which are important for running and jumping.

What You Feel: Calves

Tips

- *Use a full range of motion, rising all the way up on your toes and lowering back down below the support as far as you can comfortably flex.*

What to Do

1. Standing upright, place your toes and the ball of your foot on a raised platform.
2. Hold a rack or banister for support, and rise up onto your toes.
3. Lower back down slightly below the top of the platform, and repeat for prescribed reps before switching legs.

Dumbbell Side Lateral Raise

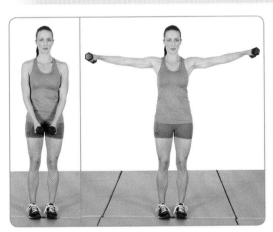

This exercise works to strengthen your shoulders. Strong shoulders help create the illusion of a narrower waist and are important in functional and athletic endeavors.

What You Feel: Lateral deltoids (middle shoulders)

Tips

- *Use a controlled movement, avoiding swinging up the weight.*
- *Keep your elbows slightly in front of your shoulders.*
- *Dumbbells should rise by shoulder abduction, not external rotation.*

What to Do

1. Grasp two dumbbells in front of your thighs, keeping your knees slightly bent.
2. With your elbows slightly bent, raise your arms to the side until your elbows are shoulder height.
3. Lower, and repeat.

Dumbbell Front Raise

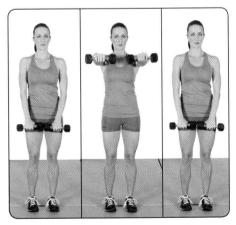 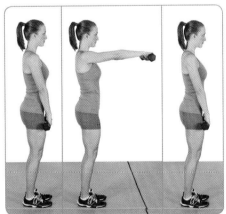

This exercise strengthens the front shoulders. Strong shoulders help create the illusion of a narrower waist and are important in functional and athletic endeavors.

What You Feel: deltoids (front shoulders)

Tips

- *Keep your elbows straight throughout the movement.*
- *Avoid shrugging the weight up.*

What to Do

1. Grasp hold of dumbbells in both hands, and position them in front of your upper legs with your palms facing in.
2. Raise the dumbbells forward and upward while rotating your arms so that your upper arms are parallel with the ground at the top of the movement.
3. Lower, and repeat.

Dumbbell Rear Lateral Raise

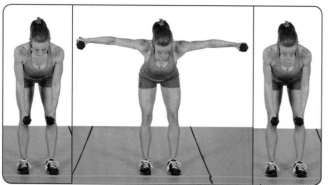 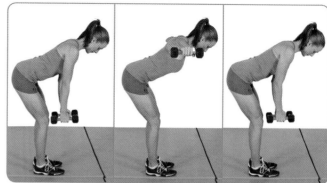

The rear deltoid helps to balance your shoulders and prevent shoulder and rotator cuff injuries. Often, front shoulder muscles are stronger than rear shoulder muscles, so this exercise helps balance out your shoulder strength.

What You Feel: Rear deltoids (rear shoulders)

Tips

- *Raise the dumbbells via transverse abduction, not external rotation.*
- *At the top of the movement, your elbows should align with your shoulders.*
- *Keep your torso close to horizontal to target the rear deltoids.*
- *Bend your knees to limit lower back strain.*
- *Avoid swinging the weight up.*

What to Do

1. Grasp hold of dumbbells at each side.
2. Bend your knees slightly, and bend through the hip while keeping your back flat and nearly parallel with the floor.
3. Position your elbows slightly bent with your palms facing in.
4. Raise your arms out to the sides until your elbows align with your shoulders.
5. Lower the weight, and repeat.

Dumbbell Upright Row

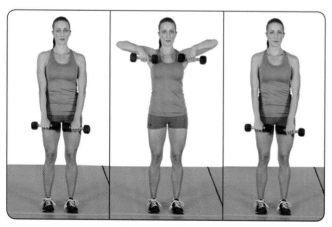 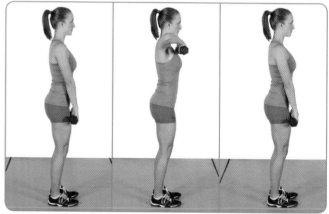

This exercise strengthens the shoulders. Strong shoulders help create the illusion of a narrower waist and are important in functional and athletic endeavors.

What You Feel: Lateral deltoids (middle shoulders), biceps

Tips

- *Keep your elbows to the side, and don't let them float forward.*
- *Don't rise up too high, and don't externally rotate your shoulders as you rise up by allowing your wrists to rise above your elbows.*

What to Do

1. Grasp hold of dumbbells at your side with your palms facing the front of your thighs.
2. Pull the dumbbells upward with your elbows leading the movement.
3. Allow your wrists to bend as the dumbbells come up.
4. Lower, and repeat.

Dumbbell Shrug

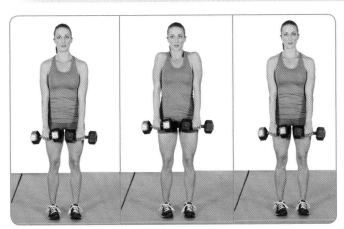

This exercise builds the upper trapezius muscle, an important scapular stabilizer. This is not a necessary exercise in most regimes for women, but I didn't want to leave it out for any reader who lacks trap development or for the men who picked up *Strong Curves* and decided to give it a go.

What You Feel: Upper trapezius

Tips

* *Do not roll your shoulders or bend your arms; think of your arms as hooks.*
* *As the weight increases, it becomes more difficult to take the weight through a full range of motion. Don't skimp on ROM at the expense of using heavier loads.*

What to Do

1. Grasp hold of two dumbbells, and place them at your sides with your palms facing in.
2. Move your shoulders straight up toward your ears as high as possible.
3. Lower, and repeat.

Prone Rear Delt Raise

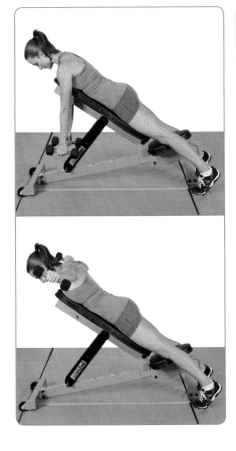

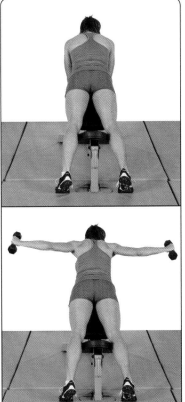

The rear deltoid helps balance your shoulders and prevent shoulder and rotator cuff injuries. Often, the front shoulder muscles are stronger than rear shoulder muscles, so this exercise helps balance out your strength in your back. By lying on a bench, you are better able to isolate the rear shoulder muscles.

What You Feel: Rear deltoid (rear shoulder)

Tips

* *Dumbbells should be raised with transverse abduction, not external rotation or extension.*
* *Your elbows may be straight or slightly bent.*

What to Do

1. Lie chest down on an incline bench at a 30 to 45-degree angle.
2. Grasp dumbbells below in each side of the bench with your palms facing each other.
3. Raise your arms to the side until your elbows reach shoulder height.
4. Lower, and repeat.

Prone Trap Raise

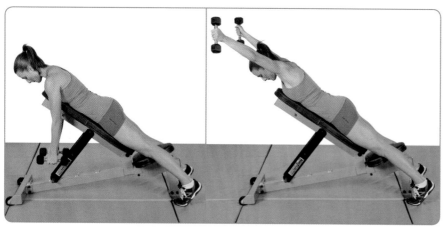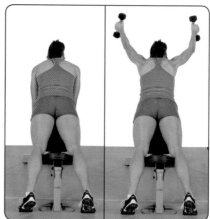

This exercise builds the lower trapezius muscle, a muscle that is commonly weak and under-activated in lifters. The low trapezius is an important scapula stabilizer.

What You Feel: Trapezius (mid and lower fibers)

Tips

- *Avoid using excessive momentum. You may find you can only use 2.5-5 pounds on this movement.*
- *Keep your arms positioned at a 45-degree angle to form a Y at the top of the movement.*

What to Do

1. Contracting the upper back muscles, raise the dumbbells over head with straight arms into a y-position until arms are next to your ears.
2. At the top position, squeeze the upper back muscles, then lower back down to starting position and repeat.

Prone Elbows-Out Row

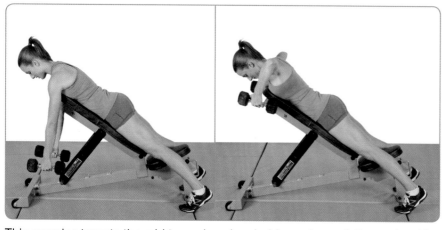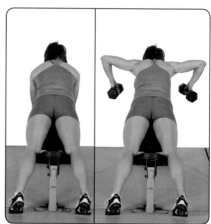

This exercise targets the mid trapezius, rhomboids, and rear delt muscles. You will not be able to row as much weight as you would when performing dumbbell or chest-supported rows.

What You Feel: Upper back

Tips

- *At the top of the movement, your arms will form an "L" with your elbows bent at 90 degrees.*
- *Squeeze your shoulder blades together up top.*

What to Do

1. Lie chest down on an incline bench at a 30 to 45-degree angle.
2. Grasp the dumbbells with your palms facing in.
3. Raise the dumbbells to the sides until your upper arms are past horizontal, squeezing the middle back.
4. Lower back down until your arms are extended, and repeat.

Prone Shrug

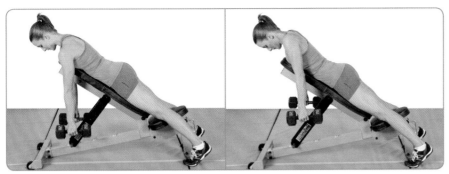 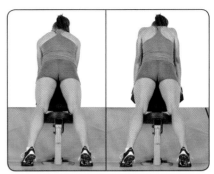

The prone shrug targets the mid-back muscles, particularly the middle traps and rhomboid musculature.

What You Feel: Scapular retractors (mid-back)

Tips

- *Squeeze the middle back and traps together to lift the weight, rather than shrugging up toward your ears like you do on a standing shrug.*
- *Don't bend the arms; keep them straight.*

What to Do

1. Lie chest down on an incline bench at a 30 to 45-degree angle.
2. Grasp dumbbells below the bench with your palms facing in.
3. Shrug your shoulders back, squeezing your middle back and traps together.
4. Lower, and repeat.

Scarecrow

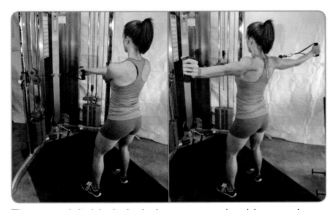

The rear deltoids help balance your shoulders and prevent shoulder injuries. Often, the front shoulder muscles are stronger than rear shoulder muscles, so this exercise is needed to achieve muscular balance. This is often a difficult exercise for women, but those who are looking for a greater challenge will benefit from adding it to their routine.

What You Feel: Rear deltoids (rear shoulders)

Tips

- *Keep your elbows slightly bent throughout the duration of the movement.*

What to Do

1. Set the cables at waist height.
2. Stand facing the cable machine, grasping the opposite cable in each hand so that the cables cross over in front of your body.
3. Pull your upper arms up and back until they align with your shoulders.
4. Lower to the starting position, and repeat.

Bent Over Cable Rear Delt Raise

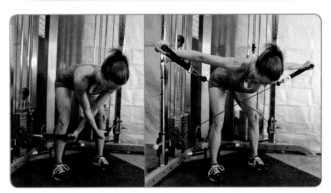

The rear deltoids help balance your shoulders and prevent shoulder injuries. Often, the front shoulder muscles are stronger than rear shoulder muscles, so this exercise is needed to achieve muscular balance.

What You Feel: Rear deltoids (rear shoulders)

Tips

- *Maintain a flat back, and bend at the hips.*

What to Do

1. Adjust the cable to a low pulley position, and set the weight on each side of the cable machine.
2. Grasp each cable handle in the opposite hands. Return to the center of the machine.
3. Bend forward holding the handles until your back is approximately horizontal to the floor. Your arms will cross over in front of your chest.
4. Raise your arms to the sides until your elbows are aligned with your shoulders. Keep your elbows slightly bent throughout the duration of the exercise.
5. Lower, and repeat.

Straight-Arm Cable Pull Down

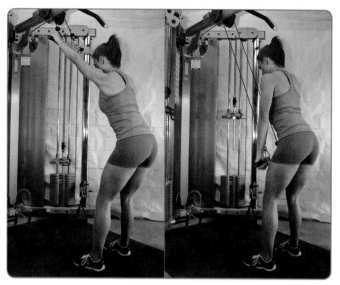

What You Feel: Back muscles, triceps

Tips

- *Pull through your back muscles rather than your triceps.*
- *Although it's called "straight-arm," you want to slightly bend your elbows throughout the duration of the movement.*
- *Aim for a large range of motion.*

What to Do

1. Set the cable at a high pulley position. Facing the machine, grasp the cable attachment, and slightly bend at your knees and hips, getting into a stable, athletic stance.
2. Keeping your elbows locked, pull the cable attachment down until your upper arms are down by your sides.
3. Rise back to the top, and repeat.

This exercise targets the lats, which are important back stabilizers. The lats are also the primary upper body pulling muscle.

Incline Dumbbell Fly

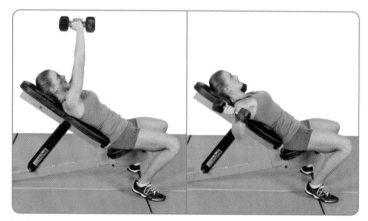 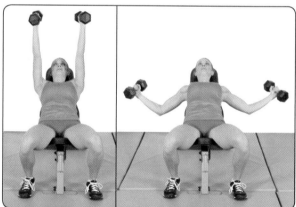

This exercise targets the upper chest. This exercise increases upper chest muscles to give greater definition above the breast tissue. Because the arms are positioned far away from the body, you won't be able to use as much weight as you would on a dumbbell incline press.

What You Feel: Pectoralis major (upper chest muscles)

Tips

- *Keep your feet positioned on the floor.*
- *Make sure your elbows track straight out to the sides.*
- *Only raise the dumbbells two-thirds of the way up to keep constant tension on the chest muscles.*

What to Do

1. Lie on an incline bench at a 30 to 45-degree angle.
2. Grasp the dumbbells, and raise them over your upper chest with your arms slightly bent.
3. Lower the dumbbells outward to the side of your shoulders until you feel a good stretch in the chest.
4. Raise the dumbbells upward, stopping two-thirds of the way up.
5. Lower, and repeat.

Dumbbell Fly

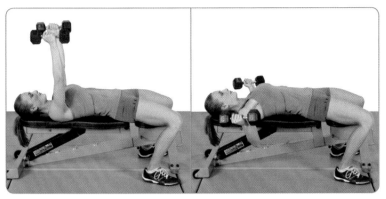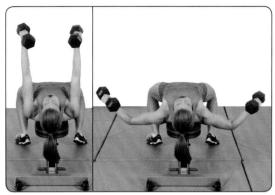

The dumbbell fly targets the pectoral muscles and places a considerable stretch load on the muscles, which simultaneously builds strength, stability, and flexibility.

What You Feel: Pectoralis major (upper chest muscles)

Tips

- *Keep your feet on the floor.*
- *Maintain a slight bend in your elbows, and keep your arms perpendicular to your torso.*
- *Only raise the dumbbells two-thirds of the way up to keep constant tension on the pectorals; don't lock out fully overhead.*

What to Do

1. Lie with your back on a flat bench. Grasp the dumbbells, and support them above your chest with your arms slightly bent.
2. Begin with your palms facing each other, and maintain this neutral position throughout the duration of the movement.
3. Lower the dumbbells to the sides until your chest muscles receive a big stretch.
4. Bring the dumbbells together in a hugging motion.
5. Lower, and repeat.

Dumbbell Pullover

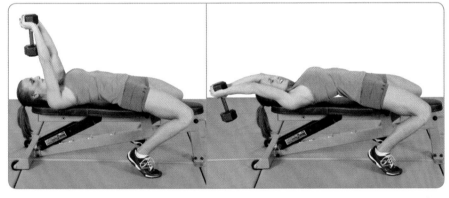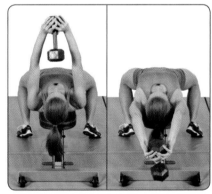

This exercise strengthens the pectoral muscles, the serratus muscles, the triceps, and the lats. The pullover is actually a great upper body exercise that works a lot of muscles and allows for heavy loads over time.

What You Feel: Pecs, lats, triceps

Tips

- *Keep your hips firmly locked and your glutes tight.*
- *Keep your elbows slightly bent throughout the movement.*
- *Don't turn the movement into a triceps extension; try to stretch your lats.*

What to Do

1. Lie with your upper back perpendicular to a bench. Grasp one dumbbell, positioning your hands on the bottom of the inner plate.
2. Position the dumbbell over your chest with your elbows slightly bent.
3. Lower the dumbbell over and beyond your head until your upper arms align you're your shoulders.
4. Pull the dumbbell up and over your chest, and repeat.

Cable Triceps Extension

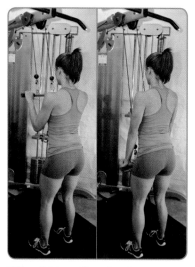

This exercise targets the triceps musculature, which is a primary area of concern for many women. Don't forget that spot reduction is a myth and that to burn fat off of a particular area, you need to lose fat all over. But again, some targeted training can improve the appearance of a region by simply building muscular shape in that area.

What You Feel: Triceps (rear upper arm)

Tips

- *Use a full range of motion.*
- *Control the load; don't heave or use excessive momentum.*

What to Do

1. Adjust the cable machine to a high pulley position. Grasp the V-bar or straight bar with a narrow overhand grip.
2. Extend the arms downward.
3. Return to the starting position, and repeat.

Rope Triceps Extension

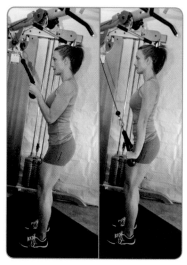

The rope triceps extension targets the triceps musculature, which is a primary area of concern for many women. Once again, spot reduction is a myth, and to burn fat off of a particular area, you need to lose fat all over. Nevertheless, some targeted training can improve the appearance of a region by simply building muscular shape in that area.

What You Feel: Triceps (rear upper arm)

Tips

- *Use a full range of motion.*
- *Control the load; don't heave or use excessive momentum.*

What to Do

1. Adjust the cable machine to the high pulley position. Grasp the rope attachment with both hands.
2. Extend your arms downward while spreading your arms out to the sides and achieving full elbow extension.
3. Return to the starting position, and repeat.

Cable Overhead Triceps Extension

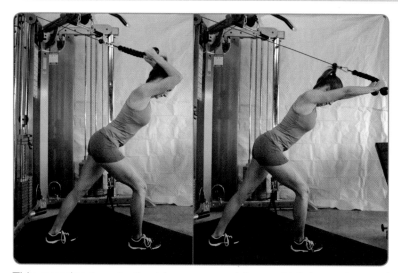

This exercise targets the triceps musculature, which is a primary area of concern for many women. You have to burn fat all over in order to lose it from a particular area; spot reduction is a myth. This exercise provides some targeted training, however, which can improve appearance by simply building muscular shape in this area.

What You Feel: Triceps (rear upper arm)

Tips

- *Don't allow your lower back to hyperextend.*
- *Keep your upper arms in position, and bend at the elbows.*

What to Do

1. Set a cable at medium pulley height with a rope attachment. Face away from the pulley system, and position the rope attachment behind the neck.
2. Lean your body forward in a split stance, placing tension on the cable while stretching your triceps.
3. Extend your arms forward until your elbows are straight.
4. Control the rope and cable back to starting position, keeping your upper arms in a stable position. Repeat.

Incline Dumbbell Curl

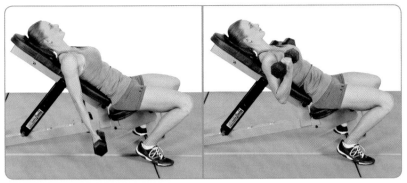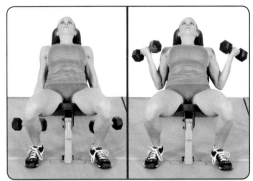

The incline dumbbell curl is one of the only bicep exercises that places the biceps in a good position of stretch. It's an amazing exercise because of the large stretch load that the biceps receive during this movement.

What You Feel: Biceps (upper arm)

Tips

- *Keep your arms positioned under your shoulders, and avoid swinging up the weight.*
- *Squeeze the end-range contraction, and hold for a brief moment.*

What to Do

1. Sit on an incline bench set at a 45 to 60-degree angle. Grasp the dumbbells, and hold them straight down at your side with your palms facing forward (supinated).
2. With your elbows positioned back near your sides, raise both dumbbells as high as possible by flexing your elbow joints.
3. Lower, and repeat.

Alternating Dumbbell Biceps Curl

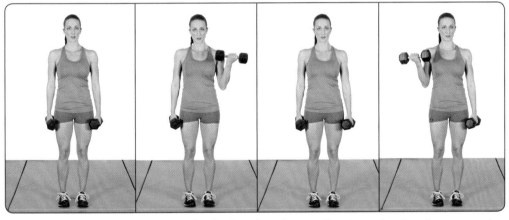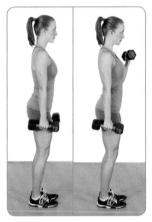

Biceps muscles are responsible for flexing the elbows. By strengthening these muscles, you increase your pulling strength for rows, chin-ups, pull-ups, and other pulling exercises. In other words, the stronger your biceps are, the more weight you can handle during many of the exercises that build your back. Plus, toned arms are just sexy.

What You Feel: Biceps (upper arm)

Tips

- *Use a full range of motion, taking the weight from a straight arm to a full contraction and back down.*
- *Keep your elbows near your sides to avoid using larger muscles to move the weight.*

What to Do

1. Grasp the dumbbells at your sides with your palms facing in.
2. Keeping your elbows at your sides, raise one dumbbell, rotating your forearm until it is vertical and your palm faces your shoulder.
3. Bring the dumbbell up to a full contraction, and lower it back down.
4. Repeat on the opposite side, alternating back and forth between arms.

Dumbbell Hammer Curl

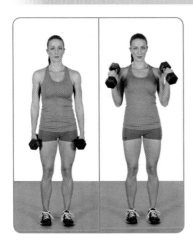

The hammer curl is similar to the alternating curl, except you will not rotate your forearm to face your shoulder and you work both arms at the same time. By keeping your palms facing inward in a neutral position, you target the brachialis and brachioradialis.

What You Feel: Biceps, brachialis, brachioradialis (upper arms)

Tips

- *Use a full range of motion, taking the weight from a straight arm to a full contraction and back down.*
- *Keep your elbows near your sides to avoid using larger muscles to move the weight.*

What to Do

1. Grasp the dumbbells at your side with your palms facing in.
2. Raise both dumbbells upward as high as you can with your thumbs facing your shoulders.
3. Lower the weight, and repeat.

Dumbbell Concentration Curl

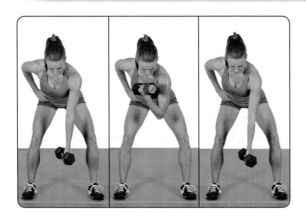

What to Do

1. Grasp a dumbbell in one hand with your palm facing in.
2. Stand with your knees slightly bent, and hinge at the hips until your back is parallel to the floor.
3. Place your arm straight by the inside of your knee.
4. Raise the dumbbell to the front of your shoulder.
5. Lower until your arm is fully extended, and repeat until the set is complete.
6. Repeat on the other side.

What You Feel: Biceps (upper arm)

Tips

- *Keep your arms positioned under your shoulders, and avoid swinging up the weight.*
- *Squeeze the end-range contraction, and hold for a brief moment.*
- *Support your weight by placing your free hand on your knee.*

Concentration curls really isolate the biceps and create a considerable peak contraction and pump.

Barbell Biceps Curl

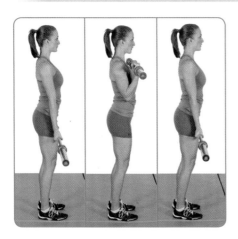

What You Feel: Biceps (upper arms)

Tips

- *Use a full range of motion, taking the weight from a straight arm to a full contraction and back down.*
- *Keep your elbows near your sides to avoid using larger muscles to move the weight.*
- *Avoid using excessive momentum.*

What to Do

1. Grasp the barbell with a shoulder-width underhand grip.
2. Keeping your elbows at your sides, raise the bar until your forearms are nearly vertical, facing your upper arms.
3. Lower until the arms are fully extended, and repeat.

This exercise strengthens the biceps. Unlike dumbbell curls, your palms remain in a supinated position throughout the duration of the movement. The barbell curl works the abdominal and lower back musculature very well; it's a challenging movement from a core-stability perspective.